The Energies of Love

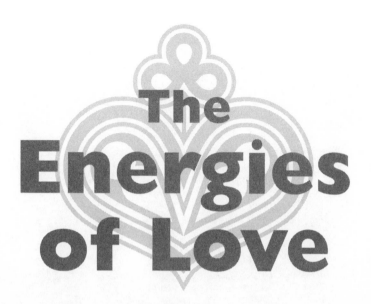

The Energies of Love

Using Energy Medicine to
Keep Your Relationship Thriving

DONNA EDEN

and

DAVID FEINSTEIN, PH.D.

Foreword by Jean Houston, Ph.D.

ILLUSTRATIONS BY ANNAMARIA PACIULLI VOLPICELLA

JEREMY P. TARCHER/PENGUIN
a member of Penguin Group (USA)
New York

JEREMY P. TARCHER/PENGUIN
Published by the Penguin Group
Penguin Group (USA) LLC
375 Hudson Street
New York, New York 10014

USA • Canada • UK • Ireland • Australia
New Zealand • India • South Africa • China

penguin.com
A Penguin Random House Company

Copyright © 2014 by Donna Eden and David Feinstein

Most Tarcher/Penguin books are available at special quantity discounts for bulk purchase for sales promotions, premiums,
fund-raising, and educational needs. Special books or book excerpts also can be created to fit specific needs.
For details, write: Special.Markets@us.penguingroup.com.

Library of Congress Cataloging-in-Publication Data

Eden, Donna.
The energies of love : using energy medicine to keep your relationship thriving / Donna Eden, David Feinstein;
foreword by Jean Houston; illustrations by Annamaria Paciulli Volpicella
p.   cm.
ISBN 978-1-58542-949-3 (hardback)
1. Energy medicine. 2. Couples. 3. Interpersonal relations. 4. Love. I. Feinstein, David. II. Title.
RZ999.E3267   2014   2014021654
615.8'9—dc23

Printed in the United States of America
1   3   5   7   9   10   8   6   4   2

BOOK DESIGN BY TANYA MAIBORODA

For our grandson, Tiernan Ray Devenyns.

May the energies of love be the hallmark of his generation.

One day after mastering the winds,
the waves, the tides, and gravity,
we shall harness for God the energies of love.
And then, for the second time in the history of the world,
we shall have discovered fire.

—PIERRE TEILHARD DE CHARDIN

Contents

PART 3 • The Mutually Created Aspects of Love

Acknowledgments

WHILE TEACHING OUR ENERGIES OF LOVE CLASSES IN RECENT YEARS, DONNA HAS become fond of saying, "Thank God I didn't leave David when I should have!" In thinking about our gratitudes and acknowledgments for this book, David's first and foremost appreciation is that Donna didn't leave him when she should have and Donna's is that David came around so it was worth the wait. Given the uncertainties and struggles we have gone through, we are as amazed as we are gratified by how many people who have watched us teach or work together in recent years have told us that our relationship is an inspiration that gives them hope. Their comments have helped push us over the line into being bold enough to write this book.

The Energies of Love, which in a true sense has been in gestation for the entire thirty-seven years of our relationship, is indebted to so many people that we aren't even going to risk naming names. Not only would that fill many pages, we would still inevitably leave out too many who have lent a guiding hand along the way. Instead, we will list categories. Guilty parties will know where they fit. First are our parents and families of origin, who inaugurated us into all that was to follow. Next, our daughters and extended family provide the foundation on which we stand. Then our closest friends, from childhood to present day. Our lovers and intimates from the past provided us with the most personal and profound instruction about what works . . . and what doesn't. Our teachers, our many magnificent teachers, formal and informal, helped shape who we are. And our therapists—we know we were tough cookies, and we thank you for giving your all to meet the challenges. Our clients and students have taught us so much by allowing us to participate in their journeys.

The actual writing, putting words on paper, was facilitated in so many ways by the support of our magnificent staff at Innersource and the hundreds of energy medicine and energy psychology practitioners who orbit around them. Our editor at Tarcher/Penguin as well as the publisher's founder, its current chief, and its staff have been gifts that few authors today can even hope for. Finally, we have sought counsel for specific sections of the book from friends and colleagues, and they have contributed generously and masterfully.

We are deeply grateful to every one of you.

Foreword

WHEN YOU FIRST MEET THEM, THEY SEEM AN UNLIKELY COUPLE. DONNA IS EXU-berant, spontaneous, intuitive. David is quietly reflective, studious, and always looking for deeper meanings. She is champagne; he is still water. She is of a tropical nature; he is most definitely northern. And yet, with all their contrasts, they have, through dint of unstinting effort and rich affection, cultivated a loving, creative, and exemplary marriage. He puts her feelings and intuition into words. She sees and orchestrates energies that enable him to enter a different universe of understanding. Together, they have done the hard work of relationship, and we are their beneficiaries.

Which is to say that *The Energies of Love* heralds a revolution in our understanding of relationships. I believe it to be one of the most important books of our time, the "Open Sesame" to new ways of being. Drawing upon their many years of work in energy medicine and energy psychology, the authors have given us a deeply original and eminently practical art and science for crossing the great divide of otherness. Theirs is the state-of-the-art understanding and utilization of the emerging science of consciously orchestrating the energies of brain and heart, body, mind, and spirit, a technology of human transformation and social evolution. They offer tools and techniques, stories, and examples that enhance ways of lifting relationships to higher bands of energy and harmony. They explore the reality of how different brains come with different energies and how to understand the structures, stages, and styles of love and romance. And their take on the traditional battle of the sexes is both unique and startling. They have found the way to end the ancient war! As they say:

> You are living in perhaps the most exciting yet challenging time in history for being on a journey inspired by love. Never before have people been beckoned so strongly to create relationships where the forces that have been traditionally thought of as masculine and the forces that have been traditionally thought of as feminine can join *within* each person and *between* two partners to form the richest relationships since the dawn of time!

The implications here are enormous. Shifting the ways we relate to one another, male and female, is an indispensable step toward the discovery of new styles of inter-personal connection, new ways of being in community, and the emergence of a global society. The movement seems to be from the egocentric to the ethnocentric to the worldcentric—a fundamental change in the nature of civilization, compelling a passage beyond the mind-set and institutions of millennia.

Critical to this reformation is a true partnership society in which women join men in the full social agenda. Since women tend to emphasize process over product, to understand the power of *being* as well as *doing*, deepening rather than end-goaling, it is inevitable that as a result of this partnership, linear, sequential solutions will evolve to the knowing that comes from seeing things in whole constellations rather than as discrete facts. The consciousness engendered by this comprehensive vision raises hope for forgiveness and healing among individuals, ethnic groups, and nations. Essential to this matured consciousness is moral and ethical growth toward the *golden rule* of human interchange, about which Donna Eden and David Feinstein know so much and give so rich a palette of information and training.

Ultimately it is about a new kind of education, of which this book is a primary text. In the places where our world truly operates interdependently and with this kind of education, old barriers can dissolve, along with the ancient fears that sustained them. What Donna and David offer in their work are the necessary tools and practices, the empathic understandings and the science that can support so great a whole-system transition. We have to learn the dynamics of getting along with each other, of coming to love and appreciate each other. They remind us that when the world is trying to coalesce into a new and higher unity for which we are seemingly unprepared, the only preparatory force that is emotionally powerful enough to prompt us to fully heed this call is found in the energies of love.

Love transforms the way we see, think, dream, act, engage the world, serve others, and even transcend our local selves. It is the source of much creative endeavor—songs, poetry, writing, dreaming, human folly, and human glory. It awakens us and keeps us going. As we love more, we honor more. We see and accept more. We honor pain, beauty, and one another's path. With love we become more intelligent and creative, for we are open to the patterns of intelligence from the whole network of life. We come to glimpse the wonder of life in its infinite forms, and the wonder that is within us. Quite simply, with love we are able to exceed our local conditions and to evolve.

The teaching of this book is to bring ourselves to a loving resonance, discovering strategies and practices of loving that then can become daily practice, constant application. This may be the most important learning of them all, the one that may hold the greatest good for life on this planet—learning how to commit to the choice of loving. As you do, you will discover that the universe is also alive and loving: as you move toward it, it moves toward you. The universe grows by its connections and its attractions: atoms to atoms, molecules to molecules, bodies to bodies, groups to groups, nations to nations, and finally the *world* as lover.

We are asked, in this epoch of cultural rebirth, to grow into the people willing and able to face, solve, and succeed in the enormous challenges that have arisen. In so huge a transitional moment of history, we require new skills and capacities as well as nurturing relationships in which our evolving selves are supported and given training that dissolves the barriers between our ordinary and our extraordinary selves.

This is all here in this remarkable work. The transformative power of the energies of love can and does evoke in us a Divine response: deep acceptance and forgiveness, profound spoken and unspoken communion and communication, the ecstasies of eros and the fires of union, a wave-tide of giving and receiving so abundant that it seems drawn from the very ocean of abundance itself, weaving together in love all of life's dramas.

—Jean Houston, Ph.D.
Ashland, Oregon
May 2014

Introduction

The Energies of Love

*Love is the pinnacle of evolution, the most compelling
survival mechanism of the human species.*

—SUE JOHNSON, PH.D.[1]

WE OFTEN JOKE, OR HALF JOKE, THAT IF WE CAN MAKE IT, ANY COUPLE CAN make it. While our basic values, mercifully, complement one another's effortlessly, our personalities, temperaments, and lifestyle inclinations don't. David thrives in dry hot weather, Donna withers. Donna's interests and attention jump like fire in a dozen different directions; David can become irritated when his plodding, intense focus is jerked from its course by one of her eruptions of enthusiasm. David organizes his life around endeavors that make him feel well utilized and worthy; Donna functions best moment by moment. Donna works most effectively within an unhurried, unscheduled, organic pace; David has been compared to a freight train when he is engaged in a project. Donna's disposition is to yield to the other person's ways, so even though David is attracted to her for her joyful nature, his more somber style sets their tone. She then feels invisible and discounted; he wonders why her friends bring out the person he wants to be with while he so often doesn't.

Having experimented with the basics of this program for more than thirty years, we went to Alex's, a restaurant in our hometown of Ashland, Oregon, with the commitment that we were not going to leave the lounge until we had completed the first sentence of this book. We finished our tempura shrimp and many refills of club soda; considered a dozen ways to begin the book; settled on the highly personal; wrote the "if we can make it" sentence; watched a young couple kissing on the restaurant's balcony overlooking Ashland's famous plaza; thanked them later for adding to the spirit of our project; joked with the restaurant's manager; who told us that she had announced to her husband that they were expecting their first child at the same table where we were birthing this project; and, finally satisfied with our sixteen-word writing spree, went on our way.

The next morning, David filled in the remainder of the first paragraph, writing as he often does in the early hours. When Donna awoke, he read it to her. She liked it very well until the last line. She said, "Do you mean to tell me you still feel that way? I thought you were over that twenty years ago." Her tone had hurt and shock. David felt discounted and unfairly attacked. Donna couldn't believe that he was accusing her of attacking him, when it was *she* whose feelings had been hurt. We were off to the who-was-wronged-worse races, both also feeling, "What an inauspicious beginning for a book on the energies of love!"

As our discouragement escalated, and after a brief period of separation as Donna bathed and David stewed, Donna said, "If we are really going to do this book and present these techniques, let's see if they can get us out of this one." David used a technique for countering the energies that can trigger his defensiveness when Donna is hurt by something he has done. Donna used a technique to counter her energetic freeze and inability to think when David reacts defensively. Why we'd never tackled this particular long-standing pattern before using these tools, we cannot say; perhaps we were saving it for demonstration purposes. The ten minutes of retrieval work not only "got us out of this one," it helped shift the pattern.

This book shows you how to work your way out of such entanglements with your partner, along with ways to turn your differences into strengths and areas of stagnation into renewal. What is most unusual in our approach is that it does not focus only on psychological differences, communication styles, and positive intentions. It also shows you how to focus directly and effectively on your *energies*, your partner's *energies*, and how they interact.

What Is This Thing Called Love?

You are reading a book whose title includes two terms—*love* and *energies*—that have baffled scientists, philosophers, and theologians for as long as their disciplines have existed. We are not arrogant enough to promise to resolve the historical ambiguities, contradictions, and mysteries surrounding either term (much as we'd like to), but we will try to give you a working feel for each that will be useful in reading this book.

Ancient Greek philosophers described four types of love: *agape* (spiritual, selfless, unconditional love), *eros* (passionate love, with sensual desire and longing), *philia* (affectionate regard or friendship), and *storge* (the natural affection of kinship, such as that felt by parents for their children). The Old Testament enumerates love's qualities: "Love is patient, love is kind. It does not envy, it does not boast, it is not proud. . . . It always protects, always trusts, always hopes, always perseveres" (1 Corinthians 13:4–8). The New Testament identifies three sources of human love (heart, soul, and mind) and suggests that we can willfully direct our love: "Thou shalt love the Lord thy God with all thy heart, and with all thy soul, and with all thy mind, and with all thy strength" (Luke 10:27). It also goes beyond the human dimension of love, equating love with God: "Whoever does not love does not know God, because God is love" (1 John 4:8). The idea of two loves—one earthly, one heavenly—can be found throughout recorded history.

For the scientist, one of the fundamental principles of the universe is the proclivity to *bond*. Within moments after the Big Bang, elementary particles began forming stable relationships of increasing complexity.[2] Brian Swimme and Mary Tucker note that "[a]ttraction between a proton and an electron is a way in which the universe gives rise to ever greater levels of complexity which, after some fourteen billion years, includes us."[3] Bonding at the subatomic level is necessary for your body to exist, and nature extended the principle so you must jump the spatial gap between you and another to create the next generation. A magnetic energy compels you to take the leap; love at its many levels, from earthly to heavenly, makes that biological leap distinctly human. Writing as a research scientist whose lab at the University of North Carolina investigates positive human emotion, psychologist Barbara Fredrickson reports that love literally changes the cell structures that affect physical health, vitality, and ultimately, "whether you'll thrive or just get by."[4] She provocatively suggests that while love is composed of many moments of biochemical, emotional, and behavioral connection, from the body's perspective, these are, "fleeting," "not lasting," just "forever renewable."[5]

The energies of love are a dynamic force between two people that transcend their personalities, their beliefs, and their backgrounds. These energies are channeled from deep in your being, meet, and merge into an alchemical fuel that transforms you. You are their container, yet you cannot contain them. As you evolve, as you expand the container, the energies of love expand along with you. This is a book about the energies of love as well as the human containers through which they flow.

The Energies within Us; the Energies between Us

Just as each of us is born with a completely unique physical structure, we are also born with a completely unique "energy structure." Electrical impulses move through our bodies. Electrical fields surround our organs. These impulses and fields control our physical growth. This was first demonstrated scientifically in the 1930s when Harold Burr, a neuroanatomist at Yale, designed equipment that could measure the electromagnetic field around an unfertilized salamander egg.[6] Burr stumbled on the extraordinary finding that the electromagnetic field of the egg was shaped like a *mature* salamander. The electrical axis that would later align with the brain and spinal cord was already present, as if the blueprint for the adult were there in the egg's energy field. The embryo would grow to take the shape of the electromagnetic field. The physiology patterned itself after the field! Burr went on to find electromagnetic fields surrounding all manner of organisms, from molds to plants to frogs to humans, and he was able to distinguish electrical patterns that corresponded with health and with illness.

Energy fields not only govern our health and biological growth but also impact our relationships. The heart and brain are each surrounded by an electromagnetic field, with the heart's field, you may be surprised to hear, having some sixty times the amplitude of the brain's field.[7] The electromagnetic field produced by your heart can be detected anywhere on the surface of your body using an electrocardiogram, and it also extends a number of feet beyond you, radiating in all directions, which can be detected by other instruments. The electromagnetic signals produced by your heart are registered by the brains of people around you. If two people are within conversational distance, fluctuations in the heart signal of one correspond with fluctuations in the brain waves of the other.[8]

Not only do your physiological responses sync up energetically with your partner's during intimate interactions, but also the field radiated by your heart can transmit emotions. Researchers at the HeartMath Institute in California have described this in measurable terms: "The rhythmic beating patterns of the heart change significantly as we experience different emotions. Difficult emotions, such as anger or frustration, are associated with an erratic, disordered, incoherent pattern in the heart's rhythms. In contrast, pleasurable emotions, such as love or appreciation, are associated with a smooth, ordered, coherent pattern in the heart's rhythmic activity. [These changes] create corresponding changes in the structure of the electromagnetic field radiated by the heart."[9] Your heart carries emotional information that physically impacts your partner.

Meanwhile, even with its smaller electromagnetic field, the brain contains some one hundred billion neurons that each connects electrochemically with up to ten thousand other neurons. The brain's electrical impulses constitute an incomprehensibly complex energy system that maintains your habits of perceiving, thinking, and responding to your world. Beyond these measurable electrical energies are more subtle energies carried by your body's meridians, chakras, and aura—concepts familiar in healing traditions across time and cultures, even if not acknowledged by Western science because they have (until recently[10]) eluded its ability to detect them. Change the energies that travel through your body and you can change your mood, your mind, and your relationships.

When David went into meltdown, the changes in his electrical system occurred in his heart as well as his brain, and measurable electrical changes in Donna's heart and brain occurred in response. Altering this electrical dissonance was our first focus in beginning to make things better. Not empathy, not analysis, not insight, not love. We turned to simple energy techniques.

We have often been painfully moved as we've watched clients and friends, as well as ourselves, ineffectually struggle to improve their relationships, using every ounce of smarts and goodwill at their disposal. Sometimes the way the energy is moving through your body keeps you trapped in a particular pattern of thought and behavior. Often the quickest way to free yourself from the pattern is to shift the underlying energy rather than to target the feelings, thoughts, or behavior.

The Tools: Something Old, Something New

Sigmund Freud, Carl Jung, and other pioneers of psychodynamic approaches to emotional healing showed how our childhood experiences—echoes from the recesses of our past—can still be affecting us today. Many of the therapies that arose from their revolutionary work have given us maps to help free ourselves from the effects of emotional injury or trauma in childhood. This resulted in a quantum leap in humanity's self-concept: Deeply embedded psychological patterns can be transformed, and tools for initiating that transformation are available.

We are now standing at another momentous threshold, one that translates these insights into practices that are more rapid and effective than ever before. Methods are available that can shift the energies that are not only at the core of your thoughts, mood, and behavior, but also of your health and happiness. The disciplines of *energy medicine* and *energy psychology*, new to Western culture yet drawing on ancient healing and spiritual traditions, are rapidly ascending in the popular as well as professional eye. We have borrowed heavily from both disciplines in writing this book.

Our own personal and professional lives have been deeply committed to advancing these methods. That commitment and the experiences that have emerged from it are our primary credentials for offering this volume. Other background about us that you may find relevant for framing our ideas:

Donna has since childhood seen energies, surrounding and moving through the body, as clearly as you see the print on this page, and she has learned that, like the print, these energies have distinct meanings and can be informative about health and healing. She is, in fact, internationally known for her clairvoyant abilities to perceive and work with the body's energies. The way people like Donna can see energies that other people can't see has been compared to the way dogs can hear frequencies that humans can't hear. The energies are there and operating, but beyond most people's awareness. More significant, Donna has taught tens of thousands of people around the world who don't see energy to nonetheless assess and shift energy flows in ways that enhance their health and vitality.

David has been a clinical psychologist for nearly four decades. In recent years his focus has, with Donna's influence, turned to the application of energy methods for working with psychological issues. Our combined six books and numerous papers and articles on these topics have attempted to bring energy medicine and energy psychology to both professional and popular audiences. With these backgrounds, we come together to present you with this practical guide for optimizing the energies that affect your relationships.

The Context: A New Age for Partnerships

While your relationship is a unique creation between you and your partner, it is not only between you and your partner. It builds on the customs and relationship patterns established by your parents and their parents and the generations before them, and it is being shaped by changes in your culture that are unfolding at a pace that could not have been imagined just a few decades ago. These changes penetrate to the ways we think of ourselves as men and women and are reflected in how we relate to one another.

Coming into Balance

In most societies, extending back to the dawn of recorded history, men have controlled property, held the central positions of political power, and retained the primary authority within the family and the community. Within this patriarchal structure, men have dominated women not only through force but more covertly through mass indoctrination into what was officially depicted as the natural order of things. Modern Western societies, for instance, assign worth to people, to a large extent, by their ability to produce wealth. Women, saddled with the tasks of child-rearing and tending the home, were, by these terms, second-class citizens. They were less valued and many of their natural ways of operating in the world were curtailed, ridiculed, or even condemned. As Laurel Thatcher Ulrich wryly observed, "well-behaved women seldom make history."[11] These constraints have, however, been imploding in recent decades.

A new valuing and empowering of women is emerging in modern societies, reflected in part by the rapid changes in women's economic status. In 1970, less than 6 percent of a U.S. family's income was brought in by women. Now it is more than 40 percent and increasing.[12] More than half of all managerial and professional jobs are also held by women, up from 26 percent in 1980.[13] Of the fifteen job categories projected to have the greatest growth in the next decade, thirteen are occupied primarily by women.[14]

Hanna Rosin explains that the inherent advantages of a man's biology no longer matter: "thinking and communicating have come to eclipse physical strength and stamina as the keys to economic success." Since "cultural and economic changes always reinforce each other . . . the global economy is evolving in a way that is eroding the historical preference for male children, worldwide."[15] In the 1980s, as sperm banks were making it possible for couples seeking artificial insemination to choose the gender of their child, it was widely assumed that there would be a universal preference for sons. Now the preference is for daughters, by as much as 2 to 1 in some clinics.[16]

While fierce backlash is still tearing at the rights and progress of women, Rosin reflects that "given the power of the forces pushing at the economy, this setup feels like the last gasp of a dying age."[17] Women have greater power, are creating new social forms and management styles, and are exercising their capacity to challenge an old order that has brought us to the brink of extinction. While that old order is characterized by patriarchal, "masculine" beliefs and values, this does not mean that masculine is wrong while "feminine" is right. What is so wrong is that we are in many ways veering even further out of balance.

Humanity's survival may depend on personal and cultural forces that have been rising to counter this trend toward the masculine principle run amok: increased domination of nature, inequitable distribution of wealth, runaway corporate power, hijacking of democratic processes, use of violence to settle disputes, and other destructive arrangements. Meanwhile, the feminine reveres nature, trusts emotion, listens to intuition, nurtures relationships, cares for every child, is embracing rather than divisive, and affirms the often messy spontaneous expressions of the soul. However much bringing balance to these qualities might lead to a better world, established orders do not yield easily. This struggle is playing out within a world where the quickening pace is dizzying, cultural beliefs and traditions are leaping social and national boundaries in an orgy of creative as well as strained cross-fertilization, and our sense of where we are collectively headed is a tapestry of unprecedented possibilities and life-threatening hazards.

The Changing Landscape of Marriage

How do these shifts in society, behavior, and consciousness impact your relationship? In a word, *profoundly*. Historians and sociologists have identified three eras in American history in relation to marriage. From the country's founding until about 1850, affection and emotional intimacy were secondary to the basics of physical survival such as food, shelter, and protection. From around 1850 through the mid-1960s, love, intimacy, and a fulfilling sex life rose in importance within the dominant model of marriage. In the current era, while love and a practical partnership are of course still vital considerations, the ability of a marriage to support each partner's personal evolution has emerged as a pivotal dimension of marital satisfaction.[18]

When women were asked, back in 1939, to rank eighteen qualities they want in a future husband, love was ranked fifth.[19] Economic support was still considered more important than love. By the 1950s, surveys revealed love to be climbing up the list until a U.S. poll in 2001 showed that "80 percent of women in their twenties said that having a man who could talk about his feelings was more important than having one who could make a good living."[20] At the heart of this new era of relationship, explains sociologist Robert Bellah, is that love has, to a great degree, become "the mutual exploration of infinitely rich, complex and exciting selves."[21]

Gallant as this may sound, the pressure has grown intense for marriage partners to be all things for one another—lovers, parents, family, friends, business partners, and now évocateurs of one another's "infinitely rich and exciting selves." Expectations about the needs a marriage should fulfill are at an unprecedented high, and many marriages do not come close to meeting them.[22] Studies of marital satisfaction present an inescapable fact: The gap between marriages that are disappointing (the larger grouping) and marriages that are gratifying (the smaller grouping) is increasing. On the one side, the *average* marriage today is weaker, in terms of both satisfaction and greater likelihood of divorce than ever before. Increased demands make us vulnerable to greater disappointment. Dissatisfaction, even in marriages that last, has become endemic.[23] On the other side, the *best* marriages today are stronger than perhaps at any previous time in history.[24]

As marriages are required to meet more of our needs, these "best" partnerships are realistic about dedicating the time and energy that is required for the new vision of marriage to flourish, and they find ways to do so.[25] You will learn in these pages some of the most effective ways for using the time and energy you do commit to your partnership. For instance, findings about the happiest marriages do not mean you are required to dote on one another during all your waking hours. Spouses who reported intense positive engagement with one another at least once each week were three and a half times more likely to be "very happy" in their marriage than those who rarely engaged one another deeply.[26]

For most of history, the models for love and family provided by the parents' generation were rarely questioned. Today they are increasingly *irrelevant*. Within our personal memories, and before that, throughout the history of Western civilization, the husband was ultimately responsible for the family, expected to be strong and dominant, treating his wife and children as his possessions. The hero's quest was the domain of the male. The woman's role was to set him on that quest, inspire him, support him, and be there to shower him with love when he returned.[27]

So it was for thousands of years. But within one generation, all of this has turned on its side for much of Western culture. Even the most basic function of marriage—producing offspring—meets the opposing force of overpopulation, opening the way for a cultural valuing of LGBT marriages and other intimate partnerships where birthing children is not a cardinal purpose. Marriages are no longer forged within a clear guiding image of how they should unfold. The roles and relative power of men and women in relationship are no longer predefined. Social arrangements that embrace characteristically female ways of being are appearing. Rising forces revaluing intuition, emotion, relationship, nature, and human welfare over the status quo shake up society as well as intimate partnerships.

Disruptive as any other fundamental change, these shifts may nonetheless be essential for cultural survival. A marriage today is more than ever a creative arrangement harboring extreme challenges and unanticipated possibilities as the maps from the past have lost their currency and the terrain itself is in continual flux. This book is designed to help you navigate your way through these perils and opportunities. You are living in perhaps the most exciting yet challenging time in history for being on a journey inspired by love. Never before have people been beckoned so strongly to create relationships where the forces that have been traditionally thought of as masculine and the forces that have been traditionally thought of as feminine can join *within* each person and *between* two partners to form the richest relationships since the dawn of time!

A Brief Overview of *The Energies of Love*

The Energies of Love shows how your energies play a *palpable* role in your psyche and your relationships, and it offers clear, practical guidance for working with these energies to enhance your partnership.

Three Aspects of Love

The book is organized around three broad themes:

- The inherited aspects of love
- The learned aspects of love
- The mutually created aspects of love

Each of these has a different dynamic, has specific requirements for effectively engaging its challenges, and has an energetic counterpart. The *inherited* aspects of love, for example, are fixed. While you cannot change them, you can influence how they express themselves and develop ways of fielding them more skillfully. The *learned* aspects of love were first acquired early in life and can be modified to enhance your ability to love more fully and relate more effectively. The *mutually created* aspects of love are an ongoing masterwork between you and your partner. This book shows you how to better understand and journey your way through each.

Part 1, "The Inherited Aspects of Love," teaches you new navigational skills for your relationship without particularly trying to change either of you. The inherited aspects of your partnership dictate that any relationship involves a coming together of the distinct energies carried by two different bodies and souls. This energetic meeting is the foundation of everything else that will unfold. From it emerges the way two people will perceive, experience, and behave toward one another. The energies that influence the way you and your partner process information and handle disagreements get special attention in Part 1. Powerful tools from energy medicine are provided for bridging your energies with your partner's and finding your way through territory where they mesh, as well as where they do not mesh.

Whereas Part 1 shows you how to flow with each other *as you are*, Part 2, "The Learned Aspects of Love," shows you how to *make changes* in learned emotional responses. Your experiences with your parents and other early intimates left imprints that impact your subsequent relationships, and since no one's childhood or parents were perfect, these imprints can be limiting and self-defeating. While the imprints that shape our relationships tend to evolve as we mature, they can become quite set in our brains, our energies, and our behavior patterns. In fact, for many people, these fundamental patterns never change. Drawing from the field of energy psychology, Part 2 shows you how to identify and transform deep learnings that no longer serve. You will be introduced to powerful self-help procedures that can heal old emotional wounds, literally rewiring the neural pathways driving outdated patterns and opening the way to more fulfilling relationships.

Part 3, "The Mutually Created Aspects of Love," is about the couple's voyage in forward motion. You take what you've inherited and what you have learned, then come together, and the rest is up to the two of you. Part 3 opens by showing how sex is "nature's energy medicine for couples" (chapter 8). Sex comes naturally, but sexual fulfillment in a long-term relationship is neither a biological imperative nor even a guaranteed outcome of deep and lasting love. The actions that keep your sexual energies engaged over the span of a lasting partnership occur outside as well as within the bedroom, and they are entwined with nature's beckoning that you keep growing as individuals and as a couple. In fact, as a relationship matures, you increasingly become "conscious partners" (chapter 9) cultivating the shared "spiritual journey" you find yourselves traversing (chapter 10).

The individuals portrayed in the case histories have granted permission to have their stories told, or their identities have been thoroughly disguised, or, in some instances, they are composites. Although we use the language of male and female partnerships throughout the book, the basic principles apply to all committed, loving relationships.

How to Use This Book

Our goal with *The Energies of Love* is to offer maps you can use to improve your partnership in relation to the inherited, learned, and mutually created aspects of love just discussed. From the explosion of scientific breakthroughs about the nature of attachment, brain development, and interpersonal dynamics, we have attempted to (1) synthesize the "best of" from all these significant developments, (2) integrate them with our own personal and professional experiences and perspectives, and (3) present them laced with our insights about the fundamental influences of the *energies* of love. Each chapter includes boxes labeled "The Energy Dimension" describing how Donna *sees* the energies underlying the principles being described. Meanwhile, the book invites you to use it as no less than a "surrogate couples coach."

You can approach the book in a number of ways. You can read it alone, read it simultaneously but separately, or read it aloud to one another and discuss as you go along. While the chapters are designed to be read from the first to the last, if you are particularly drawn to one of the sections, you can start there. After reviewing a draft of the manuscript, one of our colleagues suggested that we publish this as three books. Though we feel the three sections are too intertwined to separate, we recognize that, like the territory it explores, this is a more complex read than many self-help books. The good news is that new understanding about the invisible choreographies of the energies, hormones, and brain chemistries of love are synthesized here in a way that makes it possible to create a stronger foundation for taking your partnership to new heights of intimacy. Your parents and all the generations before them were, on the other hand, required to rely primarily on intuitive acumen or blind luck when deviating from the dictates of tradition.

Any book about couples written by a couple reflects their relationship as well as whatever it intends to present. Ours has not been a particularly easy partnership. A couples therapist we once worked with, trying to reassure us in a discouraging moment, told us that she thinks our relationship is a crucible in which the interpersonal challenges of the "collective" are being played out so we can address them ourselves and teach others what we have learned. Whether or not that is the case, we have certainly experienced some large challenges. We developed, or adapted from others, many of the techniques we present here partially because we have needed them. We have been our own laboratory. And we have been gratified when ideas and techniques that have helped us have also been valuable for our clients and students.

The twenty-first century has ushered in a brave new world for couples. Just as the challenges are unprecedented, unimagined tools for meeting those challenges are emerging. This book presents, in our experience, many of the best of those tools. We close our writing of this introduction by facing one another and, with hands clasped and eyes meeting, affirm our intention that every person reading this book be empowered on a path toward greater love and a more fulfilling partnership.

PART

I

The
Inherited
Aspects
of Love

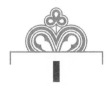

You and Your Partner See through Different Eyes

Unfamiliar Energies Attract

*Although it is nice to discover that we are liked
by a person who holds views similar to ours,
it is much more exciting to discover that we are
liked by a person whose views are different.*

—AYALA PINES, PH.D.[1]

ARLY IN OUR RELATIONSHIP, DONNA ATTENDED, AS DAVID'S GUEST, A HYPNOSIS CLASS he was teaching. The evening's session focused on the various ways people code experience. A good hypnotist works one way with individuals who organize their inner world in a manner that corresponds with how they *see* and will work another way with those who organize their inner world in a manner that corresponds with how they *feel*. Four distinct types trace to basic ways of processing information: visual, auditory, kinesthetic, and abstract reasoning.[2] At the break, David stole a private moment with Donna, hoping to hear how impressed his new sweetie was with how well he had kept the interest of this group of professional psychotherapists who were generally older and more seasoned than himself. Donna instead said, "Well, that was interesting, to learn the characteristics of each of the four types, but I can see a way to determine a person's style using a simple physical test. After all, each of the types carries a different kind of energy."

Besides the little ego twinge that she had not been dazzled enough to even comment on his teaching prowess, David was incredulous. How could a *physical* test pick up on these *psychological* differences? This was preposterous, and he was happy to share that revelation with her. Undaunted, Donna immediately turned her idea into an experiment, using the class members during the break. Sure enough, those whom David had identified as visuals tested differently from those who had been identified as kinesthetics (feelings), tonals (auditory), or digitals (abstract reasoning). By the time the class reconvened, this had become the buzz and was the only thing people wanted to talk about. So Donna wound up taking the rest of the evening, teaching a technique she calls energy testing and showing how it can be applied to determining people's style of processing information. It was an exciting evening for all involved, though the remainder of the planned agenda had to be put on the shelf. If David could have heard his guardian angels at this early point in our relationship, they would have been saying, "Get used to it, David."

That evening was our first experience in the bridging of our disciplines, and Donna's insight has held up through the decades. Identifying a person's fundamental way of internally representing the world has proven enormously useful for helping people understand themselves and for helping couples understand one another. While everyone combines all four modalities, only one of the four will dominate during the kinds of stress that evoke a survival response. And this hardly requires that a life-threatening situation has been encountered. Because humans have so strongly depended on the support of one another throughout evolution, any disturbance in our closest relationships is biologically coded as a threat to our survival. Such moments of threat are almost always found in a relationship's history, and they occur frequently in many relationships. While we each use all four modalities, it is our primary style that we viscerally trust and rely on when an intimate bond is disrupted.

Your primary way of processing information during threat is more than a mere psychological difference between you and others. It is built into your *energy structure*—a physical, measurable form—and our impression is that it is coded in your genes. Many times Donna has been present when one of her clients was giving birth, or shortly thereafter, in order to provide an energy balancing to mother and baby following the trials of childbirth. Donna, who has literally been able to "see" energy since her own childhood, can tell the parents, based on the way the infant's energy looks to her, whether they have a visual, a tonal, a kinesthetic, or a digital on their hands. This has been going on long enough now that she has substantial confirmation that by the time the newborn has reached the teen years, the primary style has not changed from the initial assessment. So a person's core way of processing information—one of the most significant differences among people and critical for partners to understand about one another—is either built in genetically or determined by prenatal experiences.

You can imagine how this might happen. Prenatal life is initially a kinesthetic journey. Everything that occurs is experienced in the moment with no sense of past or future, no sense of near or far, inner or outer, and no sensations such as sight or sound to inform the moment. All of life is a unified, undifferentiated *now*. If Mom is happy and the supporting chemistry is good, it could not be better. If Mom is sad or scared or if the nutrients are in short supply, the entire universe is a bad trip. Then Mom laughs, and it is a good trip again. The eternal moment is all there is.

By the sixteenth week of gestation, the ear has become functional and the fetus can hear and will respond to a sound pulse. Active listening begins by the twenty-fourth week. The mother's heartbeat, respiration, and intestinal gurgling form a "sound carpet."[3] The mother's voice is given special attention in relation to the "carpet" because it is so different from the amniotic sounds, and her voice establishes the first patterns of communication and bonding. No longer is the experience of the moment the sole source of information. This is a gargantuan shift in consciousness! The moment is now informed by a second way of knowing. Mom can be having indigestion. The world is a bad place. But Mom can also be singing a lullaby. The world is a good place. Which one do you trust? How do you reconcile these two sources of opposing information? Welcome to the world of interpersonal relationships, little one.

The next major shift in the sensory coding of the world occurs after birth. A responsiveness to light shining through the mother's abdomen has been developing during the last trimester of pregnancy. The newborn can see eight to fourteen inches, though at first everything is quite blurry. But vision rapidly improves and becomes a third and distinctly different way of directly experiencing the environment. While they are not the only physical senses that tell us about the world, these three—feeling, hearing, and seeing—are the ones most developed and emphasized in modern Western societies.

A fourth way of knowing your environment soon began to take form, and that was to know it by the symbols and then the words that could allow you to mentally represent your sensory experiences, form abstractions, and manipulate ideas so you could make plans and envision possibilities. For some people, this abstract reasoning becomes a more trusted way of understanding the world than their sensations. So four fundamental ways of representing experience are based on feeling (kinesthetic), sound (tonal), sight (visual), and logic (digital). Vision and logical thought are not in place at birth, yet the energies Donna sees at birth predict whether the infant will, when under relationship distress, grow up wired to rely on a kinesthetic, tonal, visual, or digital representational style. This suggests that a person's primal way of processing information is determined by genetics rather than even prenatal experiences.

We use the term *Energetic Stress Style* to describe the sensory mode you instinctively trust and favor when experiencing threat or stress, particularly when it involves your partner. This favored sensory mode is patterned after *one* of the primary ways you experience the world (seeing, hearing, feeling, thinking), and it determines how you process information when under stress. Besides influencing how you make sense of things during stressful moments, your Energetic Stress Style is an energetic state that your body enters when distressed. Donna sees each style as corresponding with a distinct type of *palpable living energies*.

Corresponding with our energy perspective are findings from modern neuroscience. As described by Dan Siegel, a Harvard-trained psychiatrist who is among the leading voices today in the application to psychotherapy of new breakthroughs in brain science:

> Brain imaging studies examine the metabolic, energy-consuming processes in specific neural regions . . . These assessments of "energy flow" are not popularized, unscientific views of the flow of some mysterious energy through the universe. Neuroscience studies the way in which the brain functions through the energy-consuming activation of neurons. The degree and localization of this arousal and activation within the brain—this flow of energy—directly shape our mental processes. . . .[4]
>
> Within the circuits linked directly to the outside world and to the body, sensory representations are created [the "kinesthetic" mode in our system]. Perceptual representations established by these sensory inputs are then processed and transformed into more complex representations [our "tonal" and "visual" styles]. . . . More complex and abstract symbols are thought to emanate from the activity of the neocortex [our "digital" style].[5]

Of the distinct modes of processing information (kinesthetic, tonal, visual, digital), you instinctively count on one more than the others when distress enters your relationship.

➤ THE ENERGY DIMENSION ←

Your Biofield Determines Your Energetic Stress Style
Here is what Donna sees when she focuses on a person's energies, including those of a newborn. Surrounding the person is a region of energy referred to in many traditions as the aura. Scientists who have detected it using electrical instruments call it the biofield.[6] Along with many other intuitive healers, Donna sees it as having several layers, each with distinct colors, textures, and other properties.

The Emotional/Mental Layer of Your Biofield
One of the layers is referred to as the emotional/mental layer. This layer is distinguished by four distinct "bands" of energy: a *feeling band*, an *emotional band* (emotions are defined as feelings interacting with thoughts), and two *mental bands*, one that is outward-focused and one that is inward-focused. The feeling band corresponds with the kinesthetic style of processing information; the emotional band with the tonal style; the outward-focused mental band with the visual style; and the inward-focused mental band with the digital style.

The Order of the Bands in the Emotional/Mental Layer of Your Biofield
The order of these four bands (from closest to farthest from the body) varies from one individual to the next. The band that is closest to the body determines the sensory representational mode the person will viscerally trust and rely on during times of distress. So, if the feeling band is closest to your body, you will instinctively rely on the kinesthetic mode under stress; if the emotional band is closest, then the tonal mode will dominate under stress; if the outward-focused mental band is closest, then the visual mode will dominate; if the inward-focused mental band is closest, then the digital mode will dominate.

How Your Energetic Stress Style
Distorts the One You Love

In an old parable, a group of blind men are brought to an elephant. Each has his hands placed on one part of the great creature and is asked to identify what he is touching. The one given the trunk determines that it is a hose. The one at the elephant's side thinks he has come to a wall. The one whose arms are wrapped around the leg knows it to be a tree. The one at the tail certifies that it is a snake. Although the parable does not account for these men's apparent olfactory limitations, it does illustrate that by focusing on only one part of a larger story you may come to conclusions that are comical at best and disastrous at worst.

This is what happens to you when you are under relationship stress. Because you are wired to treat your closest relationships and your own survival in a similar manner, such distortions are particularly strong when the stress is caused by difficulties with your partner (to paraphrase the popular song "You Always Distort the One You Love"). The closer the person is to you, the harder it is to keep the person in perspective when the relationship is having difficulties. And the way you distort the one you love has everything to do with your Energetic Stress Style. You represent the world when feeling distress according to the bias of the sensory mode that dominates when you feel threatened.

Your Energetic Stress Style is not the *act* of seeing, hearing, or feeling. Rather, your inner world is *organized* according to *principles* that most closely correspond with seeing, hearing, feeling, or the fourth mode, abstract logic. Human thought is extraordinarily flexible, and each of us normally combines all four modes. But we viscerally tend to depend and put more emphasis on one of them, and when we feel distress in our primary relationship, the other modes fade into the background. The entire elephant becomes *just* a wall or snake or hose or tree. We distort the one we love according to the principles of the sensory mode we trust the most. The other three modes simply shut down. It is not a choice but a physiological energetic response. And when this occurs, we cannot help but create mental distortions and then act accordingly (and inappropriately). It's the natural thing to do!

Energetically, You Become a Different Animal during Relationship Stress

When Donna carefully watches a couple in a stressful encounter, she will see one of four distinct energetic modes emerge in each partner. This shift in energy corresponds with the visual, kinesthetic, digital, and tonal sensory channels we've been discussing. It occurs quite consistently and is independent of intelligence, height, or political party. Yet the energy that dominates for you during relationship stress is as tangible a difference to those who see energy as is the color of your eyes, the breadth of your shoulders, or whether you have an "innie" or an "outie" belly button.

Distortions of the Visual Style

Without the other modes to round out the picture, visuals lose perspective, normally their greatest strength. Their internal take or "view" of the situation overshadows whatever actually occurred. Not only does this *tunnel vision* compellingly distort understanding and undermine empathy, but visuals can quickly assemble a vision of how things should be, or more specifically, of how *you* should be and what *you* should do. They tend to embrace this vision wholeheartedly. You, meanwhile, are feeling unseen and are experiencing your visual partner's "helpful" analysis as judgment and blame. With the energy radiating outward from your visual partner during a stressful encounter, the focus moves to you, with emphasis on how you are the cause of the problem and need to do things differently.

> ### ⇢ THE ENERGY DIMENSION ⇠
>
> #### Visual Stress Style
>
> During times of relationship stress, for people whose Energetic Stress Style is *visual*, the body's energies tend to:
>
> * Concentrate in the head and the upper chest.
> * Then move outward, particularly through the eyes and chest area.
> * Appear to tunnel *toward* the other person.

Distortions of the Kinesthetic Style

When disagreement or upset occurs, kinesthetics are more attuned to their partner's hurt than to their own needs. Whatever energies the partner is emanating are absorbed like a sponge into the kinesthetic's body. As thick painful energy accumulates in their heart and chest, kinesthetics feel like they are about to burst or drown. Their desperate impulse is to turn off the source of their anguish by *soothing the partner!* Clear thinking is not supported, as the most vital energies have left the brain and gone into the body. These energies blend with the crisis that is unfolding until the distinction between self and other is long gone. From this constellation, with their needs unrecognized by themselves or their partner, kinesthetics are thrust into the interactions that will shape their relationships.

→ THE ENERGY DIMENSION ←

Kinesthetic Stress Style

During times of relationship stress, for people whose Energetic Stress Style is *kinesthetic*, the body's energies tend to:

- Become slow and heavy, like sludge.
- Connect with the outer world and then move inward in an overpowering way.
- Concentrate at the Heart Chakra at the center of the chest (*chakras*, from Sanskrit, are energy centers).
- Move out of the hips, legs, and feet, compromising grounding and stability.

Distortions of the Digital Style

The voice of the heart is muted, yet a rich choreography of energy is unfolding within the brain. The verbal reasoning and logic of the front brain overshadow the primitive needs of the back brain, giving the digital the appearance of clarity and calmness. This seems to the digital to be the paragon of rational, civilized thought. The system is closed and encapsulated. Not only do the energies of the heart and gut have no pathways to consciousness, the energy of the partner bounces off like rubber bands shot at a granite wall. The partner's explanations, feelings, and desperate pleas do not upset the digital, who is not *consciously* trying to dismiss the loved one. The partner's concerns are just not relevant and will be put to rest when he or she grasps the logic of the digital's superior understanding.

→ THE ENERGY DIMENSION ←

Digital Stress Style

During times of relationship stress, for people whose Energetic Stress Style is *digital*, the body's energies tend to:

- Rush up into the brain.
- Move from the back brain to the cerebral cortex, the front brain, with a primal force.
- Accumulate there in the forebrain.
- Be so cut off from the body that the heart and the gut have little influence on the person's experience.

Distortions of the Tonal Style

The tonal's energies get focused in the organs involved with emotion. The vibratory rate of the outside world is also sensitively registered and reverberates in those organs as well. Under stress, the partner's comments may activate a torrent of inner emotion that is not particularly related to the actual words or intended meaning. The tonal's acute sensitivity, which under peaceful conditions lends itself to exquisite aesthetic sensibilities, leads to a roar of painful and contradictory emotions under stress. Everything begins to scream at the tonal, sound becomes extraordinarily personal, and the distinction between the sounds generated by the partner and those generated by the internal organs is lost. A rich drama of incompatible emotions may be enacted until the tonal has little choice but to escape from the bombardment.

Assessing Your Energetic Stress Style

Recognize yourself yet? You may or may not at this point, but your partner probably does. It is much harder to recognize our own distortions than those of our partner. Particularly when we are in the middle of relationship stress, our inner experiences can become quite confusing. Another complication to identifying your own style is that when not under stress, you combine all four modes, and you may have even cultivated one of the other styles so strongly that you consciously identify more closely with it than you do with your primary inborn stress response mode. But when relationship stress hits, your Energetic Stress Style returns center stage for both you and your partner to encounter. This section of the book will show you what to do when life has drawn you into such a fine mess. As you work with your own and your partner's stress response styles, the dynamics of each will become clearer and it will be easier to bridge your differences.

You can gain at least a tentative idea of your own and your partner's Energetic Stress Style by taking the following quiz. A limitation is that when you are under relationship stress, your self-understanding is at a low ebb, so your experiences of who you are at such times, as well as your memory of those experiences, may be less than reliable. That is a reason we will be asking you to rate both yourself and your partner. The ensuing discussion of differences in your perceptions may be surprising and enlightening. Expect them. Be kind to one another as you try to reconcile them. If you find that you pretty much agree from the start, do not be discouraged; you will likely stumble into areas of disagreement later in the program!

Energetic Stress Style Assessment[7]

Permission is granted to photocopy this assessment for personal use. Make two copies for yourself and two copies for your partner. First complete each item for yourself; then for your partner. Circle the letter of the response that BEST describes your experiences. If you cannot decide between two items, mark "1/2" next to each of them. The opening line, "When in major conflict with my partner," is the same for each item.

1. **When in Major Conflict with My Partner:**
   a. I can focus clearly on precisely what my partner is doing wrong.
   b. I become logical, rational, and reasonable.
   c. I become exasperated at not feeling heard.
   d. My primal feelings can take over completely.

2. **When in Major Conflict with My Partner:**
   a. My partner tells me that I can't see my own part in it.
   b. I know what I think more than what I feel.
   c. I "hear" between the lines.
   d. Feelings are facts and logic is suspect.

3. **When in Major Conflict with My Partner:**
   a. I can see what my partner needs to do to solve the problem.
   b. I want to escape until my partner calms down.
   c. I hear my inner dialogue louder than my partner's voice.
   d. I feel very lonely when my partner won't show feelings.

4. **When in Major Conflict with My Partner:**
   a. I get more irritated than I should when my partner doesn't live up to my expectations.
   b. My partner sometimes accuses me of being too calm, cool, and collected.

c. I carefully analyze my partner's behavior and have strong emotions about it.

d. I tend to be nonconfrontational and overly cautious about not hurting my partner.

5. When in Major Conflict with My Partner:

a. I tend to judge and criticize my partner.

b. My logic is one of my greatest strengths.

c. Even though my partner claims I'm not being rejected in any way, I still feel rejected.

d. I try to make my partner feel good, but eventually I may fall apart or explode.

6. When in Major Conflict with My Partner:

a. I blame my partner.

b. I am surprised because I had no clue that there was a problem.

c. I can be hurt more by my partner's tone of voice than the actual words.

d. I am more attuned to my partner's feelings than I am to my own.

7. When in Major Conflict with My Partner:

a. My partner is usually wrong.

b. I become orderly, structured, and programmed.

c. I judge myself.

d. I lose my own truth.

8. When in Major Conflict with My Partner:

a. I want to say "Look at me!" if my partner is avoiding eye contact.

b. My partner's strong emotions are a turn-off.

c. I withdraw in hurt and frustration.

d. I often just give in if my partner seems to be in too much pain.

9. When in Major Conflict with My Partner:

a. It sometimes feels like a contest that I must win.

b. My superior logic gives me comfort.

c. I am very hard on myself.

d. I lose my truth and scramble for words.

10. When in Major Conflict with My Partner, My Unspoken Position Is:
   a. "You're Wrong!"
   b. "I'm Right!"
   c. "I'm Angry at You for Making Me Feel Wrong!"
   d. "I Don't Want You to Feel Wrong!"

Although the Energetic Stress Style Assessment may lack scientific rigor or validation, it is at least easy to score. Count your total number of a, b, c, and d scores. The more a's, the more you experience yourself as a visual, the more b's = digital, c's = tonal, and d's = kinesthetic. Once you've scored it for yourself, take the test again rating your partner. Then, if your partner also took the test, compare your scores with your partner's scores on both versions.

Most people score highest in one area, somewhat less on a second, and substantially less on the other two. The top two scores reflect your primary and secondary styles. The primary is inborn, *primal*. It is what you *instinctively* rely on during primal threat. Your secondary style has been nurtured by experience and preference, is often more valued consciously, and may be how you view yourself. This will often account for the difference between the way you scored yourself and the way your partner scored you. Recognizing these differences of perception is a start for bridging them and should, for now, at least lead to some interesting discussion.

When Two Energies Dance

One of the most important insights about sex and intimacy to come from the behavioral sciences is deceptively simple. For sex to stay hot within a long-term relationship, you not only must be able to deeply bond with your partner, you must also be able to preserve a separate identity.[8] You must be able to act autonomously and sustain your own center even while deeply registering your partner's needs, expectations, and desires. This delicate interplay between *bonding* and *differentiating* is the underlying issue around which many marriages succeed or fail, and it is as much a dance of two energy fields as it is a dance of two personalities.

No matter how much you love one another, if you can't get your energies into harmony and accord, it is going to be a rough road. All people have strategies for shifting the energy when a relationship becomes tense. Yelling is very popular. So

> → THE ENERGY DIMENSION ←
>
> ### The Merging of Two Energy Fields
>
> While physical bodies are relatively fixed and stable, energy fields are fluid and ever-shifting. A relationship begins with the meeting of two energy fields. Over time, the interactions between your energy field and your partner's grow ever more intricate and complex. Some parts of your energy fields may merge, some may repel; one field may overwhelm the other, or the two may blend into a new field that surrounds both bodies with comfort and joy . . . or tension and acrimony. *The way your energy field and your partner's interact forms the framework for everything else about your relationship.* It is the invisible force that supports your intimacy one moment but may place clouds of tension between you the next.

are withdrawing, crying, or having an affair. These all work; each generates a change in the energy. But they are something like symptom-suppressing medications. They may make you feel better for a while, but they don't resolve a thing, and they often have side effects that are much worse than the original problem. The way you and your partner maintain and mediate the energies between you, moment by moment, day by day, month by month, defines your relationship.

A simple technique to get the energies of two people *dancing* is to actually dance. This can be as easy as placing your hands palm against palm and creating free-flowing figure-eight motions with one another. As your hips and bodies follow, you are weaving your energies together. Doing it to music you love brings your rhythms into an easier sync and makes it more fun. A technique to *deepen* your connection is for each partner to put one hand around the back of the other's neck and the other at the side of the waist. Do this standing while looking in one another's eyes. Let your breathing synchronize. Feel your energies connecting.

When Your Styles Get Out of Sync

Whenever your energy field and your partner's come into dissonance, primal parts of your brain perceive a threat. Something is wrong on the home front, and you find yourself experiencing the world according to your Energetic Stress Style—visual, kinesthetic, tonal, or digital. The purpose of the following discussion about this inevitable, unpleasant dynamic is not to make you less hopeful about the relationship. It is just the opposite. It is to show you just where the problem lies and to allow you to more effectively address relationship difficulties at their energetic core.

Because you handle relationship stress according to your particular Energetic Stress Style and your partner doesn't (people with the same sensory style usually don't choose one another), it is almost inevitable that you have hurt one another and will hurt one another again. There is, however, a positive twist in this seemingly absurd design. Because of the differences in your sensory styles—if you don't leave one another—you will very likely expand one another and open one another to unimagined realms of experience. Maybe that is what nature had in mind when creating the dangerous arrangement of having essentially acrimonious styles attract one another. To attain one of the most sublime states available to the human species— deep and lasting love—you are forced to expand yourself, to know a style that, without intimate contact, you might hardly have imagined.

You are required to learn that style so well that you discover, from the inside, the enormous differences in the ways two people—you and your partner—can experience the same world. Seeing through another's eyes and hearing through another's ears deepens your understanding of life, and it particularly deepens your comprehension and compassion for how and why others walk their walk and talk their talk. Two realities *are* better than one. Intimate contact with another's reality also helps in preventing you from the characteristically human pitfall of taking your own reality too seriously.

But before we get too cosmic and idealistic about the Grand Plan, we want to address the fact that differences in sensory style are *irreconcilable* differences. You cannot make your partner think like you think, want what you want, feel as you feel, or perceive as you perceive. And the differences in how you represent your world are not just psychological differences or mere tricks of perception. They are based in core energies that reflect your biological essence. These irreconcilable differences need not, however, be the grounds for divorce. The blocks they place between you can be used to build bridges. Your differences can be the foundation of a strong and juicy partnership. When the wounds they have caused are healed, and skills have been established for moving through the hazards they present, they can deepen your soul connection and maintain the spark that keeps a relationship fresh and exciting.

The differences in your energy systems and stress coping styles *cannot* and *should not* be disguised, merged, or blended. They are to be respected. Once they are deeply understood, they will be appreciated and even cherished. Some people gain this understanding through misunderstandings, skirmishes, disappointments, and shattered expectations. Others learn the essential principles by reading about them. Your call.

Sensory Style Highs and Lows

The Visual Style (For Better and for Worse)

Have you ever had the experience of being so powerfully met by another person, eye to eye, that you were swept into a vision or plan of action that was new or foreign to you, but that suddenly became compelling? Perhaps you had heard other people express similar ideas, but this person's arguments carried an energy that moved into you and took you over. You became enthralled in a different way of seeing as this fresh perspective put the world together for you in a new way. The person's strength of communication was also magnetic. If your friend was excited about a possibility, you were excited about it; if angry about an issue, you became angry; if committed to a movement, you found yourself committed to that movement. The vision became your vision. You were witnessing a force of nature in this person's persuasiveness and strength of conviction. And you were grateful somebody helped you see the underlying truth in an important but elusive issue.

This is the visual sensory style in its power and glory. However, when such a person is your life partner, particularly if the two of you are out of sync, the dynamic shifts a bit. All the energy that had been directed into a magnificent vision for humanity now becomes laser-focused onto a vision of how *you* should be and how *you* are not measuring up. Many people find this much less thrilling. *But not your partner.* Your partner is eagerly trying to help you "get the picture." This is your partner's gift to you, filled with the promise of wonderful improvements in your life and for the relationship. You are expected to appreciate every breath your partner expels in bringing these pearls your way. Meanwhile, you are drowning in the fervor of the passion that is rushing toward you. Your partner becomes exasperated, wondering how you could possibly fail to grasp the wisdom and elegance of the insights being so freely offered. And when you still do not see the light, your partner's passion has fully transformed into anger, judgment, and disgust.

The Kinesthetic Style (For Better and for Worse)

Your kinesthetic partner believes in you. Knows how you feel. Understands completely. The willingness to sacrifice in order to help you is striking. The generosity abundant. The compassion almost telepathic. You are recognized for who you are, not judged for what you do. It is your essence, more than your actions, that seems important in this relationship. And through this, you come to appreciate your own essence in a larger, clearer, purer way than you ever had before. Neither past nor future is bemoaned; each moment is lived with a presence that beckons you too into the fullness of life. Sound good? But wait, there's more.

People who are that incredibly open and who give so much pay a price. They often say "Yes" when reality requires a "No!" They are pulled by their compassion in many directions. They suffer for others and become fragmented. Their strong caring and deep understanding become the emotional glue that keeps them at the help-giving center of a sticky web of relationships. They are taken for granted. They may fall into exhaustion or disorientation or become overwhelmed. With their partners, they have a depth of compassion that prevents them from saying what would be hard for the partner to hear. The kinesthetic almost always errs toward compassion over confrontation. As a result, the partner may be operating on highly skewed information. The partner may take the unbridled acceptance and unconditional love as a sign that all is well, that the other is happy, and there is no need to make any real changes. Understandably, they usually don't. But it does not prove to be very satisfying to come up against someone whose self is being sacrificed, who will not call you on your blind spots, and who can easily be pushed over, at least until all of this accumulates to an explosive level, culminating in blowups or permanent exits. So not only are you not growing, you are somehow feeling alone despite all the love and affirmation.

The Digital Style (For Better and for Worse)

Few people are more kind, more calm, more rational. You are fascinated by this exquisitely logical mind, able to organize vast amounts of information and access it in an interesting and highly systematic manner. Not burdened with extravagant or excess feelings, and undaunted by yours, this person is as solid as an ivory tower. An individual of principle and character, there are no messy emotions cluttering this

---

→ THE DIGITAL/KINESTHETIC CONUNDRUM ←

"The facts are the facts—the feelings just confuse the issue!"

—DAVID

"The feelings are the facts—it's what you call the 'facts' that confuse the issue!"

—DONNA

---

personality. From a gift for abstraction emerges an ability to quickly understand complex situations, place them into their proper intellectual context, and serenely map out solutions for any problems they contain.

However, having your anger, grief, and pain bounce off your partner's scholarly shield, time and again, can leave you very lonely. The reasons for your feelings may be patiently explained to you, and the solutions to your problems freely revealed, but a juicy heart connection is not so available. If you do not agree—no matter, you will come around. And should you become exasperated—no matter, you will grow up. You reach in, but you can't quite touch. And you've learned that screaming is ineffective, so your choices are to become futilely hysterical or to begin to deaden yourself, in the very likeness of your kind and numbing partner. This is where you discover that calm, cool, and collected can transmute into dull, dry, and deadening.

The Tonal Style (For Better and for Worse)

No one has been able to enter your inner life more skillfully. The challenges you face, the urges you feel, and the place you occupy in your world are all intuitively grasped and precisely analyzed by this person. You are fed words and insights that help you to better comprehend yourself and appreciate your own dilemmas. You feel understood at multiple levels. You are listened to far beyond your words. Gaps between the lines that you had not noticed are filled in with wisdom and poetry. This ability to perceive at so many levels turns life into an art form. Every nuance is registered and evaluated with powerful aesthetic discernment. Whether it is music, art, or the poetry of life, you are swept into shades of experience that had previously passed by unnoticed.

Fully registering so many dimensions of experience can, however, turn life into an overwhelming cacophony. Three simultaneous conversations from adjoining tables in a restaurant cannot be ignored as they rudely intrude and overshadow enjoyment of the soup du jour. If you are the partner, please don't add to the barrage when stress is present. But even if you don't, you may be treated as if you did. The profound ability to hear between the lines, if fed by past hurts or deep insecurity, can expand into an epic ability to hear what you *never* said, felt, or thought—and to hear it as a reflection of imagined accusations, intentional unkindness, or outright punishment. You are judged not only for your own shortcomings but also for having made your partner's shortcomings evident. You are the villain in this story, and don't

→ THE FOUR ENERGETIC STRESS STYLES ←

Interpersonal Perils of Each

VISUAL STYLE

"Sees" what you do wrong.

Looks at you rather than "seeing" self.

Projects his or her viewpoint
   onto you.

Sees how things should look,
   should be.

Criticizes, judges, blames.

Dismisses you.

Nitpicky.

"Look at me when I talk to you!"

Looks powerful, not vulnerable.

Relentless, must win.

Easily moves into anger.

Disappointed when you don't fulfill
   his or her vision.

Righteous and non-negotiable.

ORIENTATION: Toward the
   future.

EYES: Looks you straight in the eye.
   Needs you to keep eye contact
   to be able to trust you.

MOTTO: "You're wrong!"

DIGITAL STYLE

Logical, rational, reasonable.

Computerlike, detached.

Too calm, cool, and collected.

The classic Mr. Spock.

Cut off from emotions.

Cut off from you.

Unaware there is a problem.

No clue why you feel exasperated.

Orderly, programmed, structured.

Tunes out the other's truth.

Can't be reached with feeling.

ORIENTATION: Moves freely among
   past, present, and future without
   fully experiencing any of them.

EYES: Looks up and to the side, left or right, as if looking into his or her mind.

MOTTO: "I'm right!"

TONAL STYLE

Sound is very personal.

Hurt more by your tone of voice than by your actual words.

"Hears" between the lines. Sonarlike.

Small specks of behavior may be exaggerated into tremendous meaning.

Easily hurt by perceived put-downs.

May withdraw, falsely feeling rejected.

Easily checks out until not really there.

Absorbed in own world.

Hears own inner dialogue louder than your words—sometimes to a paranoid degree.

Interprets, analyzes, and judges.

Judges own self harshly; hard on self.

Exasperated at not feeling heard.

Anger from frustration.

ORIENTATION: Toward the past.

EYES: Looks down and to the side, giving you an ear while trying to think without getting hit too much by your energy.

MOTTO: "I'm angry at you for making me feel wrong!"

KINESTHETIC STYLE

Over-compassion for others (suffers *for* you).

Short on self-compassion.

Acquiesces to you and your needs.

Compulsive enabler.

Not analytical or logical.

Difficulty with discernment.

So much in the now that now *seems* how it will always be (overgeneralizes from the present).

Emotionally suggestible.

Loses his or her words.

Particular difficulty putting feelings into words.

Loses his or her truth while taking in yours.

Explodes or falls apart.

Will stay in the relationship even when hopeless.

ORIENTATION: Toward the present.

EYES: Looks straight down . . . not as an evasion but an effort to cut down on sensory input and come home to self.

MOTTO: "I don't want you to suffer or feel wrong."

complain that you were misunderstood. It only proves that you care more about defending yourself than understanding your partner.

It's Not Learned Behavior

Putting these four Energetic Stress Styles into strict categories might seem too rigid, but in our experience, when people are under sufficient relationship stress, they usually become exemplars of one of the four patterns. This is not learned behavior. It is, rather, a reflection of your energy system. Recall how Donna can accurately tell the parents of a newborn which of the four styles will unfold. The quality shared by everyone, saint or sinner, is that under enough relationship stress, one sensory mode dominates and the other three fade away. The blind-man-and-the-elephant problem emerges. Significant aspects of the situation go unregistered. What *is* registered becomes distorted. The behavior that follows lacks the person's good judgment and usual attunement.

> ### → THE ENERGY DIMENSION ←
>
> #### When Relationship Stress Hits
>
> The patterns of distorted behavior are quite predictable. The energy system shifts in distinct, palpable ways. The color of the aura changes, energies accumulate in the brain and body regions described earlier, the limbic system (emotional brain) is energetically engaged, meridian flow (meridians are basic pathways for the body's energies) is disrupted, and chakra energies constellate themselves for battle.

Putting the Theory to a Public Test

In evening presentations introducing the impact of Energetic Stress Style on relationships, we sometimes ask for a couple to volunteer. We have each partner bring to mind a moment when the relationship was difficult, and we do the energy test Donna devised at the hypnosis class so many years ago to determine the Energetic Stress Style each reverts to during relationship distress. We then make predictions about how they argue. An audience member happened to tape one of these demonstrations and the following description is based on excerpts from that tape. After energy testing the couple, we determined that the husband, Dan, was tonal and the wife, Annette, was visual. When Donna simply stated, "Visuals can see very well what you're doing wrong," Dan started laughing with recognition, then Annette, then the entire audience. Donna then tried to seriously explain that "while it may feel at times that she's blaming you, for her, it's just so disappointing that you aren't seeing it in the obvious way." More laughter as Dan teasingly asked, "Were you in the backseat of our car?"

Donna finally went on, describing how she knew Annette was visual as soon as she looked into her eyes. There's a power that comes out of a visual's eyes. You *feel* it when you're being looked at by a visual. Because Annette's secondary mode is kinesthetic, Donna went on, she also has a lot of empathy. But when the distress is really bad, she goes into visual, where she desperately wants Dan to see things as she sees them.

Annette and Dan's communication difficulties illustrate how different Energetic Stress Styles, in their case visual and tonal, interact. As Annette "sees" what Dan is doing wrong, she mobilizes to try to persuade him to do it *right*. Meanwhile, for Dan, as a tonal, he is able to hear between the lines. Being able to hear between the lines can be a great skill. The best therapists we know are tonal or have a fair amount of tonal. They can hear what is meant even when it is not being said. The trouble when tonals are in relationship distress is that what they hear doesn't necessarily have much to do with what is actually being said. Tonals can also totally check out. They can be looking right at their partner while not taking in a thing.

Recognizing that these tendencies are not willful attacks or acts of sabotage can be illuminating. The dynamics at work are so basic that once you understand how they play out in your relationship, newfound empathy and more effective problem solving readily follow. For most couples, however, the differences in their sensory styles are underappreciated and misunderstood. Turning to Annette, Donna empathized, "It must be exasperating when you find yourself in the middle of an argument about having said things you never said. Next, you're watching him go into a major retreat. The whole dialogue can take place in a tonal's head, so you are not heard at all." Turning to Dan, David countered, "On the other hand, you're dealing with a visual, so all the bad things you think she is saying may be exactly what she means" (followed by much laughter). The remainder of that class focused on how to untangle the problems caused by differences in Energetic Stress Style, and that is where we are heading in this and the following two chapters as well.

Does Everyone Really Fit into Just One Category?

When Donna told Annette that her "secondary mode" is kinesthetic, what did she mean? To review, everyone uses all four sensory representational modes, but one will be more naturally dominant, trumping the other three when you encounter intense relationship stress. Life, however, provides many opportunities and incentives for developing the other three modes. Being drawn to a partner in whom an unfamiliar mode dominates is not the least of them. Different cultures and different families also reinforce different modes. Kinesthetic men are judged harshly in the United States but valued in Latin America. So most kinesthetic men in the United States develop another mode as a strong secondary mode, usually visual or digital. These two are the least like kinesthetic (feelings are more prominent in the kinesthetic mode; abstract thought is more prominent in the visual and digital modes) and are part of the role expectation for men. This is so strongly reinforced that the man's primal mode (kinesthetic) may become hard to detect. Meanwhile, south of the border, kinesthetic men walk about proudly. Although more women than men seem to be primal kinesthetic and more men than women seem to be primal digital, men or women may have as their primal mode any one of the four types. "Mars and Venus" turns out to accurately characterize some important biochemical differences and cultural influences, but each of the Energetic Stress Styles is found in both genders.

We all usually use a blend of two or more of the modes. Your Energetic Stress Style, however, is always there in the foreground or in the background. It is your first language. Most people also strongly develop a second preferred energy language, a second way of processing information. Sometimes, in fact, it is quite difficult to know which is primary and which is secondary until the person is in extreme relationship stress. The selection of this second favored mode seems to depend on a mixture of personal, cultural, and biological factors, and the channel that is emphasized will significantly shape your perceptions, preferences, and behavior. These ideas trace back at least to William James's *visual*, *auditory*, and *touch-oriented* intellectual styles and to Carl Jung's *sensing*, *thinking*, *feeling*, and *intuiting* styles. Jung believed, and a century of clinical observations have tended to support this conclusion, that people live the first part of their lives according to their innate style of processing information, but to truly flourish, you need to grow into other ways of knowing the world, into styles that seem less natural. And what could seem less natural than trying to accommodate your partner's style?

How Successful Couples Handle Conflict

Relationships are spawned by attraction but shaped by conflict. All couples disagree at times. Finding ways of managing differences in what you want, believe, or value is a basic challenge for any two people building a life together. And whatever may be going "right" begins to feel like everything is going "wrong" when dysfunctional strategies for dealing with conflict take over. A trivial disagreement can trigger your harshest judgments against your partner and escalate into behaviors that few others in your life are privileged to receive. Our most recent personal example:

We were spending the weekend with our daughter, Tanya, and her partner, Jeff. A bit before noon, Donna announces, "I'm famished, let's all just hop in the car and go to Maria's," a nearby Mexican restaurant. David had just come back from two hours in the hot tub, where he was working on this very chapter (it's tough working in someone else's space, but we try to adapt). Donna tells him to hurry and get dressed. He does so quickly, but says he can't go until he calls to finalize a radio interview that is to take place that afternoon and sends an e-mail instructing a staff member on how to handle an emergency situation. Donna, suffering from low blood sugar by this point, says with urgency, "They're waiting for us." David, feeling stressed now, says a little too loudly to conceal from those in the next room, "Don't push me, Donna, I have to do these things and I'm doing them as quickly as I can." Donna is mortified and replies under her breath, "You just announced to Tanya and Jeff that I'm pushing you. I can't believe you did that!" David snaps back, loud enough for everyone to clearly hear, "Okay, Donna, you're not pushing me. No one's pushing me. Just go without me! Good-bye!"

John Gottman, a psychologist who has studied the way couples handle conflict, comments about such interactions. If the partners just dismiss the negative emotions, "they typically will still eventually drift together again, but trust will have eroded."[9] Gottman's meticulous observational studies and follow-up with thousands of couples have produced the most reliable measures available for predicting which marriages will succeed and which will not, with 93.6 percent accuracy on a three-year follow-up in one classic study.[10] This substantial body of research corresponds with, supports, and informs our approach to working with couples, and we close this chapter with some of his most salient findings as we move into building energetic bridges between partners.

Gottman identified three different styles that successful marriages use for managing conflict.[11] *Validators*, the first style, are able to let their partners know, even in the midst of conflict, that they consider the other's opinions and emotions to be valid, despite the areas of disagreement. While this may seem the ideal, an unexpected finding was that two other strategies couples use for handling differences, which would at first glance seem to be far less than ideal, are equally effective in producing satisfying marriages that last.

These other two surprisingly successful styles are called "volatile" and "avoidant." *Volatile* couples seem to fight about everything: "Who is the best candidate for mayor?" "Whose turn is it to do the dishes?" "Whose mother is more manipulative?" Gottman notes that "such couples fight on a grand scale and have an even grander time making up."[12] Their fights are hot and full of fervor, but when not in conflict, they also laugh more and have more spark than the typical validating couple. The validating style can deteriorate into a passionless arrangement where romance and individuality have been sacrificed to maintain harmony. Volatile couples, on the other hand, tend not to censor their thoughts to avoid conflict and stay passionately engaged during the good times as well as the bad times.

Avoidant couples, the third style, minimize their differences or make light of them. Rather than resolve conflicts, they "reaffirm what they love and value in the marriage, accentuate the positive, and accept the rest. . . . It's as if the couple knows their bond is so strong they can overlook their disagreements."[13] Gottman speculates that a couple's mix of temperament, background, and personality determines which of the three strategies they will settle into.

If such vastly different styles for managing conflict can all sustain a lasting and satisfying partnership, what *does* predict whether a marriage will succeed or fail? A reliable indication is the *ratio* of positive interactions to negative ones. In successful, happy marriages—whether the couple's style for handling conflict was typified by

Validating Couples

When an area of disagreement emerges, the rupture leads to the partners energetically pulling back into themselves for a moment. This allows them to re-center and find their own strength and grounding. From that strength and grounding, a gracious energy is able to go out to the partner even during the contentious interaction.

Volatile Couples

When an area of disagreement emerges, the rupture leads to the energy field around each partner becoming huge and defiant, shooting out in all directions, including at the partner. These energies are aggressive and become enmeshed, but as they play out, the partners become deeply connected in ways that can transform into erotic passion.

Avoidant Couples

When an area of disagreement emerges, the rupture becomes a momentary frazzle in the energy field and an energetic disconnect. From this disconnect, another force emerges to smooth and reconnect the energy.

validation, volatility, or avoidance—that ratio was at least 5 to 1. If the amount of time couples spent interacting positively—touching, smiling, laughing, giving compliments, stating appreciations—was not five times the amount of time spent fighting, judging, criticizing, fuming, or skirting conflicts that have arisen, the marriage was in some trouble. If it fell below one positive interaction for each negative one, the couple was headed for divorce.

But how do you ensure that you maintain that 5-to-1 ratio? Put a chart on the refrigerator? Nag your partner about keeping a positive ratio by demanding more smiles and not tolerating expressions of frustration? Skills for creating more positive interactions and fewer negative ones can be learned. Each chapter in this book gives you some clues and concrete practices.

Going After the Best of Each Style

Is there a way of dealing with differences and handling conflict that retains the strengths of each of the three styles couples spontaneously settle into? Since each has advantages and disadvantages, is it possible to:

- Actively affirm one another even while diving into areas of intense disagreement, like *Validating* couples?
- Proceed with a level of honesty and lack of censorship that allows you to fully engage one another, like *Volatile* couples?
- Accentuate the positive, accept each other in your differences, and find encouragement from the power of your bond even during difficult times, like *Avoidant* couples?

We believe it is possible to learn from each of the styles while evolving your own. Changing ineffective strategies in the way you and your partner respond to stress requires, however, more than positive intention or even fierce determination. It requires that you:

1. Accurately understand what is going on inside each of you,
2. Develop a set of skills for effectively managing relationship distress, and
3. Use them even if you feel the urge for a more impulsive response.

Challenging though this may be, the totally encouraging news is that after some repetition, the neural networks that govern old patterns will change and reinforce a new strategy that is more gratifying.

On to Chapter 2

The first part in this sequence—understanding what is going on inside you and your partner—is greatly enhanced by appreciating one another's Energetic Stress Style, the topic of this chapter. This gives you an insider's view of your partner's experience during stress as well as perspective on your own. Chapters 2 and 3 are designed to help you develop new skills and implement them. By applying the concepts and tools that are offered, you interrupt old patterns and install new, more effective ones in their place.

2

Aligning Your Energetic Processing Styles

Turning Your Differences into Strengths

Attuned communication involves
the resonance of energy and information.

—DANIEL J. SIEGEL, M.D.[1]

T HEY HAD THE BEST OF ENERGETIC PROCESSING COMBINATIONS; THEY HAD THE worst of energetic processing combinations. So goes every couple. It is not whether your styles are compatible that makes or breaks a relationship, but how you build on your compatibilities and what you do with your differences. This chapter offers you guidelines for both.

As you saw in the previous chapter, during relationship stress your Energetic Stress Style eclipses the other modes of processing information and you tend to perceive your partner's intentions and behaviors through a distorted lens. For instance, a very kind man of the digital persuasion attended one of our relationship seminars with his tonal wife. When his wife was upset with him, he would make a list of each of her complaints and patiently attempt to explain to her why her feelings were not based on sound reasoning. This had an effect that was similar to attempting to douse a fire with kerosene. Her first impulse was to want to use a heavy object to beat him into having a feeling response, but as she would overcome her rage, she would move into the more civilized mode of fantasizing how she would leave him. "Every time he shows me one of his damn lists, I go nuts, and every word he utters makes it worse. I feel like a loose wire with no place to plug in. Everyone thinks I'm so lucky to be with such a sweet man, but he can't meet me. He cuts me off again and again. I'm so lonely, and the chances of him changing seem so remote, that I think I'd rather be on my own."

When you and your partner are headed for an "every word he utters makes it worse" type of encounter, your primal sensory systems are at odds. The Energetic Stress Style Assessment (pp. 27–29) gave you an indication about your primal sensory system, but pencil-and-paper questionnaires are limited. In addition, you use more than just your primal sensory system when you are not under stress, and the one you consciously identify with may not actually be the one you rely on during intense relationship distress. As you go through this chapter, begin with your initial impressions along with your findings on the assessment, but remain open to discoveries that expand your understanding. Also keep in mind that while your own self-appraisal may be compromised when you are in your stress mode, your partner is a leading expert in knowing how you behave at such times.

The man who made lists was using a digital coping style, but you can't really tell from the information presented if this is truly his Energetic Stress Style or if it is a secondary mode that he has cultivated and that is available to him until he is more deeply triggered. Suppose, for instance, that his Energetic Stress Style is kinesthetic. Because societal messages to men often cause them to repress their kinesthetic qualities, he may tend to use his digital system to keep from going there. Under strong enough interpersonal stress, however, his digital detachment will fall away and a muddle of feelings will become prominent and obvious.

Utilizing the Strengths of Your Energetic Stress Style

At the core of your Energetic Stress Style is a special facility with an information processing mode (visual, kinesthetic, tonal, or digital) that has strengths which give you a special window on the world, one that is not readily available to people who are not as developed in that sensory mode. Under relationship stress, however, it does just the opposite, distorting your thoughts, emotions, and perceptions. Keep in mind that these are not mere psychological differences in how you process information.

They run deep in your energy system. As already discussed in Chapter 1, we believe your Energetic Stress Style:

- is genetically determined.
- reflects one of four stress-response configurations.
- governs what occurs when you encounter a major conflict in your relationship—whether your energies concentrate more at your eyes (visual), heart (kinesthetic), forebrain (digital), or ears (tonal).

→ THE ENERGY DIMENSION ←

The energies when a person is fighting with a loved one become distorted in ways that reflect the person's Energetic Stress Style:

Visuals during an argument hurl the energies of judgment and impatience in a fast and powerful way. All the energies from the visual's eyes are focused toward the partner. Energy also seems to shoot from the chest and head. The partner on the receiving end feels attacked by this overwhelming force, which feels imposing and frightening.

Kinesthetics during an argument feel energy imploding in their Heart Chakras, as if fire hoses are forcing energy in from all directions. The pressured energy in the center of the chest is chaotic and overwhelming, making kinesthetics want to do anything to stop the feeling, to send the energy out by yelling, screaming, crying, or wailing—if the energy has not totally paralyzed them. The energies have left the head, so logic is not part of the equation.

Digitals during an argument have an artificially enlarged aura around their head, where the energy has accumulated. This biofield is a closed system, not able to flow with outside energies. The remainder of the aura becomes very thin and clings near the body, also tight and encapsulated, not interacting with the energies around it.

Tonals during an argument tend to disconnect, pulling into themselves, but vortexes at the ears draw in energies that are physically painful. The energy spirals close to their heads. It may also move into the area between the solar plexus and waist and then completely disconnect or chaotically leap out toward the partner, having become laced with anger and rage.

Understanding your own sensory mode prepares you to operate more competently from within it. This chapter provides guidelines for navigating your way through your own mode and for more effectively engaging your partner's mode.

If Your Energetic Stress Style Is Visual

Know Your Vulnerabilities

If you are a visual, your core perceptual error is to blame your partner. You distort by magnifying what your partner has done wrong. Your keen insights and compelling perspective—normally your strengths—become liabilities when distorted. Under relationship stress, you don't realize they are twisted. Your instinct is to envision how your partner should be and how the interaction should be going and to point out where your partner has an opportunity to improve. This may all occur in an instant, and you may only be aware of the part about *your partner's* opportunities to improve.

Play Your Strengths

MENTALLY:

- Remind yourself that the way you see the situation is not necessarily the only valid viewpoint.
- Expand your vision by taking in your partner's perspective.

BEHAVIORALLY:

- Drawing on your strength for painting a compelling verbal picture, state your partner's view of the situation.
- Ask your partner to confirm or correct your verbal portrayal.

This will demonstrate your desire to respect your partner's view as worthy and to embrace in your relationship your partner's truth as well as your own. Let your partner experience your determination to *see* through the eyes of love.

If Your Energetic Stress Style Is Kinesthetic

Know Your Vulnerabilities

If you are a kinesthetic, your core perceptual error is that your attention focuses on your partner's suffering and your distress about it, particularly if your partner blames you for his or her unhappiness. You distort by believing your partner may not survive without your validation and protection. You lose your boundaries in this misguided attempt to protect your partner from feeling wrong or hurt, and you lose your sense of self while pursuing a soul connection at any cost. Your remarkable empathy, compassion, and capacity to bond—normally your strengths—become liabilities as your partner proceeds with no idea about what you are needing. Your instinct is to keep your partner feeling good with whatever you must sacrifice at the slightest sign of his or her pain or unhappiness. Meanwhile, your sense of being discounted contradicts your belief that you are loved in this relationship, and your disorientation becomes immense. In each interaction building to this point, however, you may only be aware of your compulsion to validate your partner and soothe his or her pain and distress.

Play Your Strengths

MENTALLY:

- First separate from your partner energetically. Then you can tune into your body and make your suppressed needs in the situation known to yourself.
- Remind yourself that what your partner needs is your *truth* rather than overcompassion while challenging your assumptions about how desperate the situation is for your partner.

BEHAVIORALLY:

- Turn your strength of compassion toward yourself and actively rehearse asking your partner to understand your experience and help you get what you need.
- Once rehearsed, make your unstated needs in the situation known to your partner.

This will demonstrate your trust in your partner to take in your truth, your expectation that you not be discounted, and your faith that your partner can handle disagreement or disappointment.

If Your Energetic Stress Style Is Digital

Know Your Vulnerabilities

If you are a digital, your core perceptual error emerges from separating yourself from your partner's emotions. You distort with the conviction that you are completely right and your partner's perceptions, feelings, and conclusions are essentially irrelevant. Your ability to navigate brilliantly using abstract logic and reason—normally your greatest strength—becomes your weakness as you isolate yourself in a fortress built of your detached thoughts and beliefs. In distancing from your partner's struggles, you distance yourself from your own heart. Your instinct is to pull within; dismiss your partner's irrational, emotional responses; and entertain yourself in the proverbial cave of the isolated male (or in fewer cases, female). This may all occur in an instant, and you may only be aware of the *superior* truth of your position.

Play Your Strengths

MENTALLY:

- Challenge your assumption that you are completely right and your partner's differing perceptions, feelings, or conclusions are simply wrong.
- Stay present and open despite the disquieting emotions and questionable reasoning being displayed by your partner.

BEHAVIORALLY:

- Climb out of the cave, use your strong logical capacity to form the questions that will help you build a bridge of empathy, and interview your partner about the issue at hand.
- Summarize your partner's position with greater logic and caring than he or she was able to articulate.

This will demonstrate to your partner that you can use your mind to create connections, enter the realm of feelings, and establish the relationship as your priority.

If Your Energetic Stress Style Is Tonal

Know Your Vulnerabilities

If you are a tonal, your core perceptual error is to magnify the negative in what has been said and to hear reproach in what has *not* been said. You suffer over what you are sure the other thinks about you or has done to you. Your great strength—that you are exquisitely attuned to life's shades and subtleties—becomes your weakness as the slightest dissonance reverberates throughout your being, causing disruption and pain. Your instinct is to interpret tones and nuances to confirm your suspicion that the other does not hear, value, or love you. This may all occur in an instant, and you may only be aware of the part about *your partner's* reproach or negative feelings toward you.

Play Your Strengths

MENTALLY:

- Entertain the seemingly unlikely possibility that you are distorting the reality of your partner's position and challenge your assumption that your partner isn't hearing you or is disapproving of you.
- Using your aesthetic sensibilities and facility for hearing the subtleties of your partner's words, listen for what is positive rather than negative.

BEHAVIORALLY:

- Identify and put into words what you hear as the positive aspects of your partner's words and tone.
- Articulate the goodwill your partner holds for you.

This will demonstrate to your partner and to yourself that you can read positive and hopeful information between the lines and affirm your partner's love and caring.

For Everybody

These brief guidelines describe behaviors that play to the strengths of each of the four sensory modes. They contain features that can be helpful to anyone for creating more attuned, compassionate communication. These include:

- Interview your partner to help build a bridge of understanding and summarize your partner's position with strong empathy.
- Ask your partner to confirm or correct your verbal portrayal.
- Ask your partner to understand your experience and help you get what you need.
- Put into words the positive intentions in your partner's words, tone, and actions, and articulate the goodwill your partner holds for you.

Attuning to Your Partner's Energetic Stress Style

In this chapter you are learning to bring two different Energetic Stress Styles into better attunement: your own and your partner's. So far, you have reflected on the ways a person with your style is vulnerable to falling into distortions during relationship stress, and you were shown ways to use the strengths of your style to repair and reconnect. Next we turn to your partner's sensory mode, offer a map of potential hazards you may meet, and show how to move forward in ways that circumvent the hazards while building practical, trustworthy bridges. Again, your partner's secondary system may be at play, particularly before a flooding of stressful emotions occurs. So a partner who reverts to a kinesthetic sensory mode when under strong relationship stress might, for instance, be quite blaming (visual) under light or moderate stress. Before we focus on each of the Energetic Stress Styles, we invite you to learn a technique that will be useful whenever conflict is brewing.

A Powerful Communication Technique for All Energetic Stress Styles

Marital therapists have developed innumerable structured techniques for teaching attuned communication. These tend to be most effective before conflict has escalated to the point that you are in your full-blown Energetic Stress Styles (a strategy for when things have gotten out of hand is presented in the next chapter), but they can be effective in keeping you from going there. Our all-time favorite is called the *"Do you mean"* technique. It is simple, direct, and flexible enough that it can be adapted to a wide range of situations, and it is surprisingly powerful. As you practice and succeed with it, new neural networks build, increasingly making your bond sturdier.

We have been using the *"Do you mean"* technique during the thirty-seven-year span of our relationship, both personally and professionally. As a side story, David learned it from the renowned family therapist Virginia Satir in 1972, before we met. He was on the faculty of the Department of Psychiatry and Behavioral Science at the Johns Hopkins University School of Medicine, doing research on community mental health, during the year that Virginia came to the department as a visiting professor. His office was directly across from Virginia's, and he was dazzled by her abilities. They became friends and colleagues. He often drove her to her East Coast workshops, got to participate and observe her in action, and they would discuss the trainings during their leisurely drives back. He now believes that this play of good fortune was fate preparing him to meet and work with Donna, another virtuoso at inspiring people with empowering and uplifting techniques that can be self-applied, also playing on a large stage.

The *"Do you mean"* technique is applied to a single statement. If the statement has several parts, you might start with the one that is the most difficult to understand or the most loaded or simply explore your partner's overall feelings. Suppose your visual partner has said to you:

"You have made a mess of our vacation plans! You've invited Steve and Delores to join us, you've scheduled a doctor's appointment so we have to get back two days early, and I just checked Travelocity and the expensive resort you booked has a low customer satisfaction rating. Can't I trust you to do anything right?!"

You would then ask your partner a question that begins with the words "Do you mean." For instance:

"Do you mean you're angry with me for the choices I've made about Lake Tahoe?"

Your partner's response at this point can be:

- "Yes!" (1 point)
- "No!" (zero points)
- "Part right, part wrong." (½ point)
- "I believe that to be true, but that is not what I was saying." (zero points)

These are the four options. The rules for this technique are that your partner responds with one and only one of these answers and the two of you have no other discussion beyond filling in essential information that has no emotional charge. You then continue to ask *"Do you mean"* questions until you have three points (three "yes" responses; again, "part right, part wrong" is scored as half a point) or until you feel you are off track and request of your partner:

"Would you please say that again but in a different way?"

When that occurs, the game begins anew. Your partner restates and you work toward getting three points for the new statement. Suppose, in the above example, the answer to the first question was "You got that one right!" The interaction might have continued like this:

"Okay, so I have one yes. Do you mean *you* should have planned the vacation?"

"I've been wishing I had, but that's not what I meant."

"Do you mean I didn't do anything right?"

"No, that's not what I'm saying!"

"Do you mean that I made some choices that have you questioning whether I should ever make plans for both of us?"

"Yes, that's exactly what I am thinking!"

"To ask the next question, I need to give you some background. Our HMO had me waiting for that doctor's appointment for four months, and I booked the hotel because I got a great deal on it, but I hadn't looked at the ratings. Do you mean that you would like me to change my doctor's appointment and book a different hotel?"

"Yes, that would help."

After achieving three yeses, summarize with a statement in the form of "I can understand how [summary of what happened] would cause you to feel [name feeling]" and ask for a confirmation that your partner feels you fully understand the *initial* statement.[2] For instance:

"So to summarize, you are angry at me for my choices in planning our vacation; you wish you had done it yourself; and you would like me to change my doctor's appointment and the hotel booking. Given all that, I can understand why you are feeling upset with me. Did I getcha?"

This final question, "Did I getcha?" (or any version of "Is there anything more") is a particularly important element of the *"Do you mean"* technique. It is designed to ensure that you resolve each incident as fully as possible. For couples, *what is not re- solved will return.* Or as Abraham Lincoln once observed, "Nothing is settled until it is settled right."

If the answer is "Yes" and your partner feels fully understood, then it is your turn to respond to the initial statement. You either reach agreement (e.g., "You are right! I totally made a mess of our vacation plans") or you respectfully make a statement that summarizes the points of difference. Your partner then asks the *"Do you means"* about that statement.

If the answer is "No," your partner still does not feel fully understood, he or she offers a new or revised statement to convey what is apparently still not understood, and the interaction goes into another round. In this case, it might be:

"No. I can't believe Steve and Delores are coming with us!"

"Do you mean you don't like Steve and Delores?"

"No, they're fine people."

"Do you mean you don't feel close enough to them to want to spend this kind of time together?"

"Well, I feel close to them, but I don't want to share my vacation with them. So I'll give you one-half on that one."

"Do you mean you wanted this to be our vacation with no one else's needs and schedule getting in our way?"

"Yes."

"Do you mean you want me to get us out of it?"

"I'd love for you to get us out of this, but I know they've already booked their plane tickets, so that's not what I was meaning. I'll give that another half, so you're up to two."

"Do you mean I should have checked with you before including them in our plans and you're pissed with me for not doing that?"

"Yes!"

"Okay, that's three. So to summarize, you are really unhappy about Steve and Delores joining us, you wanted this to be for just the two of us, and you wish I had at least checked with you first. I can understand why you are angry. Did I getcha?"

Once the partner who made the original statement feels understood, he or she finishes this part of the exchange with a statement of appreciation to reinforce the success. You have achieved a new level of understanding about a situation that could have thrown you into an escalating mismatch. The statement of appreciation may be general, such as "I appreciate that you stayed with the instructions," or more specific, such as "I appreciate that you have greater understanding about how upset I am with the plans." The discussion might proceed this way:

> "Yes. I do feel understood. But I still don't understand why you invited Steve and Delores. So now you're supposed to tell me what you were feeling during all of this and to clarify your own position. Right?"
> "Actually, the next step is that you are supposed to tell me some appreciations."
> "Oh, okay, right. I appreciate that you seemed so interested and attentive while I was talking. I appreciate that you were looking me in the eye and didn't interrupt me. I appreciate that you seem to have understood my feelings."

While this technique is like putting the conversation into slow motion and examining each piece of it with a magnifying glass, that is exactly why it is so effective. It keeps you attuned to one another. Only now would you respond to the original statement or clarify your position or report feelings that came up during the exchange. This should again be done with relatively brief statements so your partner can clarify and stay attuned with "*Do you mean*" questions.

> "Thank you. And yes, I would like to explain a few things. I didn't exactly invite Steve and Delores. I told Delores we were going to Lake Tahoe for our vacation, and I asked her where they stayed when they went there last year. Soon she was telling me what a great time they had, that they were looking for an excuse to go back, and that joining us might just be the opportunity they were looking for. The next day she *announced* that she had talked it over with Steve, locked in her vacation dates to correspond with our trip, and was waxing on about what a great time we were all going to have. What could I do? I said, 'That's just great!'"
> "Do you mean you had no choice?"

"That's how it felt. Yes."

"Do you mean you don't want them to come either?"

"I really don't want them to come, but it's not what I was saying."

"Do you mean you got trapped into this?"

"Yes, I really want you to understand that."

"Do you mean you know you blew it?"

"No, I think you would have done the same thing. I was trapped!"

"Do you mean even I could have gotten us trapped into this?"

"Yes, dear, even you!"

At this point, your partner may still have more to say, such as, "It was very painful that you came at me with so much blame rather than giving me the benefit of the doubt," challenging your partner to look deeper at his or her behavior toward you. While it may take several rounds like these, the technique can transform daily misunderstandings into better harmony and deeper connection. Even though the interchanges can become somewhat laborious, the potential payoff is substantial, and the rules are really quite simple:

1. Short statement.
2. "Yes" to three "*Do you mean*" questions.
3. Summarize.
4. Acknowledge that your partner's initial feelings were reasonable given what you now understand.
5. Verify that your partner now feels fully understood.
6. Partner thanks you.
7. You can now make a short statement about your position.
8. Partner responds with "*Do you mean*" questions.
9. Continue until issue is fully resolved.

The "*Do you mean*" technique keeps you and your partner attuned to one another, provides instant feedback when your understanding is not accurate, and can be enlightening and even fun. Two people in the same situation, even couples—or more accurately, particularly couples—can be watching the same drama unfold but seeing totally different scenes, hearing different dialogues, and bracing for different endings. The "*Do you mean*" technique helps you slow down and reattune so you are at least watching the same movie even if your reactions to it diverge.

If Your Partner's Energetic Stress Style Is Visual

Keep always in mind that you are dealing with someone who trusts an internal vision that does not easily change. This vision projects into the future an image of what is possible, and that image carries a force that not only compels your partner forward, it collides with anything that stands in its way. Moreover, if the image is about you, it is a vision that often exceeds what is possible, and you may gently or not so gently be told how you do not measure up. While it is hard to not take this personally, you can be assisted by recognizing two things. First, your partner is dealing with genuine disappointment that you turned out to be human, fantasies during the romantic stage of the relationship notwithstanding. Don't take this personally. Second, and more important, remind yourself that your partner needs *you*, not a fantasy of who you might be.

FOR THE GOOD TIMES

If you are in a relationship with a visual, appreciate and articulate the ways this visionary capacity serves your relationship. If you aren't sure, observe closely what your partner contributes as you make plans together, how you look to your partner for perspective, and ways your partner offers you genuinely valuable guidance. Reflect deeply on the contributions your partner's sensory mode adds to your life and describe them. Do this so fully and persuasively that if at another time you are compelled to discuss how your partner is trapped in the visual sensory channel, you will have already established that you deeply recognize its value and can refer back to that discussion.

FOR THE HARD TIMES

Walk the line between knowing that your visual partner cannot easily let go of a passionately held vision *and* patiently establishing that your perspective has merit. During relationship distress:

• Look your partner straight in the eyes. Avoiding eye contact seems evasive to visuals, while direct eye contact engenders their trust.

- Maintain a respectful distance. Visuals need to see you in perspective.
- Gently share your own perspective while knowing that your visual partner cannot easily let go of a passionately held vision when under stress.
- Allow your partner time to process a requested shift in vision.
- Don't allow yourself to be bullied, since this only confirms to the visual that he or she was right.

Use the *"Do you mean"* technique shown earlier to more fully understand and articulate your partner's underlying vision. Your partner will appreciate being recognized and understood. Having connected within your partner's comfort zone, it will now be easier for your partner to hear you without judgment and blame. In the earlier sample dialogue, the opening, blaming statement was made by a visual. If your partner is visual, you may want to go back and reread that dialogue.

If Your Partner's Energetic Stress Style Is Kinesthetic

Always keep in mind that you are dealing with someone who lives in the present moment, whose first response is to give your needs, feelings, and pain an exaggerated degree of importance, and who trusts feelings more than abstract logic or reason. One of David's slowly dawning realizations in our early years was, "For Donna, feelings are facts!" This boggled his mind. For David, facts are facts. Feelings may color the facts, but the facts are the facts. For Donna, the facts that are to be trusted are the feelings. She thinks the regular facts are what David resorts to when he's dead wrong about the emotional and interpersonal realities at play but is still trying to defend himself.

FOR THE GOOD TIMES

If you are in a relationship with a kinesthetic, appreciate and articulate the ways his or her facility with feelings, deep sense of compassion, and attunement to the eternal moment serves the relationship. If you aren't sure, observe closely how your partner's spirit calls you into the here and now, invites the relationship to find an emotional alignment, and is able to meet and support your feelings when times are good. Reflect deeply on the contributions your partner's sensory mode adds to your life and describe them. Do this so fully and persuasively that if at another time you are compelled to discuss how your partner is trapped in the kinesthetic sensory channel, you have already established that you deeply recognize its value.

FOR THE HARD TIMES

Recognize the intelligence that transcends your kinesthetic partner's words. Attune to the feelings without becoming distracted by the language. During relationship distress:

- Cut the pressure. Kinesthetics can't think clearly or function well when accused, hurried for an answer, or drowned in another's words, needs, or truths.
- Remember that your partner lives in the present moment and trusts his or her feelings more than your logic.
- Give plenty of time to resolve issues. Kinesthetics need to digest and metabolize questions and requests. Without time, they are more likely to be focused on your needs rather than their inner truth.
- Notice any signs of suffering too much for you, or an inability to communicate other than to agree with you or to dissolve in emotion.
- A quick "yes" may not be accurate, even if your partner doesn't know it. Commitments made under stress can later haunt the kinesthetic.

Use the *"Do you mean"* technique to focus on nonverbal communication and identify unstated issues. The technique can also reveal whether your kinesthetic partner is giving your needs, feelings, or pain an exaggerated degree of importance. The conversation might go like this (the examples illustrating the kinesthetic, digital, and tonal sensory styles that will follow are playful excerpts of imaginary conversations that further illustrate basic principles for using the technique):

KINESTHETIC PARTNER: "Sure, you can go watch the Super Bowl with Larry and Ed. I think you'll have a great time!"

Reply: "You sound disappointed."

"Maybe a little, but I want you to do what you really want to do."

"Do you mean it's really okay with you that I leave you alone? It is our tenth anniversary."

"Well, hey, you spent the whole day with me on our fourth anniversary. That's holding me over."

"Do you mean by your sarcasm that you're going to be angry if I go?"

"I'll try not to be. I know you'll love watching the Super Bowl with Larry and Ed. It's okay!"

"Do you mean you are hoping that for our anniversary I would make being
  with you more important than the game?"
"Well, that did cross my mind, but [in tears now] I really want you to do what
  you want to do."
"I'm so relieved that you want me to watch the Super Bowl! Thank you! Bye-
  bye, honey, I'm off. Happy anniversary!"

Kinesthetic "*Do you mean*" conversation 2:

TO KINESTHETIC PARTNER: "I know that you are not answering me and I see
  that your lower lip is trembling. Do you mean by your silence that you are
  having lots of feelings but don't know what to say?"
Reply: "Yes."
"Do you mean that you do wish you had the words, but they are not coming
  to you right now?"
"Yes."
"Do you mean you felt hurt when I just told you you're not as pretty as
  Mary?"
"Wham!"
"Thanks, got it!"

While both examples are parodies, the first still illustrates how kinesthetics put
their partner's needs and desires above their own, and the second shows how words
are much harder when a complex spectrum of feelings is occurring. The kinesthetic
may seem scattered or babbling when the deeper truth is that he or she is navigating
more complex inner terrain than the partner.

If Your Partner's Energetic Stress Style Is Digital

Keep always in mind that you are dealing with someone who, when under stress, is
going to process the situation with reason and logic no matter how much you want
a feeling response. Logic and abstractions are trusted; emotions are suspect. Where
the visual is oriented toward the future, the kinesthetic toward the present, and the
tonal toward the past, the digital can readily move from one to the other without,
however, fully living in any of them. That is the upside and the downside of operat-

ing in a world of symbols and abstractions. There is a certain appeal about being able to maneuver through any situation uncluttered by emotion. Within their isolated universe, they are in control of the symbols, so, in their minds, they *always* get to be right. When Donna says in exasperation during a disagreement, "Would you rather be right or would you rather be close?" David's visceral response, which he has learned not to lead with, is "Well, that's a no-brainer."

FOR THE GOOD TIMES

If you are in a relationship with a digital, appreciate and articulate the ways this stability and access to logic and reason serves the relationship. If you aren't sure, observe closely how your partner's calmness, kindness, and organizational abilities benefit you. Reflect deeply on the contributions your partner's sensory mode adds to your life and describe them. Do this so fully and persuasively that if at another time you are compelled to discuss how your partner is trapped in the digital mode of processing information, you have already established that you deeply recognize its value.

FOR THE HARD TIMES

Recognize that your digital partner's lack of emotional contact is a coping style rather than a rejection or a premeditated way of distancing. During relationship distress:

- Digitals apply reason and logic to situations calling for delicacy and empathy. Don't expect a feeling response to an emotional issue.
- Accept that under stress, no matter how much you want a feeling response, you are instead likely to be met with reasoning.
- Raising your voice in frustration will not get you what you long for. Escalating emotional expression will generally cause your digital partner, when under stress, to become even more remote.

Stay on top of your own exasperation, using energy exercises (pp. 82–94) to keep you centered. You can, for instance, hold your stress release points (pp. 90) and breathe deeply while continuing the discussion. If you do become exasperated, you can invite your partner to do one of the exercises with you. Structured emotional expression is less threatening to your digital partner than undisciplined feeling or spontaneous outbursts.

Use the "*Do you mean*" technique to reach into your partner's logic and have it articulated more fully. Your partner will appreciate being recognized and understood. Once you have connected within your partner's comfort zone, it will now be easier to lead into the world of emotions, which your partner will also appreciate if done gently and without judgment.

"*Do you mean*" conversation:

TO DIGITAL PARTNER: "I am so upset. You know how high my last performance evaluation was. My boss told me today that the company has put a freeze on raises."

REPLY: "So you didn't get the raise after all. Oh well, you shouldn't count your chickens before they're hatched."

"Do you mean that I shouldn't feel bad about not getting the raise since I didn't lose anything I didn't already have?"

"Yes, that is correct."

"Do you mean you don't care that I won't be bringing us more income?"

"No, we really needed it."

"Do you mean that since I didn't get the raise, it doesn't do either of us any good to fret about it?"

"Yes, no sense getting emotional about these things."

"Do you mean that you care about my disappointment and that you don't want me to feel bad?"

"Yes, I suppose that was in there somewhere."

"Thank you. I think that was about the most emotionally tuned-in thing you've ever said to me."

Digitals often simply do not have ready access to their feelings or even their love and empathy, and gently helping them to recognize their deeper feelings is a gift. Notice, however, how easily "You shouldn't count your chickens . . ." could have been received as dismissive and distancing and the start of a downward spiral. As you stay centered and refrain from interpreting as rejection your partner's reach toward logic over empathy, you will find that your partner is actually capable of moving beyond the stress response and reaching into your world. Digitals actually tend to be quite kind. You know this when the two of you are not in your stress modes, and it is worth remembering when you are.

If Your Partner's Energetic Stress Style Is Tonal

Keep always in mind that you are dealing with someone who, when under stress, is not hearing your exact words but is picking up on the "vibes," both yours and those of a personal internal drama. Do not expect a neutral, empathic response. The world of sound is not casual. It is deeply intimate and impactful, with whatever is not registered as being friendly likely to be registered as hostile. Your partner is vulnerable to feeling bombarded by any stressed energy you may be putting out, to take it very personally, and to be unforgiving about what you have dished out just now or in the past. Small specks of behavior can be exaggerated into having tremendous meaning. Tonals engage intimately with life, down to the tiniest nuance. This facility with subtleties and the ability to hear between the lines can create a skewed reality under stress that tends to distort the past as well. Because stress-based distortions can become deeply encoded, tonals are particularly susceptible to being run by their past.

FOR THE GOOD TIMES

If you are in a relationship with a tonal, appreciate and articulate the ways the relationship is served by this ability to hear between the lines, deeply know what you mean, and invite you into the creative dimensions of life. If you aren't sure, observe closely how your partner is able to enter your inner world, articulate for you subtleties you had not registered, and bring you into realms of sensory and aesthetic appreciation that would otherwise pass you by. Reflect deeply on the contributions your partner's sensory mode adds to your life and describe them. Do this so fully and persuasively that if at another time you are compelled to discuss how your partner is trapped in the tonal sensory channel, you have already established that you deeply recognize its value.

FOR THE HARD TIMES

Demonstrate that you have heard what is being said. Listen well and acknowledge your partner's words. During relationship distress:

- Accept the fact that you will not easily persuade your tonal partner that the suspicions held about you are invalid. Don't even try while your partner is stressed.
- Do not expect a neutral, empathic response during stress. Your partner is not hearing your exact words but rather the tone of your voice and/or echoes from the past.

- Lack of acknowledgment is painful for anyone, but even more so for a tonal. Restate what was said to verify that you heard the words accurately, as well as the tone.
- Recognize that your tonal partner is deluged in a sea of emotion about what is happening now or what has happened in the past, with subtle nuances taking on enormous meaning. Your patient listening will be golden.

Use the "*Do you mean*" technique to demonstrate that you have heard your partner accurately and to help your tonal partner identify the assumptions he or she is making, the "reading between the lines":

TO TONAL PARTNER: "I'm sorry I'm late. Just as I was about to leave, an urgent e-mail came in alerting me to a crisis that needed to be resolved immediately."

REPLY: "I'm so tired of this! Your damn e-mails are more important to you than I am."

"Do you mean you think I'm saying you don't matter to me?"

"Well, obviously I don't!"

"Do you mean that my getting caught up at work makes you think your feelings aren't important to me?"

"Of course that's what it means."

"Do you mean that there is no other interpretation than that I don't care about you?"

"None! Any others are just excuses."

"Do you mean that it doesn't matter what I say? That you know I take you for granted and that's that?"

"I wouldn't go that far. But I can't think of what you could say that would change my feelings. What do you have in mind?"

"First of all, do you feel fully understood—that I recognize how tired you are of my getting caught up at work and acting as if you aren't as important as my e-mails?"

"I think it's obvious that that's what I'm feeling!"

"Okay, I just wanted to be sure. What I want you to know is that I never want to hurt you, but I also have a demanding job that requires me to do some things on its schedule rather than my schedule. Can you give me some '*Do you means*' on that?"

"Do you mean that your job is so important to you that you're willing to lie about how unimportant I am?"

"No! I'm telling you my truth."

"Do you mean that you feel you don't have a choice, that you have to do what your job requires?"

"Yes, it's that or the streets for both of us. We're both really lucky I have this job in these tough economic times."

"Do you mean that you're not *just* thinking about yourself?"

"Yes, that's what I mean."

"Do you mean that you try to be on time, but sometimes you just can't be?"

"Yes, I try really hard."

"You do, don't you? Sometimes I forget that."

Hearing and fully understanding your tonal partner's meaning makes it more likely that he or she will be able to take in your side of the story. Then encouraging the use of *"Do you means"* to check out whether your words and actions are being heard and interpreted accurately allows a realignment and new attunement. As your tonal partner comes back to center, you will again receive the gift of being known at your subtle depths and ushered into life's aesthetic dimensions.

Other Tools to Keep You in Harmony

We wish we could say that if you follow the above instructions, you will never again reach an impasse or have a misunderstanding with your partner. But neither life nor love works that way. Of the hundreds of self-help techniques that have emerged for couples, the following have worked for us personally and for our clients. As a group, these techniques address a range of issues that are important for maintaining positive energy in any relationship.

Notice Breath, Soften Belly, Open Heart

The following is one of David's favorite ways for quickly centering himself. When you reach an impasse, returning to your own center for a moment is an excellent strategy. The rediscovery of the healing power of meditation as used in ancient spiritual and healing disciplines is considered a breakthrough in contemporary health and mental health care[3]—for good reasons, including a more relaxed physiology, enhanced ability to meet stress, increased power of concentration, reduced vulnerability to a range of problems from anxiety to heart disease, and greater spontaneity, creativity, peace of mind, and happiness. While this book does not teach a deep, committed, daily meditation, you can still use basic meditative methods to shift your energies in highly beneficial ways.

When you evoke emotions like love, appreciation, caring, and compassion, your heart produces coherent rhythms that get your brain to resonate with them. According to scientists who have investigated the workings of the heart, the heart is able to learn and make decisions independent of the brain. In fact, laboratory experiments have shown that "the signals the heart continuously sends to the brain influence the function of higher brain centers involved in perception, cognition, and emotional processing."[4] Your heart has its own "brain" and "nervous system," and the *brain in your head* dutifully obeys messages that are sent from the *brain in your heart.*[5] As you bring your awareness into a "heart space," your perceptions shift toward compassion and caring, the opposite of the focus that is invoked during flooding. As simply put in Rumi's mystical poetry, "The way to heaven is in your heart." A simple technique that brings your focus into your heart can be particularly valuable during relationship stress.

The three-step instructions for the practice contain six simple words: *Notice breath. Soften belly. Open heart.*[6] Set an intention of opening your heart to your partner's feelings. Then let everything drop away except the six words: *Notice breath. Soften belly. Open heart.* Say each pair of words with a deep in-breath and a deep out-breath.

- With "*Notice breath*," your mind concentrates on your breath.
- With "*Soften belly*," your whole body relaxes.
- With "*Open heart*," an expansiveness emanates from your chest area.

Repeat this three-breath sequence at least three times. Return to the business at hand. It may seem to have become a different situation altogether. The energies surrounding the situation may have already been transformed.

Gentle Start-Up

One of John Gottman's most practical single findings is that the way a delicate topic is introduced has a strong influence on whether it will lead a couple on a path toward

Notice Breath

Because energy follows attention, there is an immediate shift, with energy moving from your brain to your lungs. The energy becomes more rhythmic and coherent as your awareness focuses on the movement of your breath.

Soften Belly

As your focus shifts down to your belly, the energy literally softens. It becomes less dense and more fluid, moving out beyond the confines of your belly. The energies of your abdomen also align with the energies of your breath.

Open Heart

Even with people who seem to have "closed hearts" or armoring across their chests, Donna sees the energy literally open and become more receptive during this part of the meditation. It looks like a large French door in the front of the chest opening outward. It expands and extends out much farther from the body as the heart, belly, and breath come into a resonance.

resolution or toward emotional flooding. The amount of accusation, blame, criticism, and negative voice tone and facial expressions in the early phase of a conversation allowed him to predict the outcome of the conversation with 96 percent accuracy![7]

A habitual communication style that distinguished happy and lasting marriages from failed relationships was what he calls the "soft start-up." If you are going to make a request or bring up a disagreement, you are at a choice point. Whether you introduce the issue in a soft or harsh manner is up to you.

It is easier, however, to lead with a soft start-up if you've not been stockpiling negative feelings until they finally burst out of you. Research confirms this. While women are more likely to be the ones who bring up difficulties for discussion, the most successful couples tend to deal with conflict as it comes up rather than let it build.[8] That means that they are not already overloaded by the time they raise an issue and can take the time to formulate a gentle start-up. Gottman's guidelines for a gentle start-up and for introducing complaints in a constructive manner follow,[9] along with some typical harsh start-ups and how the situations might have been approached more constructively:

1. **Begin with a positive rather than negative reflection of your relationship.** Harsh start-up: "When was the last time you left space for us to have some fun and connection time on our work trips? It's work, work, work, and more work! If we leave it to you, we'll never have any fun together." Gentle start-up: "I remember the first concert we went to—Crosby, Stills, and Nash. We sang in the car all the way home. Let's find a concert we'd both enjoy when we're in San Francisco next week. Wouldn't that be fun!"

2. **Express appreciation and gratitude.** Harsh start-up: "You never help me with the housework." Gentle start-up: "I appreciate your having brought in all the gardening tools now that autumn is almost over. Would you help me move the furniture in the living room this weekend so we can make room for my new desk?"

3. **Start with "I" instead of "You."** Harsh start-up: "You always find something more important than being with the kids. You hardly know them!" Gentle start-up: "I was sad this morning when Janie asked you to help her with her math and you had to go off to work. Was that hard for you?"

4. **Don't stockpile complaints.** Harsh start-up: "You never reach out to me anymore. We haven't had sex in months, and you probably haven't even noticed." Gentle start-up: "I've been missing our intimate time. I know we're so busy that we're exhausted by the time we could even cuddle, but let's make our time together more important."

5. **State your feelings and needs without attacking or blaming the other person.** Harsh start-up: "I can't believe that you forgot Jimmy's birthday. You are the most self-centered person I know!" Gentle start-up: "I'm angry and disappointed that you forgot Jimmy's birthday. Will you tell me how that happened?"

6. **Describe your side of the story as your perception rather than as the absolute truth.** Harsh start-up: "I'm no fool. Let's face it, you're bored with me." Gentle start-up: "I've been feeling lonely lately, and I'm afraid you're bored with me. You've looked at your watch three times just since we started talking."

7. **Focus on specific behavior, not global judgments.** Harsh start-up: "You are the sloppiest person I've ever had the misfortune to know." Gentle start-up: "I know it's a bummer to have to tidy up the bathroom after you shower, but hanging up the towel and putting your stuff in the hamper would make a real difference to me."

> ## → THE ENERGY DIMENSION ←
>
> **A harsh start-up** causes the receiver's energies to pull back into the body, disconnect, and become ready to move back out aggressively. The sender's energies look exactly the way this start-up is named: harsh. They are fast and forceful.
>
> **A gentle start-up** invites the energy of curiosity, responsibility, and receptiveness. These energies appear to Donna to have a rolling and engaging quality as they move toward the partner. The sender's energies move out slowly and softly, with colors that remind Donna of faith and hope.

Making a conscious choice to use a gentle start-up when bringing up a request or expressing a difficult feeling sets the direction of the interaction. The way a start-up is received, even a gentle one, also of course evokes an energy that will influence all that follows. The counterpart of the gentle start-up is nonjudgmental listening.

Nonjudgmental Listening

The *"Do you mean"* technique is a set of training wheels for nonjudgmental listening. It keeps you attuned so you take in your partner's feelings, experiences, and meaning before you take action. It gives a structured way for successful conflict resolution, and it puts first things first. Before you try to get your partner to come to your point of view, be able to state your partner's position to his or her satisfaction. There is tremendous power to listening with an open heart, signaling with your eyes and facial expression that you are completely present and attentive, and offering periodic non-intrusive verbal encouragement with utterances such as "Yes," "I hear you," "Uh-huh," "Go ahead," "I see why you would feel that way," and "That must be hard."

When your partner has the floor during a disagreement, make nonjudgmental listening your priority. Receiving your partner nonjudgmentally is powerfully affirming, though it may be difficult if your partner is exuding anger, judgment, or blame. Before you yourself begin to flood, remind yourself that your partner's anger is (in most instances) a measure of investment in the relationship, a reflection of caring. A complaint is a bid for connection and, even if this is a hard moment, it is only a moment in a relationship that contains many strengths and that has seen and will almost certainly see many brighter moments. Your job right then is to (1) accurately take in your partner's feelings and (2) offer verbal and nonverbal evidence that you understand. Particularly important (and challenging) is to remind yourself that your job is *not* to change your partner's feelings, fix the situation, or further your own agenda.

Like the gentle start-up, active, attuned listening is a choice that is available to you that can have a transformative effect on the direction of the interchange. It is also a simple and direct way of "turning toward" rather than "away from" or "against" your partner's bids for connection. Gottman found that the newlywed couples who would still be together on six-year follow-up turned toward each other's bids for connection an average of 88 percent of the time, while those who would be divorced six years later turned toward each other's bids an average of only 33 percent of the time.[10]

Cultivating Gratitude

Expressing appreciation is not just for the soft start-up. However much tension may (or may not) pervade your relationship, your partner has chosen you for building a shared life. This puts you in an exclusive position as a primary source of affirmation and "mirroring." Your partner's sense of self is influenced by what you reflect back. Genuine appreciation is incredibly reinforcing, and what is reinforced tends to be repeated. In a very real sense, "what you see is what you get." The more you appreciate your partner's favorable qualities and convey that appreciation, the more those qualities are likely to be expressed. Most people, however, begin to take for granted what is always there. The tendency to scan for what needs to be fixed rather than for what is right can also overshadow an appreciative outlook. Regularly delivering appreciations is powerfully affirming for your partner, and it also keeps you on the alert for what you truly appreciate in the everyday flow of your lives together.

AN APPRECIATION VOLLEY

While expressing gratitude and appreciation is valuable any time, if you do it in a structured manner, attending to this vital need to say and to hear what is positive won't get lost in the busyness of your lives. You can do it as a "volley," giving your partner three "I appreciate . . ." statements, or you can alternate, one of you making the statement, then the other. Receive the appreciation with a "thank you" or other positive acknowledgment. We will set our writing aside right now and do this, recording what we say:

DAVID: "Donna, even though it was hard to take it the other day when you told me that you were mad at me because I wanted to fire Lina, I am realizing right now that I got over it so quickly because I thought of the thousands of times you have been there backing me in my choices. I *really* appreciate that."

DONNA: "Thank you, David. I appreciate how you come around after something difficult with me and how kind you are when you do."

DAVID: "Thank you, Donna. Donna, I appreciate the way that even when you are having difficulty with something, you will switch into moments of absolute joy. Yesterday you were so stressed trying to get ready to leave for our conference, and then you suddenly said, 'Look at these blue shoes, they make me *so* happy!!!' Things like that just dissolve the tension and make my life so much more fun."

DONNA: "Thank you! David, even though you're a pretty in-your-head kind of guy, I really appreciate how you are so often able to put my feelings into words when I can't."

DAVID: "I couldn't have said that better myself, Donna! Thank you. Donna, I appreciate the way you invite me to help you word things when you are writing a hard letter or trying to express a difficult concept. That is so affirming, and it brings out a part of me that I really like."

DONNA: "Thank you. David, I appreciate how well you do that for me. You have a big heart, and you're able to be right there for me."

DAVID: "Thank you . . ."

We invite you to experiment with creating regular, dedicated time together for "volleys" like this. Making structured appreciations a regular practice trains you to keep yourself attuned for what you truly appreciate about one another in a way that helps the love between you to blossom. A note on protocol: While there is no rule against using the same statement more than once, and some qualities or acts deserve to be acknowledged many times, you will find it embarrassing if the best you can come up with week after week is "I appreciate the tennis racket you gave me for Christmas three years ago." Attuning yourself during the week so you notice what is worthy of your appreciation can quickly upgrade the quality of the energy that flows between you.

AN APPRECIATION SANDWICH

Another valuable use of the power of appreciation is coming to be known in couples therapy circles as the "Appreciation Sandwich." It is actually a structured approach for the soft start-up. It gently brings your focus to a problem that needs to be solved, sandwiching your concern between two appreciations. When you wish to raise an issue that may be touchy, announce to your partner that you would like to offer an Appreciation Sandwich. This becomes a way of signaling to your partner that you are planning to gently enter difficult territory and hope he or she will be receptive.

1. From this invitation, move right into the Appreciation Sandwich or agree on a time for you to deliver it.
2. Begin by expressing a sincere statement reflecting something you genuinely value about your partner, in the form of "I appreciate . . ."
3. Your partner listens attentively and responds with a "Thank you."
4. You then express your area of concern or a request with a carefully worded statement that begins "I have difficulty with . . ." or "I would like you to . . ."
5. Again, your partner listens attentively and ends with a "Thank you."
6. You complete the "sandwich" with another statement that begins "I appreciate . . ."
7. This is received with another "Thank you."

> ### → THE ENERGY DIMENSION ←
>
> #### Expressing Gratitude
>
> The more you state genuine appreciation, the more you activate your body's *radiant circuits*—the energies of joy, gladness, awe, wonder, and generosity. Because of the stresses in our lives, this energy system has gone dormant for many people, but by exercising it you rebuild it. So expressing gratitude not only serves you as a couple, it builds stronger muscles for joy within you.

8. Your partner's first response is to clarify the "I have difficulty with . . ." statement using the "*Do you mean*" format, continuing until receiving "yes" responses to three questions.

Once your difficulty or request has been fully received and understood, tell your partner that you appreciate that your meaning was taken in. At that point, any subsequent discussion about the issue will proceed on a more solid foundation.

Tell Me What You Want to Hear!

Sometimes appreciations that come out of a structured exercise fall flat. You just can't quite find the words or the focus or the passion to ring your partner's bells with your appreciation statements. You can instead ask your partner to *role-play* being you and to state the appreciations he or she would like to hear you say. It is often astounding not only how well he or she can do it, but how your partner's sincerely saying what he or she longs to hear may boost your empathy and become highly instructive for you. In fact, this is a powerful technique in many situations. If your partner is not giving you the response you long for, simply pretending you are your partner and saying your own name and then what you would wish to hear can sometimes clue your partner right into giving you what you are wanting. Usually it is not that your partner doesn't want to tell you what you want to hear but that he or she doesn't have any idea about what that is. This often traces to your sensory modes and other differences far more than any insensitivity or lack of caring. If you have established the technique as part of your repertoire with one another, it can be a powerful tool.

In our relationship, Donna is most likely to be the one who feels the responses she is receiving are not on the mark. At such times, she may say to David what she would like to hear, such as (Donna speaking): "Donna, I so appreciate how you take care of requests that come in to both of us. I sometimes find out that you have handled requests without me even knowing about them. And you handle them so gracefully, even when we can't accommodate them. You really protect my time and space that way. It is a very loving gift you give to me." David, often oblivious to the whole matter, may only manage to utter back a wimpy reply like, "Yeah, what you said!" As we were writing the last sentence, with David poking fun at himself, Donna commented, "But I treasure the look of recognition and empathy on your face!" And more often, when David recognizes the truth of Donna's words, he is likely to restate it in his own words, in a way that touches us both. At a minimum, Donna's overture tunes him in to a whole new slice of the relationship and Donna isn't having to sit on her resentment about how oblivious David has been.

High-Band It

Another technique we've been using in our own relationship for more than thirty years is to invoke the phrase "High-band it" to invite each other to lift the discussion to a "higher band" of energy. Like the Appreciation Sandwich, it is a simple technique that can quickly improve the energies between you and your partner. At any moment, you can be placing a more positive interpretation on the circumstances in your life or a more negative one. Each tends to be self-fulfilling. High-banding means that positive perceptions become the lens through which events are viewed. You place the most favorable interpretations possible on the situation, however much of a stretch it may seem in the moment. When one of us sees the other spiraling down in the stresses of daily life, the other will gently and with compassion say, "Let's high-band this one." We've each learned that when the other offers this invitation, we are at a choice point.

Often, that simple reminder can create a shift from being immersed in the emotional misery of the moment to becoming aware that our interpretation of the situation is bringing us down as much as the situation itself. Simply remembering that this is a fleeting moment and placing it in the context of all that is right will be enough to lift you from the "low-band" path to the high band. Talk about this concept and try it. If you can't get there, if your negativity is too strong to let you high-band it, use one or more of the energy exercises on pages 82–94 and then give it another try. One more caveat. Take care not to use this as a way of criticizing or blaming: "Would you please HIGH-BAND IT, dammit!" Repeatedly for us, a compassionate and loving "Let's high-band it, David" can be a marvelous gift. Combining it with an offer for a Spinal Flush (p. 94) is the lover's meow.

How to Instantly Stop an Argument

The most vulnerable moment in couple communication is generally the point where you (or your partner) are becoming flooded with anger and are sure you are right and your partner is wrong. When we go into our energetic stress response mode, the first thing lost is our ability to respond to the situation creatively and the next is any sense that a higher path is possible. If you are the one who is becoming flooded, there is a quick two-step process you can do at this point that may instantly bring you back into attunement and connection.

The first step is an energy technique; the second step refocuses your mind. Immediately take a deep breath. Place one hand on your belly just beneath your navel. Place the base of the palm of your other hand above your nose between your eyebrows with your fingers facing up and resting easily as far as they reach toward the top of your head. Take another deep breath and ask yourself to find the fear that is beneath the anger or blame. The physical posture has several advantages. First of all, it shifts your attention from the disharmony to your body. It also energetically connects three chakras: the second chakra, beneath your navel, is the chakra of creativity; the sixth chakra, between your eyebrows, is the chakra of higher perception (known as the "third eye" in yoga practice); and the seventh chakra is the chakra of higher purpose. The posture is called the Three Chakra Hook-Up. The hand on your head also stimulates reflex points that keep the blood from leaving your brain for the fight/flight/freeze response. So you are immediately interrupting the stress response and at the same time bringing creativity to your faculties of higher perceptions and higher purpose.

But you don't stop there. Now that you have shifted your focus from the disagreement to your body and brought the energies in your body into a more favorable state, you are able to ask yourself a vital question: "What is the fear in me that is driving this anger or blame?" Gay and Kathlyn Hendricks—who have been teaching couples about "conscious loving"[11] since the early 1980s and are high up among the couples who coach couples whom we most admire—point out that beneath anger and blame is usually fear. You may be afraid that your partner is doing something that will make your life harder, is blaming or judging you, is never going to change a behavior that is hard for you to tolerate, is losing interest in you, or is going to leave you. One of Gay and Kathlyn's favorite techniques, which helps couples instantly shift from argument to connection, is to ask them to go beneath the anger, find the fear that is driving it, and state it. For instance, "Every night you sink into the TV and every night I feel angry about it. Deep down I'm afraid you are getting bored with me." Saying what you are afraid of connects you with your partner at a more vulnerable level and shifts you out of a confrontational space. Doing the energy posture first makes you more likely to be able to tune into the underlying fear with self-compassion. Your partner's compassion will, in turn, be beckoned. Try it. It works!

Cultivate Positive Thoughts About Your Partner and Your Relationship

Thought and energy influence one another. Your thoughts follow your energies, but your energies also follow your thoughts. Make a list of ten qualities you deeply appreciate about your partner or your relationship. Carry it with you. At least once during your workday or another time that you are apart, stop, consult your list, select one of the qualities, and for fifteen seconds mindfully immerse yourself in it while doing the Three Chakra Hook-Up or simply placing both hands over your Heart Chakra. Savor this. Enjoy it fully. Imagine you are breathing the positive thought into every cell of your body.

Physical Connection Stimulates Loving Energies

Caring physical touch keeps loving energies flowing between you. A simple conscious hug can initiate a shift when your energies are out of sync. Couples, even in strong relationships, tend to touch less over time, and when partners are feeling alienated from one another, hugs and other caring touches are often first to go. For most couples, even if the hugs seem forced in the beginning, they will usually have become genuine by the fourth or fifth second. Relaxing into a full-body embrace for

---

→ THE ENERGY DIMENSION ←

Positive Thinking

When you immerse yourself in a positive thought, the energy of your aura becomes large, expansive, takes on a halo look around your head, and tends to connect with natural energies in the environment. Meanwhile, the energies of your heart and your head come into greater sync. When you repeatedly hold positive thoughts, this energy becomes more habitual—easier to access and present more of the time.

---

even six seconds increases serotonin, leaving you feeling closer and less irritable, edgy, or sad.[12] One thing we have done right is that even in the hard times, we hug one another. Sometimes we just hold on to one another as the upset dissipates. Daily heartfelt hugs are a wonderfully simple way to facilitate and maintain closeness (unless so much contempt has entered the relationship that prescribed hugs are not the place for you to start rebuilding).

A particularly good time for hugs is at moments of separation or reuniting. The part of us that longs to bond tends to become activated during partings and reunions, so you are, at a deep level, both more vulnerable at such times and more open to the power of a connection such as a conscious, full-bodied hug.

A deep embrace each evening can invite and dissolve the energies of fear, anxiety, shame, sadness, or resentment that may be left over from the day. Without even talking about the feelings, your body will quickly learn that in this safe haven, your vulnerabilities can be soothed in the simple enjoyment of a heart-to-heart embrace.[13] Your relationship is your port within the storm.

Heaven Rushing In

In one of Donna's favorite exercises to teach in an energy medicine class, you stand, open your arms toward the sky (best done outdoors, but you can visualize the heavens above you no matter where you are), and feel the energies come into your hands, arms, and body (see Figure 2-1). Even if you can't quite feel them, they are there, moving into you as you hold this receptive posture. As the energies gather, you are likely to at least feel a tingling in your hands. Whatever you register, you can know that the heavens do respond when you are open. As a child of both the earth and the sky, you spontaneously receive healing energy and even information and guidance when you hold this position. Take in all you want. It is also a great technique to use when you don't know what else to do.

When you are ready to continue, gather these energies into your hands and bring them over the center of your chest, a vortex that is known as "Heaven Rushing In." The healing energies and guidance you have gathered rush into your body. Breathe them in.

This technique can be adapted to uplift your relationship. Begin by facing one another and with the open posture, look up toward the heavens (see Figure 2-1). As you bring your hands to your heart, make eye contact with your partner. Feel

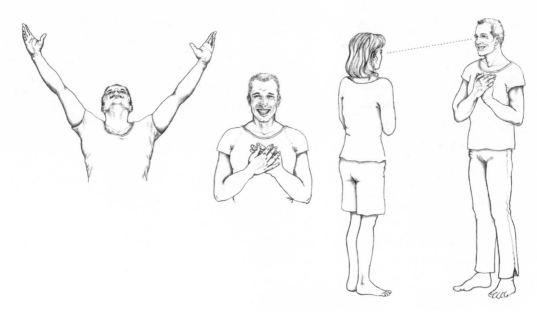

FIGURE 2-1 *Heaven Rushing In*

the energies you have gathered not only going into you but also building a bridge between you. Breathe into this bridge. Let it connect and enrich you both. This simple practice can be a lovely way to open or close any important encounter between the two of you.

On to Chapter 3

Understanding your own and your partner's Energetic Stress Styles can keep you attuned in ways that head off many difficulties. When emotionally charged disagreements do arise, as they do in all relationships, what do you do? Many couples feel helpless as they watch themselves being taken onto an ugly course. Again. Is there a way to reliably turn conflicts into opportunities for deeper understanding and the affection that usually follows? Chapter 3 presents a step-by-step process for constructively engaging conflict. We call it "The Pact."

3

When Your Energies Collide

A Pact for Setting Things Straight

Use can almost change the stamp of nature.

—WILLIAM SHAKESPEARE, *Hamlet*

A DEEP LOVING PARTNERSHIP IS A BOND, A *COLLABORATIVE ALLIANCE.* THIS BOND involves friendship and union that brings out the best in each of you. When it is broken or threatened, you are pulled into your Energetic Stress Style and may fall into fear, rage, or retreat. Sustaining a collaborative alliance, according to David Schnarch, author of *Intimacy and Desire,* requires you to work together for mutual benefit *"even when this is difficult, anxiety-provoking, or painful."*[1] More than analyzing what went wrong, it requires a willingness to align with one another in service of the relationship even when every instinct in you wants to strike out or retreat. While a successful marriage may be measured in years, the collaborative alliance ebbs and flows, able to be "made or lost in a split second."[2] Even within a strong relationship, partners aren't able to stay in a state of collaborative alliance every moment. But the more you can maintain that state, the better your relationship will fare. Positive practices *can* "almost change the stamp of nature."

Chapter 2 closed by promising you a Pact that can help you encounter relationship conflict constructively and creatively. This Pact will be able to serve as a means for repairing your collaborative alliance when it has become disrupted. It has four parts, each named for the action it requires:

1. **S**top
2. **T**ap
3. **A**ttune
4. **R**esolve

The acronym *STAR* will help you remember these four parts. Begin by emblazoning in your mind the first and most elusive step: *Stop!*

Part 1 of the <u>S</u>TAR Pact: Stop

It can happen while you are watching TV, describing a precious event that occurred during your day, sharing a candlelight dinner, or, in the grand tradition of marital conflict, talking about money, sex, or raising the kids. Adrenaline pumps into your bloodstream, your heartbeat accelerates, and your ability to take in and process information diminishes dramatically. You lose your empathy, compassion, creativity, and sense of humor. Your defensiveness is on the rise. Your primal sensory channel takes over, and the sensory modes that usually balance it turn off. John Gottman wryly notes that when such "flooding" occurs, couples may wonder what they ever saw in one another in the first place. You feel overwhelmed by your own reactions and shocked by your partner's. "You go into 'systems overload,' swamped by distress and upset. You may become extremely hostile, defensive, or withdrawn. Once you're feeling this out of control, constructive discussion is impossible."[3]

Yet stopping the discussion, even if you know it has taken a sharp downhill turn, may also seem impossible. Your partner has just assaulted your sacred bond and doesn't care enough to apologize on the spot and begin to repair it. You've been insulted, blamed, or dismissed; fight, flight, or freeze hormones are surging through your arteries; you are caught in your Energetic Stress Style; and an accelerating momentum has taken on its own life. It may feel dreadful, but it is compelling. Stopping at such a moment is usually the hardest part of the Pact, which begins with an agreement to *stop* at the moment you are aware that defensiveness or anger toward your partner is building:

"If *I* recognize that a conflict is escalating, I will immediately *stop* and suggest we do a pre-agreed technique designed to shift our energies. If *you* make this suggestion, I will immediately interrupt the conversation and join you in the technique you suggest."

This is so difficult to do because every fiber of your being is engaged in a rapidly escalating conflict. Marriage counselors know that it is critical to prevent people from reenacting the destructive, harmful confrontations that brought the couple into the office.[4] Failure to do so not only erodes hope for the relationship and confidence in the therapist, it further establishes the neural pathways of threat and distrust. An effective couples therapist will intervene by providing a structure to the session that does not allow the couple to go into a negative freefall, but instead points them in a constructive direction. The purpose of the Pact is to provide that kind of structure at precisely the times it is most likely for the brain chemistry of threat and distrust to become more deeply established. It is designed to intervene during an interaction that is taking a harmful turn and to put it onto a constructive track. While it requires more determination to implement than if a couples therapist or coach is there in the room telling you to do it, your Pact is much cheaper. It is also on call 24/7.

But for the Pact to work, you need to give it the power you would give to a therapist! If a therapist whom you are paying a substantial fee interrupts your argument and suggests you instead begin to do a relaxation technique, you are likely to obey. The Pact gives you exactly this kind of instruction, and its success rests on an ironclad agreement (made between the two of you during a calm time) that you will implement it to head off a storm at the point when the weather seems to be turning. You won't be able to create the Pact during the storm, and it will be harder to apply if you have waited until you are in full battle, though it can still be effective even in the midst of full battles—just harder to set into motion.

This first part, *Stop*, is, in theory, the easiest one to do—you just apply the brakes—yet it is, paradoxically, the hardest phase to initiate. As the intensity of negative emotion rises, you are caught between wishing the altercation would just go away and hearing the nastiest and most provocative words in your repertoire come out of your mouth. It is hard to pause when you would rather righteously drive your point home. Slamming on the brakes despite your biochemistry propelling you forward is, nonetheless, the maneuver you need to establish as your default in order for the Pact to be effective. Unlike communication techniques that are often useless during the height of couples conflict, however, your Pact provides a dependable structure for shifting your agenda from pursuing the *conflict* to changing the *energy* (Part 2 of the Pact). Couples can become practiced and capable of switching to an energy technique that breaks the spell that was keeping them in a negative spiral. Changing the energy becomes a shared achievement that is in itself empowering and bonding.

Part 2 of the S**TA**R Pact: Tap

Gottman suggests that the pauses couples take in the face of emotional flooding last at least twenty minutes because that's the time required for adrenaline and other stress chemicals that were released into the bloodstream to break down. In fact, most people in his research *believed* that they had completely calmed down after a fight even though their pulse rate was still ten percent above its normal resting rate, leaving them primed for quicker re-arousal. For the break to serve its purpose, (1) it must not be an excuse to avoid the issue, (2) there should be a specific plan for returning to the discussion, (3) it should not be a time to simply rehearse your arguments or relive your sense of betrayal, and (4) the break should be relaxing. This is not, however, easy to accomplish at times of intense interpersonal conflict. To collect yourself when your emotions are raging requires you to swim against a fierce internal tide. Energy techniques quell the tide so the break can be effective.

Introducing simple energy techniques can actually reduce the twenty-minute cooling-off period Gottman prescribes because they help the body process stress more effectively. Of the hundreds of energy medicine techniques we have used in our work, certain ones seem universally powerful and so flexible that they can serve many purposes. Of those, we've selected eight that are easy to learn. They have been taught widely, and they are particularly potent for re-centering after coming into an explosive moment in your relationship. When your energies have become disorganized and your mind is in defense mode, you can restabilize body and mind with some or all of the following simple techniques. They begin very simply, by *tapping* on your body.

The first step of the Pact is to STOP!
The second step is to immediately begin to TAP.

Just as your Pact includes an agreement to stop the discussion the instant either of you recognizes that one of you has become emotionally hooked, the second agreement is that you will immediately tap on four sets of points on your face and torso. If you can make this your reflexive response, it will immediately begin to balance the energies in your body. You will have these points memorized after just a few run-throughs, so you will be able to do them with little thought. To further balance and stabilize your body's energies, you can then proceed through some or all of the additional techniques listed here. This will center you energetically, which calms your body and refreshes and refocuses your mind. The centering techniques are:

1. The Four Taps
2. The Blow-Out/Zip-Up/Hook-Up
3. The Crossover Shoulder Pull
4. The Crown Pull
5. The Stress Release Hold
6. The Wayne Cook Posture

7. Connecting Heaven and Earth

8. The Cross Crawl

It is often a losing battle to try to will yourself to stay centered in the midst of escalating conflict with your partner, but you can will yourself to do physical movements that will calm and align your energies. Your mind will then follow, your coping abilities will return, and it will become possible then to creatively reconnect. Instructions for carrying out each of these eight techniques follow.

The Four Taps

Certain points on your body, when tapped with your fingers, affect your energy field in predictable ways, sending electrochemical impulses to specific regions of your brain and releasing neurotransmitters. By tapping the following sets of points (see figure 3-1), you can activate a series of internal responses that will restore you when you are stressed or simply tired. You can also tap these points at any time you need a boost. The Four Taps include:

STOMACH MERIDIAN POINTS

On the top of the cheekbones directly beneath each eye are acupuncture points on the Stomach Meridian.

KIDNEY MERIDIAN POINTS

Place your fingers on your collarbone and move them toward the center until you come to the corners of the collarbone just below your throat. Move your fingers down beneath the bone. Most people have an indent there. These points beneath the collarbone knobs are the location of the paired "K-27 points," the twenty-seventh acupuncture points on the Kidney Meridian.

THYMUS POINT

The point at the middle of the sternum stimulates the thymus. Tapping it not only helps center your energies but also helps boost your immune system, which is compromised by relationship stress.

SPLEEN POINTS

The points one rib below the "bra line" (fellas, use your imagination) and directly beneath the nipples are the neurolymphatic reflex points for the Spleen Meridian.

Tap each point firmly for the length of one deep in-breath and out-breath, but never so hard as to risk bruising yourself. Do not be overly concerned about finding the precise location of each point. If you use several fingers to tap in the vicinity described, you will hit the right spot.

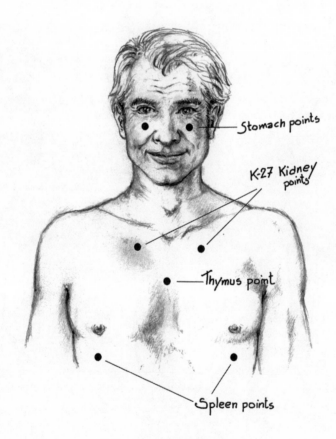

FIGURE 3-1 *The Four Taps*

The Blow-Out/Zip-Up/Hook-Up

THE BLOW-OUT

Blow out the energetic residue of accumulated feelings by (1) making fists as you bring your hands and arms in front of you, (2) swinging your arms down and around behind you, (3) lifting them above your head, and (4) rapidly and with some force sending your fists down to your sides (see Figure 3-2). Purse your lips as you blow out the emotion. Open your hands when they have come all the way down. Repeat this several times. End by doing the movement once more, but this time, slowly and deliberately. Now with some of the energies cleared, do a Zip-Up.

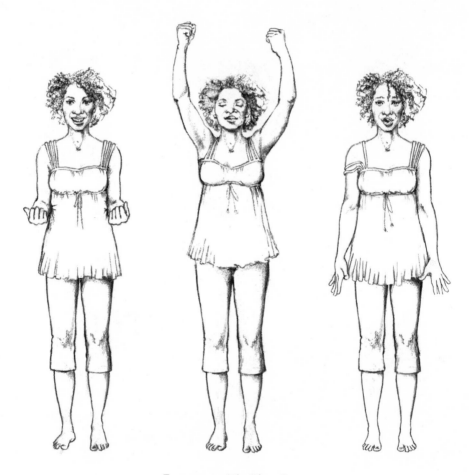

FIGURE 3-2 *The Blow-Out*

THE ZIP-UP

Zip up by placing either or both hands at your pubic bone and taking a deep in-breath as you move your hand with deliberation straight up the center of your body, to your lower lip (see Figure 3-3). Repeat two or three times. Breathe deeply each time. Your hands emanate an electromagnetic field and, with this movement, you are tracing your Central Meridian, one of the body's major energy pathways. This strengthens the meridian and tends to stabilize your energies, centering and empowering you.

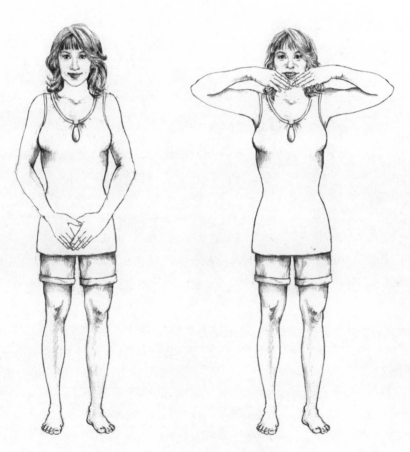

FIGURE 3-3 *The Zip-Up*

THE HOOK-UP

Hook in this calm and clarity by placing the middle finger of one hand on your third eye (between your eyebrows above the bridge of your nose) and the middle finger of your other hand in your navel. Gently press both fingers inward, pull them upward, and hold there for at least three deep, full breaths (see Figure 3-4).

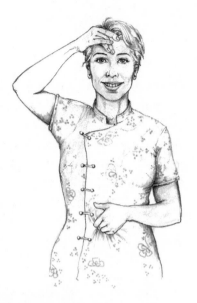

FIGURE 3-4 *The Hook-Up*

→ THE ENERGY DIMENSION ←

When a person is emotionally flooded, the energy within becomes compacted and crowded. It can feel thick, slow-moving, and even painful. Each of the energy exercises presented in this chapter impacts your energy field in ways that are beneficial for processing stress, calming your emotions, becoming centered, and thinking more clearly. Here is what the Blow-Out, Zip-Up, and Hook-Up do energetically:

The Blow-Out moves toxic stressed energy out of your body, counters feelings of being overwhelmed, and allows the energies to flow more freely. Meanwhile, your aura expands, giving you more energetic "elbow room."

The Zip-Up moves your life force up through the energy fields within and surrounding your body. Having just emptied discordant energies with the Blow-Out, the Zip-Up also stabilizes you in that calmer state.

The Hook-Up connects the energies going up the front of your body with the energies going up your spine and over your head, strengthening a force field that energetically surrounds and protects you, leaving you more resilient and confident.

The Crossover Shoulder Pull

Several meridians run through the shoulders and tend to become clogged at the shoulders when we feel stress. This also interferes with natural left-right crossover patterns. All this can be quickly reversed with the Crossover Shoulder Pull.

Place either hand on its opposite shoulder and press in hard behind the shoulder with your fingers (see Figure 3-5). Drag your hand over your shoulder, maintaining the pressure. Continue, with less pressure now, to your opposite hip. Repeat two or three times. Shift to the other side.

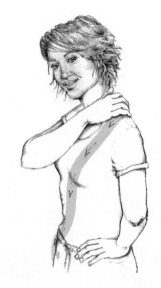

FIGURE 3-5 *The Crossover Shoulder Pull*

The Crown Pull

While doing the Crown Pull, breathe deeply, in through your nose and out through your mouth.

1. Place your thumbs at your temples on the sides of your head. Curl your fingers and rest your fingertips just above the center of your eyebrows (see Figure 3-6).
2. Slowly, and with some pressure, pull your fingers apart so that you stretch the skin just above your eyebrows.

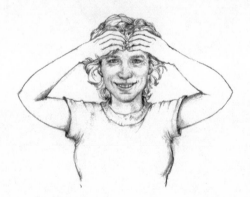 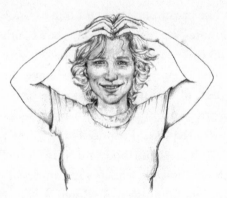

FIGURE 3-6 *The Crown Pull*

3. Rest your fingertips at the center of your forehead and repeat the stretch.

4. Rest your fingertips at your hairline and repeat the stretch.

5. Continue this pattern, fingers curled and pushing in at each of these locations:

   a. Fingers at the top of your head, with your little fingers at your hairline. Push down with some pressure and pull your hands away from one another, as if pulling your head apart.

   b. Fingers at the center of your head, again pushing down and pulling your hands away from one another.

   c. Fingers over the curve at the back of your head, again using the same stretch.

   d. Continue down your neck, fingers at the center of your neck, pushing in and then pulling around to the side, finally hanging your fingers on your shoulders.

When you are ready to release, push your fingers into your shoulders, drag them across the tops of your shoulders, and finally drop your hands.

The Stress Release Hold

While we have placed this as the fifth technique in this series, it is a gem that you can use any time you feel emotional distress.

Place the palm of one hand lightly over your forehead and the palm of the other around the back of your head (see Figure 3-7). If you hold them there while breathing deeply for one to three minutes, the energies from your hands and the contact with areas of the skin called "neurovascular points" have the effect of shifting the neurochemistry of stress, turning off the fight/flight/ freeze response. First doing the Crown Pull makes your body more receptive for this posture, which you can do sitting, standing, or lying down.

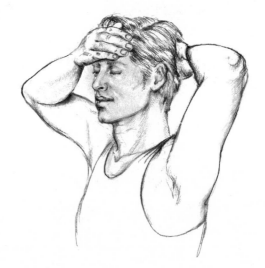

FIGURE 3-7 *The Stress Release Hold*

The Wayne Cook Posture

This is one of the most powerful techniques we know for restoring clarity of mind. Originally developed by Wayne Cook for working with people who stutter, it has been effectively applied now with a wide range of issues, from helping people with learning disabilities to improving the performance of athletes. The technique involves three postures:

1. While sitting, place your right foot over your left knee, wrap your left hand around your right ankle, and wrap your right hand around the ball of your right foot (best done with shoes removed). Your wrists will be crossing over one another (see Figure 3-8a). Breathe in slowly through your nose, lifting your body as you breathe in. At the same time, pull your leg inward, creating a stretch. Exhale slowly out your mouth, letting your body relax. Repeat this slow breathing and stretching four or five times.

2. Switch to your other foot. Place your left foot over your right knee, wrap your right hand around your left ankle, and wrap your left hand around the ball of your left foot (see Figure 3-8b). Lift your body and breathe as described above.

3. Uncross your legs, place your fingertips together to form a pyramid, and bring your thumbs to rest on your third eye, just above the bridge of your nose (see Figure 3-8c). Breathe slowly in through your nose and out through your mouth about five times.

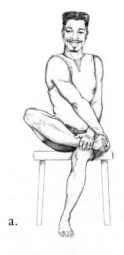

a.

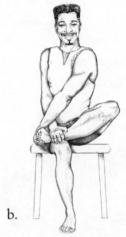

b.

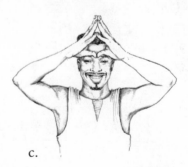

c.

FIGURE 3-8 *The Wayne Cook Posture*

Connecting Heaven and Earth

Stretching is one of the most natural ways to keep the body's energies moving, which is in turn one of the best ways to keep your mind clear. From watching cats and dogs upon waking to practicing disciplines that have made stretching into an art form, such as yoga and tai chi, many models are available. Versions of the following exercise have been found in numerous cultures, and it is not only an excellent way to get energy flowing throughout the body, it is formulated to help integrate the brain's left and right hemispheres and to activate the *radiant circuits*, the energy system that supports joy.[5] To "Connect Heaven and Earth" (see Figure 3-9):

1. In a standing position, rub your hands together and then shake them out. Place them on your thighs, with your fingers spread. Then with a deep inhalation, circle your arms out, and on the exhalation bring your hands together into a prayerful position.

2. With a deep inhalation, stretch one arm high above your head and flatten the hand palm up (as if pushing something above you); stretch the other arm

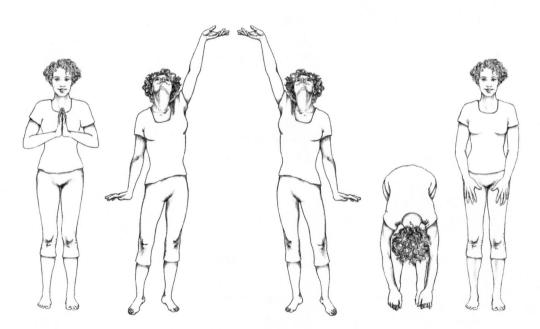

Figure 3-9 *Connecting Heaven and Earth*

down and flatten the hand palm down (as if pushing something toward the earth). Stay in this position for as long as is comfortable, then release your breath through your mouth, returning your hands to the prayerful position.

3. Repeat, switching the arm that raises and the arm that lowers. Do one or more additional lifts on each side.

4. Coming out of this pose the final time, bring your arms down and allow your body to fold over at the waist. Hang there with your knees slightly bent as you take two deep breaths.

5. Slowly return to a standing position, ending with a backward roll of the shoulders.

The Cross Crawl

We are designed to replenish our energies through activity. Energy crosses over from the left hemisphere of the brain to the right side of the body and from the right hemisphere to the left side of the body. Figure-eight crossover patterns operate throughout your body, from the biofield that surrounds you down to the double helix in your DNA. When you are stressed, this energy may go into a homolateral, up-down pattern instead of the crossover rhythm that supports your health and vitality. Any activity that involves a crossover motion (e.g., left arm moves at the same time as the right leg, right arm moves with left leg)—such as walking, running, or swimming—tends to boost and balance your energies. One of David's favorite mood-changers is a vigorous swim. The simplest technique to obtain these benefits, called the Cross Crawl, is in essence simply walking in place (see Figure 3-10).

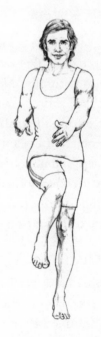

1. While standing or sitting, lift your right arm and left leg simultaneously.

2. As you let them down, raise your left arm and right leg.

3. Repeat, this time exaggerating the lift of your leg and swing of your arm across your midline to the opposite side of your body.

FIGURE 3-10 *The Cross Crawl*

4. Continue this exaggerated march for at least a minute, breathing deeply in through your nose and out through your mouth.

These exercises are not only valuable for re-centering after an argument; they boost your physical health and mental well-being and bring you home to yourself. We encourage you to do them with your partner when you are *not under stress* so you familiarize yourself with them and get a glimpse of their general benefits. You will also get a sense of which techniques are likely to provide the best first aid for you.

Part 3 of the STAR Pact: Attune

By this point in the Pact, you have realigned your own energies. Your partner has done the same. This third part of the Pact will help you reconnect. Your bond has been strained or perhaps even feels ruptured. So you now face not only the task of resolving the disagreement but also of repairing the bond. You can start to repair the bond by realigning your energies with your partner's.

Attuning Energetically

Doing a few of the centering exercises described above in unison with your partner, such as the Four Taps or Connecting Heaven and Earth, gives your energies a chance to realign naturally. No discussion is necessary. Or take a brisk walk, the classic Cross Crawl activity, with an agreement that you will comment only on what you observe during the walk rather than reenter the discussion just yet. Attend particularly to objects of beauty or interest. While it takes some discipline to stay focused on the here and now of the walk rather than to reengage the argument, you begin to bridge with one another energetically as you together exercise your powers of observation and description during a joint Cross Crawl activity. Our *all-time favorite* energy medicine technique for wordlessly reattuning is to give one another a Spinal Flush.

THE SPINAL FLUSH

The Spinal Flush is a brief massage along the spine, a kind act you can do for your partner even before you are *feeling* kind or able to say kind things. It is a gift you can give to one another as an act of good faith. First, it is easy to give and feels great to receive. Second, it releases toxins that are generated by the fight/flight/freeze response back into the lymph system, where they can be eliminated. Third, it brings balance to each of the major meridians, the body's energy pathways. Deep, caring touch is good for your partner's health and mood, as well as your own. In fact, University of Miami psychologist Tiffany Field reports that receiving fifteen minutes of massage each day from their husbands was as beneficial for women suffering from postpartum depression as receiving antidepressant medication.[6] By focusing on your back instead of the more emotionally vulnerable front of your body, you are more able to receive a caring gesture even while still closed off or feeling defensive. To do the Spinal Flush:

- Have your partner lie facedown or stand three to four feet from a wall and lean into it with both hands. Either position stabilizes your partner's body so pressure can be applied along the spine. When David sees Donna starting to flood, his code phrase for initiating a Spinal Flush is "Up against the wall, Donna."
- Massage the points down both sides of your partner's spine (but not directly on the spine), using the thumbs or middle fingers and using your body weight so strong pressure is being applied. While most people can tolerate and will enjoy considerable pressure on these points, check to be sure you are not using more than your partner wishes. If your partner has any kind of back injury or vulnerability, be particularly diligent about checking in, though deep pressure along the sides of the spine will still usually be safe and beneficial. You will be massaging from the bottom of the neck all the way down to the bottom of the sacrum.
- Go down the notches along the vertebrae and deeply massage each point. Staying on each point for at least five seconds, move the skin to and fro or in a circular motion with strong pressure.
- You can stop when you reach the sacrum or repeat the downward flush once or twice more.
- When completed, "sweep" the energies down your partner's body: With either one long swipe or several brushstrokes, use the palms of your hands to sweep the energy from the shoulders all the way down the legs and off the feet. Repeat the sweep two or three times.

→ THE ENERGY DIMENSION ←

The Spinal Flush

The toxic energy of distress gets clogged along the spine, interfering with the function of major nerves and energy pathways. As the fingers press on these points, the clogged energy becomes dispersed into the lymphatic system, which empties it out of the body.

Giving the Spinal Flush When You Are Angry

Interestingly, if the partner giving the Spinal Flush is angry, as may occur after an argument, the anger does not get absorbed by the person receiving the Spinal Flush. While angry energy certainly can be transmitted through touch, the anger gets dissipated rather than transferred during a Spinal Flush.

THE DESIRED STATE

When you are arguing with your partner, "flooding" is a physiological state in which you are feeling overwhelmed by your own and your partner's negative emotions while you focus on an issue.[7] Any relationship has many such moments. During flooding, people are likely to become defensive, pursue conflict, and at the same time wish to get away. This is *not* the desired state, but each time it occurs provides an opportunity for emotional reconnection. Stations on the path to reconnection include self-soothing, soothing one another, and attuning to one another's feelings. The underlying tone of your relationship becomes a bit more positive with each successful reconnection, and a bit more negative each time a flooding incident does not lead to reconnection. At this point, your Pact has given you tools from energy medicine for self-soothing and for connecting energetically with your partner. If you or your partner are still feeling flooded, go back to the exercises. If you are both feeling calm, though perhaps still pessimistic about resolving the issue, you can proceed.

Attuning Emotionally

Stopping when you are flooded, centering yourself, and energetically reattuning with your partner is like pressing the reset button on your interaction. What you do next is critical. If you just pick up where you left off, you are likely to find that one of you, and then both of you, may soon be feeling flooded again. But in centering and reconnecting energetically, you have primed yourself for a shift.

SHIFTING YOUR FOCUS

Rather than focusing on your side of the disagreement, or all the reasons you are right and your partner is wrong, or all the ways you have been unfairly perceived or dismissed, this is a moment where the most constructive choice available to you is to attune to your partner's feelings. It is not that you discount or disregard your own reality, but rather that you establish an ability to hold both perspectives at once. You don't need to make yourself wrong to attune to your partner, but attunement shifts your attention. It puts you on a path that veers away from flooding or blaming and toward repairing the bond.

At times, our Energetic Stress Style tends to seize control, distorting our perceptions as reliably as the blind man who is able to perceive only one part of the elephant. While all couples fight and a relationship can weather many arguments that go unresolved, Gottman's research shows that a couple is headed for divorce when criticism, defensiveness, contempt, and stonewalling escalate over time.[8] Consistently responding to sadness or anger with criticism, dismissal, or contempt intensifies negativity and becomes cumulative. Attunement, on the other hand, enhances intimacy. Rather than abandoning your truth for your partner's, attunement means opening to your partner's experience, even vividly imagining how it feels to be him or her, and proceeding with compassionate awareness of your own as well as your partner's position.

Your Pact has had you (1) force an interruption in an escalating argument, (2) center yourself using energy techniques, and (3) do a Spinal Flush or other energy exercise that is soothing for your partner and begins to energetically reestablish your connection. In the next crucial step, you will proceed into a deeper, heartfelt awareness of your partner's emotional state.

PUTTING YOUR PARTNER'S THOUGHTS AND FEELINGS INTO WORDS

Place your hands over your Heart Chakra (the middle of your chest). Breathing deeply, center your awareness in your heart. Visualize your partner as a child: young, fresh, innocent, undamaged. Absorb this for a few moments. Next bring your attention back to the argument. Breathing deeply and "seeing" through your heart, see that pure version of your partner, even during the argument. Attuned to your partner in this way, mindfully step into his or her shoes. Experience the argument as if you were your partner.

Inevitably your own opinions, anger, or hurt will intrude into the scene. Do not try to stop them or judge them. Instead, bring your focus to your hands over the center of your chest and observe your own feelings from this heart-centered space. Thoughts and feelings may pass or simply dissolve as you meet them with curiosity and acceptance. If they do not dissipate, or if they intensify, rather than dwelling on them further, use the Blow-Out/Zip-Up/Hook-Up exercise (pp. 86–88) to dispel their energies.

When the feelings have passed, return to the image of your partner and to imagining the argument through your partner's eyes and heart. Sense your partner's likely feelings, thoughts, and hopes during the interaction. Write your insights in a paragraph or two in first-person present tense, describing the experience as if you are your partner. You will be able to verify the accuracy of your account in the final part of the Pact.

Part 4 of the STA<u>R</u> Pact: Resolve

It is now time to return to the original issue and *resolve* it. Teaching active listening, much to the dismay of many conventionally trained couples therapists, has been found to be relatively ineffective in improving marital satisfaction or stability.[9] While active listening is great in theory, it is difficult to be constructive listeners when the hostility, anger, and defensiveness of flooding have been evoked. On the other hand, shifting to an activity that changes your energies can be done in a mechanical manner and still be effective.

You are about to enter Part 4 of your Pact, the phase of effective communication—reengaging and *resolving* the issue that propelled you into flooding, disconnection, and discouragement. You have already centered yourself, reconnected energetically, inwardly attuned yourself to your partner's feelings and position, and written your insights. Now you are at the phase where the rubber meets the road. Decide who will read first. Before you begin, simultaneously and in unison do one more brief centering technique. David's favorite is the Crossover Shoulder Pull. Donna is most likely to use the Wayne Cook Posture. If your preferences are also different from one another's, use both. A favorite for both of us is simple hands–over–heart breathing.

Sharing Your Empathic Statement

Read the piece you wrote at the end of Part 3 of the Pact. Your partner listens and receives your attempt to tune into his or her experience. Your Pact is still providing the structure of an invisible surrogate "couples coach."

Responding with Appreciation

Once you have read your account of your partner's side of the story, your partner is to respond with three sentences that begin with the words "I appreciate . . ." Knowing this assignment is coming up will help your partner scan for your genuine effort, accurate insights, and enhanced empathy. The appreciations can be simple and basic: "I appreciate that you know how hard I tried." "I appreciate that you are wanting to understand me." "I appreciate that you understand that I didn't mean to overreact."

This does not mean your partner is saying that every statement you uttered was on target; only that your partner acknowledges and appreciates your efforts. You will also be receiving feedback about how accurate your statements were according to your partner's experience. Sometimes the statement being read will totally miss the mark. Appreciations can still focus on the partner's intentions in writing and sharing the piece. After each appreciation statement, respond with an active acknowledgment: a "thank you," a smile, or a request, such as "Help me understand that better."

Further Inquiry

Next you ask, "Is there anything else you would like me to understand about your experience regarding our disagreement?" If your partner feels fully understood, this round is completed and it is your turn to hear your partner's statement. More likely, however, your partner will have at least one area to expand on or correct. Your partner selects only one at this point, so the response is one or two sentences describing or clarifying *one* aspect of the situation, such as: "I wasn't angry that you were busy; I was angry that when I asked you to help me, you looked disgusted." Or, "My feelings got hurt at the party when you were bragging about our garden and didn't mention how much work I put into it." Or, "I felt discounted when you still punished Susie [their seven-year-old daughter] after I'd explained why I thought we should let her off the hook this time." The statements should be brief and descriptive of what happened rather than any interpretation of the meaning of the events except to state how they impacted the speaker. Use "I statements" about your feelings, thoughts, and reactions.

Bringing in the "*Do You Mean*" Technique

Your partner has just expanded on or corrected your write-up. This may be a perfect time to use the "*Do you mean*" technique (p. 51). Drawing from the earlier example, suppose your partner's comment was:

> "I felt discounted when you still punished Susie after I'd explained why I thought we should let her off the hook this time. You always discount me!"

Looking for where to focus, "You always discount me!" provides much that is worth exploring. So you might put this into the "*Do you mean*" format. For instance:

> "Do you mean that I ignored what you were saying?"
> "Yes."
> "Do you mean by saying I *always* discount you, that I never take in what you are saying?"
> "No."
> "Do you mean by saying *always* that you feel discounted a lot of the time?"

"Yes!"

"Do you mean that you don't trust me?"

"There may be some truth in that, but that is not what I am saying."

"Do you mean that I run my agenda while ignoring yours and that it is because I'm insensitive and selfish?"

"The first half of that is what I mean, so you now have two and a half yeses."

"Do you mean you want to leave me?"

"No."

"Do you mean that you want me to be influenced more by what you say?"

"Bingo!"

Even the four-word sentence "You always discount me" can have multiple meanings. It could easily be misinterpreted. After achieving three yeses, summarize what was just established to the extent that you can acknowledge your partner's initial meaning or feeling and check for accuracy:

"So you felt I ignored what you said—it reminded you of other times you have felt ignored—and you stated this so strongly because you don't want that to keep happening. Given that, I can understand why you were feeling discounted. Did I getcha?"

If the response was, "Not completely. I thought we should have let Susie off the hook this time," your *Do you mean* questions could try to capture your partner's meaning about the entire statement or any aspect of it. For instance:

"Do you mean I should always just obey you?"

"No."

"Do you mean Susie is such an angel that we should never punish her?"

"No."

"Do you mean you felt I was too harsh?"

"Yes."

"Do you mean Susie didn't deserve to be punished this time?"

"Yes."

"Do you mean that you are smarter than me?"

"While I do believe that is true, it's not what I am saying."

> ## → THE ENERGY DIMENSION ←
>
> ### Missing a "Do You Mean"
>
> What happens energetically when your partner's "Do you mean" statement is dead wrong? It was not what you meant at all. Does this cause the energies between the two of you to repel further? It usually doesn't. In fact, the bond that had been broken tends to repair whether the partner's response is right or wrong. The energy reconnects. The fact that the partner was curious and trying to understand energetically trumps the fact that the guess was wrong.

"Do you mean that you are oversensitive about not being taken seriously?"

"NO!"

"Do you mean that you were hurt that I didn't give your opinion more weight?"

"Yes."

"I can understand how my punishing Susie after you explained why you felt we should let this one go would leave you feeling discounted. Now do you feel fully understood?"

"Yes. Thank you for making the effort!"

Accepting the Outcome

Often the discordant feelings will have dissolved or the disagreement will have been settled before you even get to the first "Do you mean" in Part 4 of the Pact. But sometimes the outcome is simply, "We agree to disagree." In fact, one of John Gottman's most unexpected findings was that, more than two-thirds of the time, couple conflict was about "perpetual issues in the relationship that never got resolved."[10] If you come to fundamental differences in your characters, values, or beliefs that you cannot settle, you may wonder what you are doing on the same train. All couples, however, have issues they have been unable to resolve.

Many couples "make peace" with such perpetual problems by going into denial about them. But if deep problems become permanently buried in the foundation of your relationship, your footing with one another becomes unsure. Or, in the other direction, unremitting complaints and nagging build barriers and ill will without doing anything to constructively resolve the issue. The solution that happy couples reached around their irreconcilable differences "was to establish a 'dialogue' around the perpetual problem—one that included humor and affection and communicated acceptance of the partner and even amusement. In this way happy couples coped with the irresolvable problems rather than to get trapped in 'gridlock.'"[11] Your pact helps you accomplish this.

Whether guiding you through the inevitable bumps of building a life together or helping you establish a constructive dialogue around irresolvable issues, your Pact calls to the best in each of you. If the issue is resolved, you can happily celebrate your accomplishment. If, on the other hand, a problem persists after you have submitted it to the rigors of your Pact, you can recognize that you have come into territory all couples encounter. You will know you have done all you can, at least for the time being. In Part 2, you will learn an approach from energy psychology for getting at the heart of and transforming some "perpetual" problems, but for now, you will have brought your goodwill, caring, and most effective communication skills for coming to terms with a stubborn difference in a loving and mutually supportive way.

Making the Pact a Reality

If nothing else, shifting a disagreement from automated but unproductive knee-jerk reactions to the relatively laborious steps in the Pact is an affirmation to yourself and your partner that your relationship and its well-being are at the top of your priorities.

Perhaps the hardest times for us to invoke the Pact were in premenstrual moments when, at least as David experienced it, there was no right response. Whatever he would do or say seemed to make matters worse. Every cell in his digital brain wanted to pull away, separate, take time apart. This is similar to the "Stop" phase of the Pact, but it isn't quite on the mark because when done abruptly or with anger, it breaks emotional contact in a manner that feels like punishment or abandonment. It doesn't feel like an affirmation of the agreed-upon steps in the Pact. David learned, however, that he could bridge his impulse to withdraw into a constructive scenario by saying something like: "Donna, we're both upset right now and having a hard time. Let's follow our Pact, take a few minutes apart, get ourselves centered, and then how about I give you a Spinal Flush." That extra step was the kingpin to success. Sometimes all was well following the spinal flush. Other times, the remainder of the Pact was still needed.

A Commitment

Giving your Pact the power of a contract is not an idle choice. Before you *commit* to the Pact, try it. Experience the structured steps of *Stop*, *Tap*, *Attune*, and *Resolve* (*STAR*). Then evaluate. How well did this work for you? Did the experience give you hope? What did you learn for next time? Does it feel promising enough that you *want* to commit to making the Pact a part of your relationship? If you decide to do so, be prepared to deeply honor your commitment. When you make a promise to one another, particularly when it concerns the well-being of your relationship, keeping that promise affirms your partnership; breaking it erodes trust.

When you are acting in accordance with the Pact, you are diverted from the downward spiral of relationship conflict and are instead establishing new patterns. With your first success in using the Pact to transform a conflict into enhanced intimacy and understanding, you have created a prototype, a model of successful attunement during a challenging time. The principles of attunement you are developing for difficult moments will echo throughout your relationship, but you don't have to wait until you are devastated or furious to use them. The more you use them, the less frequently or urgently you will have to invoke your Pact.

It is not whether you argue or are triggered into flooding with one another that determines stability and satisfaction in a marriage, but how you repair the ruptures to your connection when they do occur. The resolution of each incident involving a breach in your bond has a cumulative impact on your sense of safety and on the way you view one another. It can increase your appreciation and add to your shared trust and bonding—or it can add to a backlog of hurt, negativity, and discouragement, and an escalating focus on what seems wrong with your partner and the relationship while minimizing what is right. Each time you invoke your Pact, you are affirming your intention, right then and there, to resolve this challenge in a manner that restores your connection and enhances your mutual understanding and affection.

A Weekly Meeting for Appreciation and Taking Stock

We have one more clause to add to your Pact. Relationships, like any other living entity, require care and feeding. Rather than waiting for encounters that lead to flooding to use the Pact, make it part of your Pact that you set aside an hour per week of protected, sacred time to reflect on (1) how you have enjoyed one another during the week, (2) how you have supported one another, and (3) any problems or resentments that may be brewing. Consider it a date with your surrogate "couples coach." Have your Pact ready in case you need it to work your way through problems that are identified. Doing this kind of preventive maintenance with your Pact at your side will, paradoxically, mean that you need to invoke your Pact less frequently.

In a Nutshell

While you may need to review the detailed instructions provided in this chapter a number of times before the Pact is internalized, here they are in outline form. As you use the Pact, you will no doubt see ways to adapt it to make it more appropriate to your own personal styles, but internalizing this basic structure is a powerful starting point. The Pact, stated as an agreement, is as follows:

1. **Stop!** When either of us is becoming upset or flooding during an interaction, we will interrupt the conversation and invoke the Pact.
2. **Tap.** We will each immediately do the Four Taps and draw on other energy medicine centering techniques presented in this chapter, or others we know to be effective, and use them. We will agree on a time that we will come back together for the next step.
3. **Attune.** Following these exercises, we will energetically attune with one another through a shared activity such as a "here and now" walk, a Spinal Flush, or other energy technique. We will then, from a heart-centered space, review the interaction that just occurred with a strong intention of understanding the other's emotions, experience, and position. This does not mean that we agree, but that we will step into the other's shoes with an attitude of curiosity and respect. We will each write this understanding in our partner's voice.
4. **Resolve.** We will share our written passages about each other's experience with a firm intention for heart-centered communication, taking opportunities to ar-

ticulate genuine appreciations along the way. We will continue the dialogue—using the *"Do you mean"* technique if necessary—until we reach agreement or respectfully agree to disagree.

Final Piece of the STAR Pact

We will dedicate at least an hour each week to creating protected, sacred time for appreciatively reflecting on our lives together that week.

On to Chapter 4

Your desire to maintain intimacy and a collaborative alliance with your partner is in itself a beautiful intention. It can be powerfully supported by understanding your own and your partner's Energetic Stress Styles (chapter 1), effective strategies for working with your own style and your partner's style (chapter 2), and the Pact (this chapter). Next, we shift our focus to the brain chemistry of love, the stages of love, and the yin and yang energies that shape a relationship.

4

Different Brains—Different Energies

Structures, Stages, and Styles of Love and Romance

Romantic passion harmonizes with myriad other feelings, drives, and thoughts to create different melodies in different keys.

—HELEN FISHER[1]

ONE OF THE LIABILITIES FOR DAVID OF BEING MARRIED TO A PARTNER WHO SEES energy is that when we would go to a conference or anywhere else where new people entered our worlds, Donna knew if David was attracted to someone before he even had a chance to process the experience, sometimes before he fully recognized what he was feeling, digital that he is. "It's in your Root Chakra, dear, and it comes straight up to your Heart Chakra and out to her. Your energies and her energies were doing a dance right there during the group lunch for anyone to see." David, usually quite discreet and private about such matters, quickly learned in the early days of our relationship that there was no place to hide. Donna, accustomed to seeing a million energies dancing among people, did not take it personally, did not view it as a threat, and did not interpret it as anything other than simply the way a healthy, young heterosexual male's energies connect, merge, and begin to interact with an attractive female's energies. She was not above teasing David about what she saw, but she held him accountable only for what he did with such energies and the feelings they evoked—not for the fact that they existed.

David's energetic response to attractive women was just as inborn as the Energetic Stress Styles discussed in the previous three chapters. This final chapter of Part 1, "The Inherited Aspects of Love," examines several additional qualities of love and romance that seem built into human nature. It begins by exploring (1) the neurological underpinnings of love, lust, and romance, (2) the stages by which love seems to evolve, and (3) the way that differences in male and female brains and energies impact relationships.

When we were in college, the word *love* was not even in the index of most psychology textbooks. Biologists and social scientists have since discovered a great deal about love's mysteries. We will present pertinent highlights from what has been scientifically established interwoven with our energy perspective. The chapter then sets aside Western science and delves into the energetic forces, described in ancient healing traditions, which operate within each individual and are at the foundation of every relationship. You are familiar with terms like *yin* and *yang*, but you may not know that each has five "flavors" or that the interaction of these forces within you and between you and your partner invisibly shapes the way you treat one another.

This is a chapter of maps more than techniques. Learning about the inherent forces at play when you are in a particular stage of romance or when your partner's yang seems to be trumping your yin helps you navigate your way through the high adventure called love with greater insight about yourself and empathy for your partner.

The Brain Structures of Love, Lust, and Romance

Your brain is designed to work in tandem with your energies. When David was attracted to someone—when his Root Chakra's energies involuntarily rushed up to his Heart Chakra and surged out of his body like a heat-seeking missile speeding toward a near-stranger—his brain initiated a series of pre-programmed sequences as well. The urge to mate is a powerful drive for species survival, and nature designed your energy system and your brain to work in sync to be on the ready, with or without your volition.

Helen Fisher, an anthropologist at Rutgers University who has studied the dating profiles of tens of thousands of people across cultures and has also conducted brain imaging research on couples in various stages of relationship, has identified three potent, independent, but interacting *behavioral systems* that govern love. A behavioral system grows out of *separate brain structures* that *work together* in harmony to *produce specific behaviors*. Different parts of the brain team up to motivate you to do nature's bidding. By coordinating neural pathways, hormones, and neurotransmitters, behavioral systems regulate:

* *Lust*—the craving for sex and the drive to pursue it
* *Romance*—the rapture, pining, and obsession for one special person
* *Deep/Enduring Love*—a calmer, more secure lasting union with a partner

Lust

Lust serves our deep design to find a partner by keeping us "on the prowl." Sexual urges pique an interest in mingling with potential partners and cause people to consider many more possibilities than they could ever consummate. Lust in men is directly related to testosterone levels, while in women it is a mix of estrogen, progesterone, and testosterone. Men produce far more testosterone than women, but women are much more sensitive to its effects. Meanwhile, oxytocin promotes the desire to bond in men as well as in women.

Men and women differ, however, in the conditions that will *stimulate* the chemistry of lust. Men tend to be turned on by visual stimuli, fantasies of beautiful bodies, novelty, and scenarios that involve conquest. A woman's desire and sexual interest are aroused more by romantic words, images, and themes, by affection, and by fantasies that involve active surrender, though Fisher also points out that this does not mean coercion. In a survey of 3,432 American men and women between ages eighteen and fifty-nine, less than half of 1 percent of men reported enjoying forcing a woman into sex, and less than half of 1 percent of women wanted to be coerced into sex.[2] In addition, humans can override or redirect their sexual impulses, regardless of the levels of sex hormones surging through their veins. But once the brain system for *romance* is fully engaged, it is virtually impossible to ignore.

Romance

Romance keeps you focused on one person instead of many potential partners, allowing you to begin to build a relationship. Whatever your selection process in coming to prefer this individual above all others—whether wise or foolish, instant or gradual, impulsive or considered—you are wired to pursue the relationship with extraordinary intensity. Nature pulls out all the stops and laser-focuses your energies. Your bloodstream is injected with a cocktail of powerful chemicals—including the stimulant norepinephrine, the mood elevator phenethylamine, and the motivation enhancer dopamine—whenever you see, smell, hear, or even think about this object of your desire. Your fixation is fueled by powerful feelings such as elation and hope. Potent motivational centers below the limbic and cortical regions of the brain are engaged while parts of the prefrontal cortex shut down, making you less capable of logical decisions. The same systems responsible for the rush of cocaine are, in fact,

---

✦ THE ENERGY DIMENSION ✦

Lust vs. Romance

How is a person in lust energetically different from a person in romance?

In lust, the person's energy moves outward, focusing itself on the desired one. This energy is a strong force coming out from the eyes and face (even when the person is trying to act demure) and, at the pelvis, from the Root Chakra. When the person begins to maneuver or strategize, the energy comes out from the Third Chakra (solar plexus). This energy of the Third Chakra—which governs power and pursuit—seems "loud." Donna can almost "hear it." Lust activates the Root Chakra, the Third Chakra, and the *Penetrating Flow*, one of the body's radiant circuits. The Penetrating Flow is an intense, insistent force that penetrates deeply into our primal energies and moves them out into the world.

In romance, the energy is very different. It originates in the Heart Chakra in swirls and spirals and figure eights, with all these patterns merging in a unique harmony. It is a higher, uplifting vibration. The energies of each partner seem to surrender to one another in a swooning sort of manner, weaving their way through the person's entire energy system and tapping into the other person's aura. Romance drops you into the deepest layers of the radiant circuits, which are the energies of joy, passion, thrill, excitement, and awe. These energies exist only in the present moment but are accompanied by a shift in the sense of time, "for in a minute there are many days" (Shakespeare's Juliet lamenting Romeo's imminent departure).

activated. Marion Solomon and Stan Tatkin explain that in this state the brain "produces a wonderful sense of timelessness and euphoria that involves little thought but intense emotion. Millions of neural networks are activated and the brain centers that mediate emotions, sexuality, and the self begin to expand and reorganize."[3]

The brain regions that regulate obsession are also involved in romance.[4] When these brain areas are low in the neurotransmitter serotonin, the mind begins to obsess. And indeed, in the early stages of romance, serotonin levels drop, causing you to obsess about your beloved, about how happy this person—and *only* this person—makes you, and about what you can do to please or impress or attract this enchanter of your soul. Fisher likens it to "someone camping in your head," and obsession is indeed one of the hallmarks of romance. Beyond all of that, the brain region involved in mystical experiences is activated so that a sense of a love that is larger than life is invoked. Nature mobilizes every biological and energetic resource available to get you to give your all to the task of establishing a relationship with this new potential mate.

Deep/Enduring Love

The neural networks involved in a deep/enduring love are designed to keep you in your relationship long enough to raise your children (nature's evolutionary imperative) and ideally to grow old together (nature's retirement gift for you). Over time, love becomes deeper and more serene. "No longer do couples talk all day or dance till dawn," observes Fisher. "The mad passion, the ecstasy, the longing, the obsessive thinking, the heightened energy: all dissolve. But if you are fortunate, this magic transforms."[5] And another kind of magic emerges. Deep feelings of calm, security, and connection are fulfilling joys for your soul. A third neural system has become activated. The prefrontal cortex, the most rational part of your brain, is now in full gear, weighing your thoughts and feelings and modulating your basic drives. Meanwhile, two closely related hormones, vasopressin and oxytocin, which are produced primarily in the hypothalamus and the gonads, keep chemistry-driven passion active even in the calmer delights of a deep and lasting union.

Experiments with prairie voles illustrate the role of vasopressin in males.[6] Prairie voles stay bonded with a single partner for life. But when researchers blocked the production of vasopressin in male prairie voles, the bond with their partner deteriorated immediately. The male lost his devotion to his mate, failed to protect her from new suitors, and would copulate and then abandon her for the next mating opportunity. Louann Brizendine, a neuropsychiatrist at the University of California–San Francisco, describes vasopressin as "the hormone of gallantry and monogamy, aggressively protecting and defending turf, mate, and children."[7] While we like to think that there is some evolutionary distance between male voles and male humans,

---

→ THE ENERGY DIMENSION ←

The Physics of Human Bonding

One of the strangest findings from quantum physics is that if two subatomic particles interact and are then separated, what happens to one of them after they have been parted influences the other. For instance, if the rotational spin of one of the particles is changed from clockwise to counterclockwise, the other particle's spin will instantly change as well. Physicists refer to this mutual influence as "entanglement"; Einstein called it "spooky action at a distance." Once believed to operate only with subatomic particles, such entanglement has been shown to occur with humans as well.

"Spooky Action" between People

For instance, in an experiment conducted by Amit Goswami and then independently replicated, two people were taught a meditative exercise where they were instructed to establish a direct communication so they would be able to feel one another at a distance. When they were separated, one was exposed to a strobe light, which evoked a specific EEG pattern in the brain. At that instant, an identical pattern was evoked in the brain of the other person. Imagine what happens after years of intimate communications!

The Energy of "Spooky Action"

As partners develop an enduring relationship, not only do they begin to complete one another's sentences, this entanglement looks to Donna like the partners are complementing one another energetically. They become energetically linked and harmonized, with unbroken figure-eight patterns weaving their energy fields together.

---

human sexual practices are influenced by vasopressin as well. The gene for vasopressin comes in two versions, and men who have the longer version of the gene are more likely to be monogamous. As Brizendine notes, "when it comes to fidelity, the joke among female scientists is that 'longer *is* better.'"[8] Oxytocin is also involved in deep feelings of attachment for men as well as women. At the most primal level, it stimulates bonding between a mother and her infant, but it builds magnetism between adults as well. At the moment of orgasm, both oxytocin and vasopressin levels increase dramatically. Nature makes a bid for sexual enjoyment to transmute into deep bonding from the get-go.

In fact, while the brain systems for lust, romance, and deep/enduring love are distinct from one another, they may be stimulated in any order and one may activate another. People who have been close friends for many years, deeply attached but romantically uninvolved, may one day fall in love and only then become sexually interested in one another. Lust often accompanies romance, but the romance circuits may light up in new acquaintances before sexual desire is kindled. Different circuits can also, inconveniently, become simultaneously involved with different people. As Fisher points out: "You can feel profound attachment for a long-term spouse, *while* you feel romantic passion for someone in the office or your social circle, *while* you feel the sex drive as you read a book, watch a movie, or do something else unrelated to either partner."[9] But, as she also observes, "as romantic love matures, it often expands into hundreds of complex and fulfilling feelings of attachment that produce an enormously intricate, interesting, and emotionally rewarding union with another living soul."[10]

The Stages of Love

O, how this spring of love resembleth
The uncertain glory of an April day,
Which now shows all the beauty of the sun,
And by and by a cloud takes all away.

—WILLIAM SHAKESPEARE[11]

The neural networks for lust, romance, and deep/enduring love express themselves in three basic stages of love:

- **The first stage** centers on the exhilarating processes of falling in love and beginning to build a partnership. It is dominated by the brain systems for *lust* and for *romance.*
- **The second stage** is the challenging path from the first stage to the third stage. Strewn with hazards and triggers that bring out your worst behavior and your meanest or most pathetic ruminations, it doesn't seem to have a brain system involved at all. At least it may feel that way as you and your partner are moving through it.
- **The third stage** reflects the achievement of a rich, fulfilling, lasting partnership. It is dominated by the brain system for *deep/enduring love.*

Such stages are, of course, generalizations. Not every love relationship passes through all three stages or passes through them in this order. In fact, in cultures where arranged marriages are commonplace—including parts of Asia, Africa, and the Middle East—a different sequence is typical. "Love starts hot in the West and cools down," goes the saying, "but it starts cool in the East and heats up." This is promising news for couples who have lost or never had great passion. Still, understanding the stages that typically unfold for those of us in cultures that hold romance as an ideal can provide a useful map for a volatile landscape.

Stage 1: The First Breaths of Love—Romance!

In fabled tales of new love, you see passion, determination, high spirits, sparkle, idealizing, obsession, loyalty, possessiveness, gratitude, courage, hope, and joy. Romance and lust energize one another. The chemicals of romance (dopamine and norepinephrine) trigger production of the chemicals of lust (such as estrogen and testosterone), but the chemicals of lust also trigger the chemicals of romance. You may spend hours every day thinking and pining about your new love, with imaginings that are rich with passion, creative vision, and poetic expression. Fisher describes how "the brain network for romantic love melds with many more brain systems . . . as well as with many emotions, memories, and thoughts. All these ingredients add fantastic depth, nuance, and spice to our feelings of romance."[12]

On the inside, you are powerfully focused on this new being who has entered your psyche like a wild horse running free. But something else is happening as well.

The boundaries that restrain your spirit seem to fall away. You know yourself as a larger force, feel more joy, and sense—perhaps more fully than ever before—how profoundly connected you are not just to your partner but to every human who has ever lived and loved and even to the cosmos. You love being in this loving space, but even more important, you feel complete.

Stage 2: Disappointment and Reckoning

Being seen through the eyes of a treasured someone who perceives your true, beautiful nature is among the sweetest and most uplifting pleasures a person can enjoy. However, the higher the pedestal, the greater the drop. The more powerful the merging, the more challenging to find your way back to yourself as a complete and separate individual. In Stage 1, a glimpse of possibility fueled by deep longings propelled you into a sense of glorious fulfillment. But its foundations were weak, its staying power limited. Stage 2 is nature's way of forcing you to come to terms with the illusion, to reclaim your deeper self, and to evolve. It accomplishes this in part through an insidious perceptual shift, changing the lens through which you view your partner—from rosy to dark. Disorienting though this can be, Stage 2 seems, for many couples, a necessary passageway to a Stage 3 where two people build a relationship that transcends each of them yet embraces both in their weaknesses as well as their strengths. It is most often not an easy passage.

When your beloved's focus shifts to mere behavior, personality, and the tasks of

Stage 2: Disappointment and Reckoning

How do your energies look when you are in Stage 2? Your auric field and your partner's auric field tend to repel rather than to overlap. Your field spirals around you, alone, disconnected, and self-absorbed, unless you are actively engaged with one another, as in a fight. In calmer times, when you are together, your energies are no longer joyful or expansive. They look somewhat wilted as they weave around you, sometimes seeming rigid or retreating from the energies of the other in fear or anger.

daily life, the magic fades, the shine tarnishes, and disappointments and resentments grow. This is the stage where the person who seemed so stable is now simply boring. The one who was wildly exciting is now erratic and volatile. The one who was so romantic and persistent is now intrusive and smothering. Compared to the shiny promise of Stage 1 you may have shared, the letdown can be heartbreaking. Yet compare you do, and the realities of the reckoning stage are depressing. The psychic boundaries that had fallen away—giving you each vastly expanded appreciation, apprehension, and a deepened, perhaps spiritual connection with all of life—have somehow sprung back into place. An independent brain system turns out to be involved after all, the biochemistry of fight/flight/freeze and the "diffuse physiological arousal" that precedes it.[13] Your emotional centers are on the ready for evidence that the relationship your biochemistry is wired to find—and that your soul has been investing itself in—is failing. Even the most subtle signs of criticism or withdrawal can propel your primal sensory system into a threat response.

You were on a magical ride and you don't know why it stopped. The bond that thrilled your heart and sent your woes quietly into the background is rupturing. You find faults in your partner that you are sure are the reasons your relationship has become difficult. Where you had each magnified the other's virtues, you now minimize them and magnify the flaws. You also come face-to-face with your own vulnerabilities and shortcomings. Like a person who has had a spontaneous mystical experience, you long for the profound connection and the bliss that went with it. So you are willing to do everything you can think of to get it back. Through this effort you may break through to Stage 3 or you may, ultimately, wind up deciding it is hopeless and leave the relationship. Stage 2 impels you and your partner to reckon with difficult realities in one way or another. But all this is somehow surrounded by a lingering sense of possibility. Echoes of what you once shared together or long to share now call to you through the fog, beckoning that you try to find your way back to one another.

Stage 3: Deep and Flowing

Stage 1 is built on fantasies, and Stage 2 requires coming to terms with the distortions contained in those fantasies. Commenting on romance, George Bernard Shaw once quipped that love consists of overestimating the differences between one woman and all the others. Stage 3 is based on reality. It is built on shared experiences, honest appraisals, earned trust, acceptance, and jointly acquired skills for fostering your unique relationship. The energies in you and your beloved become fluid within that secure base, contained within you yet readily merging into the larger field that is your partnership. The adrenaline and dopamine that drove you with addictive power toward the goal of establishing a secure partnership has receded. The low serotonin that was causing you to obsess about your partner is back to its normal levels. Even without these biochemical propellants, the relationship moves forward on its own power. Meanwhile, oxytocin and vasopressin pepper your highest brain functions as you mold a partnership that has never before existed and will never exist again. When at their best, couples in Stage 3 find ways to keep restimulating the brain systems for lust and romance while building a soul-deep partnership, the topics of Part 3 (chapters 8–10).

As the two of you in tandem paint your unique journey together onto a life-size canvas, you are able to reach for not only the more mundane colors of daily existence but the magnificent shades of love that—in a stable, evolving partnership—manifest in ever-fresh ways. Lasting love is a shared achievement whose beauty reflects your souls. Less euphoric but more deeply gratifying, Stage 3 is the culmination of all that has gone before—the romance and the reckoning now integrated into a larger context that is even more fulfilling.

We are, of course, not suggesting that every love relationship passes through these stages in some neat order, or that couples don't move back and forth among them, or that when you are in one stage, elements of the other stages won't also be present. But at its core, the three-stage model does seem to represent an organic direction and design, with each stage having its own set of required tasks, neural networks, and energy configurations. No one in Stage 1, however, is particularly interested in understanding its ephemeral nature, so if you are in the heat of romance, just enjoy it and set this book aside until you need it. But if you are in the reckoning of Stage 2 or the challenges of maintaining a vital Stage 3, this book is for you.

Men's Brains/Women's Brains

We will explore yin and yang—the energies of the female and male principles—later in this chapter, but any discussion of heterosexual marriage would not be complete without having addressed the gender differences that are rooted in the brain and the hormones. Contemporary scientific understanding offers greater detail and nuance about brain physiology and chemistry than existing language allows when speaking of energies. Keep in mind, however, as you read the following that the body's energies are always operating in concert with the brain and hormones.

As shown earlier, we each have distinct brain systems for lust, romance, and love, and there is some neurological rhyme and reason to the way each unfolds. Another inherited set of traits that impacts the way you love and want to be loved is whether your brain has male or female wiring. Consider, for instance:

HER DIARY: I think Bob is planning to leave me. We got together tonight at a restaurant for dinner. I was a bit late and he seemed upset, but he made no comment about it. Conversation wasn't flowing, so I suggested we go somewhere more quiet so we could talk. He agreed, but he didn't say much. I asked him what was wrong. He said, "Nothing." I asked him if it was my fault that he was upset. He said he wasn't upset, that it had nothing to do with me, and not to worry about it. On the way home, I told him I loved him. He smiled slightly and kept driving. I can't explain his behavior. I don't know why he didn't say, "I love you too." When we got home, I felt as if I had lost him completely, as if he wanted to have nothing to do with me anymore. He just sat there quietly and watched TV. He continued to seem distant and absent. Finally, with silence all around us, I decided to go to bed. About fifteen minutes later, he came to bed. But I still felt he was distracted, that his thoughts were somewhere else. He fell asleep. I cried. I don't know what to do. I'm almost sure that his thoughts are with someone else. My life is a disaster.

HIS DIARY: Motorcycle won't start . . . can't figure out why.[14]

While men's brains and women's brains are far more similar than different—over 99 percent of the genetic coding is identical—where they are not the same, *vive la difference!* A boy, by the time he is seven months old, is able to tell when his mother is angry or afraid by the expressions on her face, and this will focus his attention.[15] By the time he is twelve months old, however, he has developed an "immunity" that allows him to *ignore* those expressions. For a girl, her mother's subtle look of fear will rivet her attention. Even within the womb, girls' brains are outpacing boys' in the development of brain circuits for communication, gut feelings, emotional memory, nurturing, and social nuance, while boys take the lead in circuits that will support rough-and-tumble muscle movements, exploration, and sexual pursuit.

Until eight weeks old, the fetal brain has the characteristics of a female brain. At the eighth week, if a Y chromosome is part of the genetic coding, testosterone begins to surge, developing more cells in the brain's aggression centers while killing off cells in the communication centers; if there is no Y chromosome, the communication centers develop unimpeded. This particular dichotomy in male-versus-female fetal development apparently holds true regardless of the individual's eventual sexual orientation.[16] We each occupy our own special place on the spectrum of having more yin (female) or more yang (male) energy, and there are great differences in degree from one person to the next, but some characteristics come with your gender.

The Relative Size of Brain Structures

The differences in male and female brain structures lead to different behaviors and different realities. Louann Brizendine explains common misunderstandings between women and men by comparing the female brain to the male brain:

What if the communication center is bigger in one brain than in the other? What if the emotional memory center is bigger in one than the other? What if one brain develops a greater ability to read cues in people than does the other? In this case, you would have a person whose reality dictated that communication, connection, emotional sensitivity, and responsiveness were the primary values. This person would prize these qualities above all others and be baffled by a person with a brain that didn't grasp the importance of these qualities.[17]

After birth, your brain structure continued to develop according to a genetically programmed plan. A girl's ability to maintain a mutual gaze will increase by more than 400 percent during her first three months of life, while a boy's does not increase at all. The parts of your brain that grew larger in relationship to other parts govern specific functions that are linked to your gender. Women have larger brain areas for language, hearing, feeling, observing emotion in others, and remembering the details of emotional events. This translates into abilities and behavior. Girls can, for instance, discern nuance in the human voice that boys simply cannot hear, which leads to great accuracy in reading another's emotions. Brizendine summarizes that the female brain is hardwired for "outstanding verbal agility, the ability to connect deeply in friendship, a nearly psychic capacity to read faces and tone of voice for emotions and states of mind, and the ability to defuse conflict."[18]

Men, meanwhile, are hardwired to prioritize problem solving and physically supporting and protecting their family. They have larger brain centers than women for muscular action, aggression, mate protection, and territorial defense. When a man's partner is in emotional distress, the areas in his brain devoted to problem solving light up. Another area that creates an emotional boundary between his experience and his partner's is activated, strengthening his ability to use his analytic and cognitive capacities to find a solution. He focuses on finding a way to fix things in situations where a woman would first be inclined to attune to her partner's emotions and foster interpersonal connection. Another important brain difference is that the hypothalamus, which regulates visceral responses, allots two and a half times as much real estate to sexual drive for men as it does for women. As a result, sexual thoughts enter a man's consciousness with considerably greater frequency.

Experience

In addition to the relative sizes of specific brain structures and the impact of hormones, experience further wires the brain. An adolescent girl's obsession with her sexual attractiveness is reinforced by powerful cultural messages and personal experience—relentlessly delivered by media, peers, and boyfriends. These encounters add to an expanding network of behavior-shaping pathways in her brain, while a boy's built-in propensity toward competition and protection is reinforced by messages that he must be strong; must hide his fears, pain, and softer emotions; and must meet challenges bravely and with confidence. As boys and girls carry out their culturally prescribed roles, neural pathways are formed that further support those roles.

Maturation

Brains change with age and experience, and in many ways for the better. A man's brain is transformed in a number of important ways as his mate's first pregnancy progresses. His testosterone levels decrease and his prolactin levels increase. Prolactin stimulates neural connections for paternal behavior while decreasing sex drive. The father's pheromones also "waft through the air and into the mother's nose and trigger her to make more prolactin [which] increases the growth of maternal brain circuits."[19] During the pregnancy, men often find themselves becoming obsessed with "nesting" behaviors—painting the baby's room, putting up shelves, fixing up the house.[20] They often gain weight right along with their pregnant wives. During the three weeks prior to the birth, their testosterone levels drop 33 percent and their prolactin levels increase 20 percent.

While these levels adjust back after the birth, dads who are actively involved in child-rearing keep lower testosterone levels than those who are not. When the infant cries, the same brain areas become activated in the dad as in the mom—areas for worry, threat detection, and gut feelings—and the baby's smile also activates reward centers in the father's brain. Then holding the infant releases hormones that dramatically increase the number of connections in the brain for paternal behavior, increasing *synchrony*, the easy nonverbal understanding between parent and child. Beyond parenting, as men move on to their later years, their focus tends to change from pursuits for their own personal gain to those that benefit their community and the coming generation.

As women move past menopause, the "surges and plunges of estrogen and progesterone" that are part of the menstrual cycle are replaced by a "constancy of the flow of impulses through her brain circuits. . . . The hair-trigger circuits in the amygdala that rapidly altered her reality" are no longer there.[21] She has stopped producing copious amounts of the hormones that had "boosted her communication circuits, emotion circuits, the drive to tend and care, and the urge to avoid conflict at all costs."[22] Nor is she getting the dopamine rushes or oxytocin rewards that had kept her focused on communicating the nuances of her emotions, keeping the peace, or taking care of others. Her brain circuits are less reactive to stress and less emotionally labile. Her interests shift from the needs and desires of those she loves to her own needs and desires.

Misunderstandings Rooted in the Brain

As with our Energetic Stress Styles, we tend to interpret our partner's behavior according to our own equipment, and this is a source of much ill-conceived, injurious judgment. For instance, women change their mind far more than men, and men become frustrated, disoriented, and judgmental about this propensity. Brizendine explains that because a woman's brain may change the way it functions up to 25 percent over the course of a month, her "neurological reality" will not be as constant as a man's. His reality "is like a mountain that is worn away imperceptibly over the millennia by glaciers, weather, and the deep tectonic movements of the earth. Hers is more like the weather itself—constantly changing and hard to predict."[23]

Men are often accused of being driven by the "brain below the belt." It in fact takes a man only a fraction of a second to "classify a woman as sexually hot—or not," and his genetic programming tends to be "driving him to seek sex and encouraging him to pursue a variety of partners."[24] This traces to his ancestors' evolutionary advantage for impregnating as many females as possible. While other brain structures mitigate this drive, many women vigilantly scrutinize their partner's behavior for any sign of attraction to another woman and interpret it as evidence of their own unattractiveness, of his having lost interest, or of his being a philanderer and a scoundrel. Providing a neurologically sophisticated take on the situation to a client who was upset that she caught Ryan, a man she was seriously dating, "checking out a girl with big boobs at the car wash," Brizendine explained to her:

> The lust center in the male brain automatically directs men to notice and visually take in the details of attractive females. When they see one that lights up their sexual circuit board, their brain instantly produces a quick sexual thought, but then it's usually over. To Ryan's mating brain, the buxom woman

was like a bright, colorful hummingbird. She flew into his line of vision, caught his attention for a few seconds, and then flew off and out of his mind. For many men, this can happen several times a day. Ryan couldn't have stopped his eyes from looking at her breasts even if he tried. But he could learn to be more discreet. Because this is an autopilot behavior for the male brain, men don't think it's a big deal, and they can't understand why women find it so threatening.[25]

Grasping the enormous differences in the workings of a man's brain and a woman's brain can help your relationship immensely. You can feel compassion for a partner you might otherwise feel like strangling. Understanding the inborn and cultural differences between the two of you can replace fierce judgments with empathy and appreciation. This kind of deep understanding can bring a balance to the two of you that can also radiate out to a world in dire need of greater understanding and balance between men and women.

His Hormones/Her Hormones

Your mood, your behavior, your energies, and, more than you may realize, the way you respond to your partner, are all profoundly yet invisibly influenced by your hormones. While hormones potently impact the lives of both men and women, they operate in contrasting ways for each. Estrogen, progesterone, and oxytocin build brain circuits that lead to characteristically female activity, while testosterone and vasopressin cause the brain to build circuits associated with male behavior. Beyond the impact of these and other hormones on brain development, their production influences day-to-day behavior. As estrogen floods the brain of a teenage girl, Brizendine explains, interest in communication and romance skyrockets and her "entire biological raison d'être is to become sexually desirable."[26]

Meanwhile, testosterone turns on different genes than estrogen. The genes it activates in a boy "trigger the urge to track and chase moving objects, hit targets, test his own strength, and play at fighting off enemies."[27] With increased concentrations of testosterone bathing the brain of a male adolescent, he grows less communicative and more competitive.

In his book *Venus on Fire, Mars on Ice: Hormonal Balance—The Key to Life, Love, and Energy*, John Gray opens by focusing on how stress is, biochemically, a totally different matter for men than for women, and that much of our behavior is in response to the stresses we face every day.[28] For instance, in a situation that is even moderately stressful, the emotional part of a woman's brain has eight times the blood flow of a man's. A woman's body copes with stress by utilizing oxytocin; a man's consumes testosterone. When oxytocin levels go up in women, their stress levels go down. When testosterone levels go up in men, their stress levels go down. Women also produce testosterone and men also produce oxytocin, but with different effects. Testosterone can feel good to a woman—it can be empowering and cause her to feel sexy—but it doesn't do a thing to lower her stress level. In fact, too much testosterone can increase her stress level. Oxytocin can feel good to a man—causing him to feel more generous and communicative—but it doesn't do a thing to lower his stress level. Too much oxytocin can, in fact, increase his stress level. Beyond their roles in managing stress, "fully feeling love, passion, and desire is directly linked to an abundance of testosterone in men and oxytocin in women."[29]

To be at his best, a man needs thirty times as much testosterone as a woman, and without it he loses his stamina and tends to become depressed and dejected. For a woman, with the shift in roles from homemaker to homemaker *and* co-breadwinner, her stress levels are twice those of a man when she is at work, and they become even more elevated as she attempts to care for the kids and manage the home with the limited time that remains. Nurturing activities produce oxytocin, but activities that involve urgency, problem solving, and sacrifice for a noble cause produce testosterone (up to the point that the situation is stressful enough to produce cortisol, which inhibits the production of testosterone). For most women today, activities on the job as well as at home produce testosterone rather than oxytocin, leaving them deprived, frustrated, and unhappy. To make it worse, finding the time to receive nurturing is often the last thing a woman will do when she is under unrelenting pressure. Gray summarizes the dilemma:

> Forty years ago or more, a woman had the time and the financial support to fill her day with an oxytocin-producing balance of nurturing and woman-to-woman support. Today's women enjoy the freedom of creating a career for themselves outside the home, but it has cost them the nurturing and support that rebuilds oxytocin and counteracts the testosterone they build up during a workday.[30]

Many of the activities our grandparents did routinely supported the biochemistry of love in ways our current lifestyles do not. Our lifestyles, rather, deplete the supplies of oxytocin in women and of testosterone in men, with serious costs to our ability to thrive as well as to bring out the best in our relationships. Other hormones such as estrogen, serotonin, dopamine, and cortisol, as well as blood sugar and blood flow, further confound our biochemical challenges.[31]

For instance, a woman's large supply of estrogen enhances the bonding effects of oxytocin, while a man's large supply of testosterone tends to inhibit oxytocin's bonding effects. In fact, many gender stereotypes reflect biochemistry. Women produce oxytocin when talking about a goal or a problem; men produce testosterone when achieving a goal or solving a problem. Women use up oxytocin when they are dealing with stress; men use up testosterone when encountering stress. Women restore the oxytocin they have consumed during a stressful day through quality relationships and pleasurable activities such as shopping or a pedicure or lunch with a girlfriend. Men restore the testosterone they have consumed by retreating within or chilling out watching a sports event on TV.[32] By understanding the cause-and-effect relationships involved, we can better bolster the chemistry of both romance and love.

Energy Techniques That Support Oxytocin and Testosterone Production

The eight energy techniques presented in chapter 3 (Crossover Shoulder Pull, Four Taps, Cross Crawl, Crown Pull, Stress Release Hold, Wayne Cook Posture, Connecting Heaven and Earth, and Blow-Out/Zip-Up/Hook-Up) can be done in the order listed here as a set that will bring balance to your energy system. Carried out as a daily practice, they will require only about six minutes once you are familiar with them, and they will begin to build positive energy habits into your body. This daily energy routine is the most effective simple procedure we know, not only for optimizing the flow of your energies to promote your health and mental clarity, but also for keeping your hormones in good balance. We recommend it highly.[33]

In addition to a daily routine, techniques are available that create an internal energetic landscape that stimulates or inhibits the production of specific hormones. For instance, when you are feeling distress, shifting your attention to taking five deep in-breaths and out-breaths has been shown to decrease the production of adrenaline and other stress hormones. Techniques that enhance oxytocin production and testosterone production follow. They can be done on a daily or as-needed basis.

Oxytocin Hearts

The *Bridge Flow* is a radiant circuit (see p. 278) that surrounds the heart and entire torso. One of its several functions is to energetically connect with other people, supporting harmony and receiving intuitive information. Because oxytocin is the hormone of loving connection, when you stimulate the Bridge Flow, you stimulate the production of oxytocin. This one-minute technique for stimulating the Bridge Flow simply has you tracing its natural path with your hands. Interestingly, the path of the Bridge Flow is shaped like a valentine heart.

Breathe in slowly and deeply as you draw your hands up from your pubic bone until you get to the center of your chest. Before you exhale, move your hands up and out toward your sides as if you were tracing a heart above and around your breasts. Slowly exhale as you bring your hands back toward your pubic bone, completing the tracing of a large heart over your torso. Repeat a few times. You are stimulating your Bridge Flow and triggering the production of oxytocin.

The Testosterone Cave Hold

Men renew their supply of testosterone when they retreat into their proverbial cave, becoming absorbed in a pleasurable solitary project, vegging out in front of the TV, or relaxing on an easy chair. Each is a way of reducing tension so that the testosterone consumed during stressful activities can be replaced. A quicker way to reduce tension and initiate the production of testosterone is to simply hold a set of reflex points that reduce stress and support testosterone production.

Place the heels of your hands on the bottom of your cheekbones, let your thumbs lie over your temples, and flatten your hands so your fingers fall easily over your hairline. Your eyes will want to close. Hold for at least five deep breaths. You are relaxing your entire energy system and stimulating the production of testosterone. End by pushing your fingers into your forehead and, with a deep inhalation, dragging them toward your temples.

Tending to Your Hormones Is
Also Tending to Your Energies

You can use energy techniques to directly stimulate the hormones of love and relationship, or you can take actions within your relationship that produce hormones that stimulate the energies that foster bonding. Some interactions rebuild the woman's supply of oxytocin and the man's supply of testosterone. This is good for each partner and good for the relationship. When oxytocin and testosterone supplies are restored, the energies of love are nourished.

If Mama Ain't Happy Ain't Nobody Happy

This time-honored observation has biological underpinnings. If the wife is chronically unhappy, the husband's deep impulse to keep her happy will be continually thwarted. If her stress levels are high, his stress levels will be high. While this challenging arrangement seems an inconvenient quirk of nature, on the good-news side, the steps he can take to increase her supply of oxytocin (read on) will at the same time increase his supply of testosterone.[34] It's a win–win after all!

You Can Keep Romance Alive over the Years

Romance is one of the most powerful ways to produce oxytocin. To keep Mama happy, keep romance alive. This, however, requires a different formula once Stage 1 is no longer producing the chemical cocktail that knocks you off your feet. For one thing, production of the "gotta have it" hormone, dopamine, is triggered by fresh discoveries, not by a familiar face. Whether you feel it is merciful to regain control of your brain or tragic to descend from the euphoric heights, Stage 1 does not last forever.

But because romance was once automatic, the expectation that it will always be effortless deflects us from finding new ways to feed the spirit of romance, and we then confuse the dimming of passion with the fading of love. We long for romance to visit us again or sadly accept our fate that its season has passed. Just as love matures over time, so does romance, but both require cultivation. For romance to continue to nourish us, Gray points out, we need to "find new ways of getting our feel-good hormones made."[35] Women and men have surprisingly stereotyped requirements, yet most have no idea of what they must do to keep romance alive.

Put the Man's Propensity for Problem Solving to Good Use

Particularly important on the man's side of maintaining romance is the act of planning special times together. Where taking her out on a date had once been part of the thrill of courtship, what back then was spontaneous now requires deliberate intention. Obstacles to supporting enduring romance include not knowing what to do, not having the time or energy to do it, or previous failures. If he is able to simply make a plan and put it into action, his testosterone levels go up, her oxytocin levels go up, and the embers of romance are fanned. Gray is very direct about this: "A man should think of this as a requirement of his husbandly job. . . . At work a man doesn't think twice about doing things he doesn't 'feel' like doing. He does them because it's necessary to get the job done. His reasoning goes, 'I don't want to do it, but if it's necessary, I'm happy to do it.' . . . If he wants to keep the passion and attraction alive, he must do certain things that have been proven to work, even if at first he doesn't feel like it."[36]

His Propensity to Fix Her Problems Is Born of Empathy

For men, repair and protection is not only part of their cultural role, it is part of their biology. Two separate empathy systems have been identified, and each uses different brain mechanisms. One is based on neurons that resonate with other people, resulting in one person feeling what another is feeling. This is what we usually think of as empathy. Another system, however, which is more dominant in men, is based on an area of the brain that recognizes and registers another person's feelings but immediately sends the information to the part of the brain that analyzes and fixes things, motivating him to correct any problem that has been discussed.[37] You've heard the plaintive song. She feels emotionally abandoned when he puts all his focus onto trying to fix the very problem she has just brought to his attention. She was hoping for nothing more than empathy about her dilemma and a chance to talk about it. She can learn that his scurrying into problem solving *is* his empathy in action. He can learn to recognize that the first "problem" needing his attention is her need for emotional contact.

Little Things Count

In the man's mind, the need for little acts of courtship—like bringing flowers and candy or planning a special date—are replaced by major acts like bringing home a good income or landscaping the yard. He figures that now that he is doing the big things, the little things don't matter anymore. But small gestures that would not be particularly meaningful to a man stimulate oxytocin in his partner, reduce her stress, and put a smile on her face. In terms of his hormones, a smile on her face caused by his actions is a powerful catalyst for his testosterone. After discussing all of this, Gray advises, "even if he's not in a romantic mood, if a man makes the effort to take action—a kiss, a squeeze—these small moves will raise his testosterone levels"[38] as well as increase her oxytocin.

Action Is Needed for Him to Cultivate Romance, but Attitude Is the Key for Her

Initiating romantic activities raises a woman's testosterone levels but not the oxytocin levels that would satisfy her romantic longings. So when she takes on the responsibility of trying to light the spark, she often winds up feeling disappointed and frustrated. Assuming both partners are in alignment with the desire to have a happier relationship, the most powerful actions available to her are sometimes simply to reinforce what he does right. Where a woman needs to receive ongoing messages that she is loved (and little things *do* count), a man needs to hear that he is being successful in his efforts to make her happy. Scanning for what he does that she appreciates and expressing that appreciation raises her oxytocin levels as well as his testosterone levels.[39] This also makes him more likely to do more of what she likes. Rather than focusing on what she is not getting, she can focus on the smallest things he does for her. Simplistic as it might sound—that he needs messages that he is being successful in the same way she needs messages that she is loved—this is a very practical insight: "A woman doesn't have to offer a standing ovation. She must simply appreciate the things he does."[40]

Combining Appreciations with Requests That Are Direct, Brief, and Positive

Expressing appreciation creates an atmosphere in which she can take steps to further ensure his success with her by making it clear what she wants. Men often have no idea. In this atmosphere, it is much more efficient to be transparent about what she is asking him to do than to leave him to guess. The strategy of using complaints or bringing up past hurts to justify asking for what she needs can be replaced with simple requests that are "direct, brief, and positive."[41] Combining appreciations with direct requests puts Mama back on the path to happiness.

The *Energy* of Male/Female Differences

The differences between men and women are not just in their brains, hormones, and sex organs. Each gender has its own energy. In traditional Chinese philosophy, the terms *yin* and *yang* are used to describe the qualities of feminine and masculine energy. Women are considered to be more yin; men more yang. But unlike fixed differences in the brain, yin and yang are dynamic energies that both flow within each of us in an active interplay that defines how we experience and relate to the world. Every relationship, straight or gay, is a dance not just between two people but between the yin and yang energies within one and the yin and yang energies within the other. Yin has been characterized by adjectives such as *slow, soft, yielding, cold, damp, contracting, sinking, internal,* and *passive.* It is associated with earth, moon, nighttime, and femininity. Yang, by contrast, is characterized by words such as *quick, hard, solid, hot, dry, dispersed, rising, external,* and *aggressive.* It is associated with sky, sun, daytime, and masculinity.

These two primal forces operate within all of us, and they explain some of the conflicts in our inner natures and in our partnerships. While yin (receptive, deep, mysterious) and yang (active, surface, evident) are seemingly contrary forces, they are interconnected and interdependent. Like night and day, they give rise to one another. Rather than mere opposites, they are complementary forces that compose a dynamic whole.

While aspects of one of these forces will be more developed in you, and the corresponding aspects less so, knowing that both are latent within you is a mind-expanding way of understanding your potential and your partner's potential. We are attracted to people who manifest qualities that are not as well developed in ourselves.[42] Not only does this expand our range of experience and provide balance in our lives, but the less-developed parts of ourselves resonate with our partner in ways that evoke the evolution of those parts.

For instance, David finds Donna to be wonderfully feminine. She is a girlie-girl who loves sentimental stories, romance, and fun clothes. Highly maternal, her caring and compassion can be disarming. She puts other people first, to a fault actually, and feels very deeply about them and about virtually everything that commands her attention. She loves receiving—people's stories, their pain, their gifts. When she is with a client, she goes inward and deep. Her yin energy is very strong.

When she is teaching or in front of a group or in a social situation, however, you might not realize that she can readily access such depths. The quality she is known

---

→ THE ENERGY DIMENSION ←

Yin in Action

When a person is in a yin state, the aura becomes soft, movement slows, and energy spirals easily into the body in a counterclockwise motion. Yin energies get you to "smell the roses." You are taking in the life around you. You are sitting on your porch, drinking tea, enjoying and appreciating the trees and view in front of you. You are relaxed, in deep reverie. In a relationship, you follow your partner's lead. You are a warm hearth for your partner to come to. You are open, inviting, and alluring.

Yang in Action

Yang energy moves out from the body, rather than into the body, spiraling out in a clockwise direction. Where yin energy is slow, yang energy is fast. If the person is particularly active, the energy shoots out rather than spirals out. Yang energy is animated, busy, making things happen. In a relationship, it makes the plans, provides the leadership, and runs the show. Sometimes it is so powerful a force that the partner retreats, becoming more inward and yin. When this occurs, the partners can become fixated and polarized in their respective yang-dominant and yin-receptive temperaments. As a relationship matures and becomes more vital, we usually see the yin and yang forces in each partner coming into better balance and the yin and yang forces between them finding greater harmony.

Yin Goes Yang; Yang Goes Yin

With age and the natural hormonal changes programmed into the human body, the energy in men becomes more yin and the energy in women becomes more yang.

---

for in these contexts is her effervescence—an exuding, sociable energy that reaches out and touches people. This expansive, emphatic energy is yang. Both her yin expressions and her yang expressions are completely authentic. People who first know Donna by being her client are often baffled by her exuberance when they see her teach; people who first know her from one of her classes wonder if it is the same person when she is working on them.

Poor David has to put up with all of this, not really knowing who he married or who will be there tonight. Fortunately—although he is emphatically yang in his intellect and professional risk taking—he is highly receptive to Donna's shifting energetic states, very yin in that regard. This works for both of us. Donna's flights into excitement and journeys into the depths expand David, whose customary range is more limited. All couples have areas where they balance and expand one another in these ways as well as areas where the yin-yang chemistry presents challenges. If you assess yourself, your partner, and your relationship through this yin-yang lens, it will become clear to you that no one is purely yang and no one is purely yin.

To muddle things further, the influence of testosterone on yin or yang energies is very different from the influence of estrogen or oxytocin. So Donna's yang qualities express themselves in a manner that is markedly different from the expression of yang qualities in David. David's yang onstage is focused and intent, in contrast to the force of Donna's yang exuberance. Their yin characteristics are similarly colored by their hormones. Testosterone is a yang hormone, so it "masculinizes" a man's yin energies. Estrogen and oxytocin are yin hormones, so they "feminize" a woman's yang energies. Thus as it is with all things human, even this yin-yang dichotomy does not play out in simple categories.

The Five Flavors of Yin and Yang

Yin and yang energies are the complementary aspects of your *life force*. Their polarities find expression in your feelings, thoughts, and actions, as well as in your health. Though they are polarities, they are related to one another as fundamentally as the front and back of your hand. One hand, two aspects (front and back); one life force, two aspects (yin and yang).

Carefully observing how illness and health manifest in different individuals, physicians in ancient China divided a person's life force first into yin and yang and then further divided each into five categories or types of vibration. Yin energies have five types of vibration and yang energies have five corresponding types (of course, within each type are infinite variations—just as no two voices are identical even though they can be put into categories such as bass, tenor, alto, and soprano). In brief, your yin energies are not identical to your partner's yin energies; nor are your yang energies just like your partner's. And these are not gender-related differences. Your life force, with its yin and yang aspects and the five unique vibrations of each, is different from the life force of anyone else.

The distinct vibration of your life force is reflected in the way you walk, talk, feel, think, and act. It is particularly evident in health and illness. For a person of one vibrational type, for instance, stomach is the organ that is most vulnerable to illness, while it may be liver for a person of another vibrational type.

Because a person's life force and its unique vibration are not generally visible to the human eye, metaphors are used to describe the types. The most well known of these are the *Five Elements*—water, wood, fire, earth, and metal—and the *Five Seasons*—winter, spring, summer, and fall, as well as the solstice/equinox (transition periods between seasons). The Chinese sometimes called these elements or seasons the *Five Walks of Life*.

Each Element has its own vibration or rhythm. Observable traits and behaviors are generated by a person's essential rhythm. You will find that the description of one of the Five Elements, or a combination of two or three of them, is instructive for understanding primal forces within yourself and your partner.

Exploring Your Element

While your Energetic Stress Style (visual, kinesthetic, tonal, digital) is activated in response to threat or distress, your Element is always active. To gain a more visceral understanding of the Five Elements:

1. As you read the following descriptions of each of the Five Elements, look for what resonates with what you know about yourself and with what you know about your partner.
2. Make a list for yourself and another for your partner.
3. Have your partner do the same.

> ➤ THE ENERGY DIMENSION ←
>
> **Your Element and Your Personality**
> You may think the following descriptions are personality types, but personality is just an outward manifestation. The traits described are, rather, expressions of your core energies. Your Element and its rhythm underlie your personality, but many other factors also form it. Your Element simply expresses itself according to one of five basic themes or a combination of themes.
>
> **The Seasons of Our Lives**
> The seasons were also used to illustrate the Five Elements, and your life moves through phases that correspond with the seasons. Your Element may, for instance, be metal, which corresponds with autumn. But you move through periods that are typified by the energies of winter, spring, summer, and autumn, in that order, as well as the transition periods of the solstice and the equinox. So even if your core energies correspond with autumn, you might be going through a season of your life that corresponds with summer. The interacting qualities of the rhythm of summer and the rhythm of autumn will be prominent in your thoughts, feelings, and actions during this phase of your life. This may seem complicated, but it brings order to your world when you understand it.

4. Compare lists only after you have each read the following and completed your own list.
5. Discuss where you agreed and where you disagreed.

Since two or more Elements may combine in a particular individual, it is likely that neither of you will fit neatly into any of the categories, but that you will find clusters of traits that describe the fundamental "rhythm" by which you each move through your world.

WATER ELEMENT: EMBRYONIC POSSIBILITY[43]

Water Element carries the rhythm of winter. It embodies the seed, the embryo, potential. The time of long nights and little light, winter holds the promise of the future. While life appears to have ceased, it is growing decisively under the ground, waiting to burst forth. Waters, when in their strength, embody a fresh spirit that is infused with childlike enthusiasm because their season is about beginnings. Rooted in nature's embryonic time, this Element has a babylike quality.

When Waters feel safe, they utterly trust their surroundings, and they laugh and play with an infant's spontaneity. They know how to envision a project and joyfully get it under way. Their energies may be limited since their season has little sun, but like a hibernating polar bear, they are able to retreat into themselves and regenerate. Winter marks not only the beginning of the solar cycle but also its end. For this reason, it is symbolized by both the baby and the wise old philosopher. Waters are not only spontaneous in their play but also deeply reflective about the meaning of life.

As with each of the rhythms, the Water's potential weaknesses are the polarity of these strengths. The playful energy of the infant or the all-consuming reflections of the philosopher are not so well suited for going the full distance of completion. Waters may have little motivation for the long haul. Just as special care and protection are required to survive in winter, people who move to winter's rhythm often need and demand special attention, so they are particularly vulnerable to narcissism. Waters may be unable to recognize how they are affecting others, focusing only on what others are doing to them. They can have difficulty feeling loved unless love is showered on them. Needing the mother's succor like the seed needs the unfailing sustenance of the earth, Waters who feel unloved tend to retreat within, becoming cold, isolated, fearful, or depressed. Your first cycle of winter's rhythm extends from conception through about eighteen months. But if stress or trauma or circumstances prevented you from sufficiently meeting the requirements of this phase or garnering its lessons, its issues can become fixated into a lifelong pattern where you behave out of the need to feel as if you are the center of the world. Your development can become arrested while moving through any of the rhythms.

The talk of a Water is a slow, flowing kind of groan from deep within. The walk is unhurried and paced, like a rolling wave, almost a swagger, knees slightly bent with the body lowered toward the ground. The characteristic mental state is the longing to feel safe. Under stress, this longing may become fear, which is the stress emotion of a Water. Because the future is hard to see from winter's embryonic shadows, Waters are often afraid to move forth, afraid to make a commitment. They reflect deeply, sometimes motivated by their fear of what is to come. In the wild, a newborn animal is utterly vulnerable and must quickly learn to distinguish between what is dangerous and what is safe. During your first eighteen months, your first cycle of winter's rhythm, fear alerted you to that which was dangerous. Through fear you learned to establish boundaries. You defined a zone of safety. Dangers, both real and imagined, can tend to paralyze a Water's rhythm, making it more immobile, more hidden, more pulled toward hibernation. With maturity, however, a Water's fear becomes a wise and discerning caution.

If You Have a Water Partner

By understanding these traits and tendencies in your partner, you are able to set your expectations more realistically, meet your partner's imperfect behaviors with grace and compassion, and be a force for evolution and positive change that comes from understanding rather than judgment and irritation. For example, your partner may draw into his or her own world, paralyzed in fear or hopelessness, and shutting you out. Understanding this helps you to not take it personally, to leave space that it may occur, and will also help you be more skillful when the timing makes it possible to beckon your partner to come out of mental hibernation and meet you again. Because your Water partner loves to produce ideas and generate a shared excitement about them, but is weak on implementation, you may find that helping your partner with follow-through adds a needed balance. Your partner will want to be mothered when in the infant end of the infant/wise-philosopher spectrum, and your understanding of this dynamic can help you stay centered and able to provide valuable guidance instead of mothering that reinforces infantile behaviors.

WOOD ELEMENT: NEW GROWTH

Wood Element carries the rhythm of spring. Spring embodies the power and insistence of new life and change. The earth becomes warm, and the hours of light begin to outnumber the hours of darkness. Life bursts forth as the landscape explodes with color and exuberance. The energy of a Wood is reminiscent of a seedling you might see bursting forth through hard ground after a March rainstorm. The rhythm is staccato and unstoppable, like a marching soldier, an awesome power that vanquishes resistance. Spring yearns for expression as life pushes forward.

Woods take a strong stand. They unabashedly claim their space, as if proudly announcing, like a budding rose, "I am here. Deal with me, thorns and all!" Their strength is in the power of their vision. They see inequities and gather forces of justice. They see the truth. They see the way. Their vision inspires others and can marshal them into action. They are sure of themselves and shine in a crisis. Their sense of timing cuts to the quick. Their ability to assert themselves and organize efforts is characterized by sound goals, good judgment, and carefully formulated decisions.

The Wood's self-confidence, however, carries the risk of becoming arrogance while the assertiveness can become an inflexible, self-indulgent force. Woods may come into a narrow and rigid vision that causes them to harshly judge those who do not subscribe to their truth or follow their direction. They may righteously hold to this position and become easily and vocally frustrated about the beliefs and actions of others. Or they may lose their vision and be left disorganized, hopeless, and despairing.

The talk of a Wood is choppy and syncopated, almost a shout. The walk is also choppy, hitting the ground decisively, with clear, concise movements, like percussion. The characteristic mental state is assertiveness. The stress emotion is anger. In nature, the energy that has been accumulating beneath the ground in winter explodes forth above the earth in spring. Ideas or opinions that took root in winter now grow and are expressed with potent force. During the "terrible twos," your first cycle of the rhythm of spring, you were exploring, expanding, moving outward, and whoever or whatever blocked this energy knew your fury. If you are a Wood, your disposition is to push forth. Your roots are firm, your territory well marked, your purpose strong. You meet obstacles decisively. If they do not give way, your anger is quick and forceful. With maturity, however, Wood's anger becomes a wise and healthy determination.

If You Have a Wood Partner

Emotions build swiftly and intensely, pushing for determined action. If these emotions are pent-up, the pressure can become unbearable. If there is no release, this pressure cooker can lead to physical symptoms (headaches are common) or illness—or a measured explosion (often, against you). Understanding this helps you create space for the valve to release without taking it personally. It encourages you to set aside time to talk about whatever is building up and to have compassion for your partner's struggles with these forces. Wood partners also tend to polarize and lack sensitivity when handling differences. They can be too direct, too blunt, so you may feel that your alliance has dissolved. If this occurs, shift the focus to reaffirm your alliance so it becomes clear that you are both on the same team and need to find a solution that doesn't make either of you wrong. Woods also tend to push onward, even after they have run out of gas. Once they pass a certain point, they become less flexible or effective. Ask yourself what would help your partner to step out of this obsessive determination to race to get closure. Related to this is the urgency, almost a physical necessity, to deal with issues as they arise. This may not be convenient or practical, but knowing its pull on your partner makes it more palatable, plus it should be comforting to know that rather than sweeping things under the rug, your Wood partner will insist that they be handled. Your partner is also independent and will want to be in control of the relationship. Understanding this does not mean you should cave in and put your own authority in the backseat. However, it helps you negotiate more effectively when you recognize that the tendency is in your partner's natural rhythm and includes gifts—benevolence, kindness, truthfulness, protection—that can serve the relationship.

FIRE ELEMENT: FULFILLMENT

Fire Element carries the rhythm of summer. Summer embodies fruition. The earth becomes warm and the days long. New light bursts forth in the early morning. The fruit on the tree has matured, ripe and luscious. Summer holds the radiance and joy of youth in all its glory. It gives delight in the richness of the moment. The energy of a Fire blazes up and out, creating the impression that the person is everywhere at once. Like wildfire, which jumps ravines and spreads in every direction, its rhythm is rapid, random, and rising.

Fires move from their heart, open and vulnerable. Their strengths are in their warmth, empathy, joy, and exuberance. With passion and radiance, they are able to draw out the positive and the hopeful in others, communicate with them in their uniqueness, and elicit cooperation. With charisma and a grasp of the whole picture, they ignite the actions of others with insight, compassion, and clarity. In recognizing what is possible, they are the magicians and catalysts who help others believe in themselves, free themselves of self-imposed limitations, and move with confidence to a better future.

Fires may go into a panic of frenzied activity, trying to make everyone happy. They often have difficulty with discernment and setting priorities. They may become junkies for love, for the "high"—whether through parties, drugs, sex, or spirituality. They may give from their hearts until they have no more to give. Fires often burn themselves out, overcommitted and exhausted. They are so drawn to the bright side of life that they may not register the dark, the negative, or the dangerous and become innocently embroiled in another's dark side. To those who look to them for leadership, their optimism and enthusiasm may set up expectations that were never meant and are rarely met.

You can hear laughter in the talk of a Fire. The walk is like a skip, with an up-and-down movement, arms rising and falling like flames. The characteristic mental state is fused with joy and passion, which under stress can escalate into panic or hysteria. In summer, the light is dazzling, the fruit is abundant, and the fish are hopping. Excess is all around. During adolescence, your first cycle of summer's rhythm, you lived for thrill and exhilaration. Joys and sorrows were laced with passion and taken to excess. If you are a Fire, you want to enjoy, not strive. The present is all that matters, and as you bask in its warmth, you radiate your excitement. Others may find your Pollyanna optimism contagious, exhausting, or irritating. With maturity, a Fire's wild enthusiasm, passion, or infatuation becomes discerning love and discriminating involvement.

If You Have a Fire Partner

Know that your partner's panic and hysteria do not mean what it would mean if *you* were experiencing it. Lightning fills the summer sky but quickly passes. It is part of a Fire's rhythm. Contagious though the panic may be, remain calm instead and, most important, don't try to "fix" it. Allow it to pass. Another point to remember is that your partner's first instinctive response to an opportunity or invitation is a big "yes." The excitement about the probable joys overwhelms consideration of the costs. If your Fire partner has enthusiastically agreed with you about a plan or new venture, ask again a few hours or a few days later to be sure yesterday's truth is still true today. And if your partner has said yes too many times to too many people, have compassion as the costs of these misjudgments come due. Fires burn out. They need to come back to themselves to restore, even though they are magnetically drawn to be involved with others. So encourage them to take time alone. Forcefully confronting them is usually not the best approach for helping them see the errors of their ways. When cornered, they cannot think. Your judgments can weaken the Fire's glow more effectively than almost anything else you could do. People who were drawn to the carefree joy of a Fire are often left wondering what happened to that joy and spontaneity, having no idea of their role in extinguishing it. Lead with understanding, compassion, and appreciation of the sparkle your partner is capable of bringing into your life.

EARTH ELEMENT: TRANSITION

Earth Element carries the rhythm of the solstices and equinoxes, the times of transition. As the midpoint between two seasons, the time of transition is governed by a balance between opposing forces, holding both the past and the future in the present moment. Most familiar as Indian summer, its colors are bright and glorious, a last burst of the waning summer. This rhythm creates stability amid transition, assimilates change, and coordinates between the season that is ending and the season that is arriving. The energy of an Earth can harmonize potential conflicts when other elements meet. The rhythm sways with a side-to-side roll, as if the person is moving to the rhythm of the earth itself.

Earth people know about holding steady. Like the balance scales that are the symbol for justice, they embody fairness. At the center of the cyclone, their strength is to stay stable while nurturing the changes happening around them. Like a midwife, they bring support, compassion, and confidence to times of transition. They hold the center, staying in the present moment as they add their tranquil touch to life's changes. Keeping a fresh perspective as the old order passes, they pave the way for stable change, rarely seeming rushed or stressed. Because they exude compassion, people feel safe with them. They bring equilibrium to chaos, peace to the threatened, and shelter to the displaced.

With a compulsion to help others stay in a comfort zone, Earths may hinder others' transitions. This aversion to rocking the boat, combined with their characteristic desire to support the other, may also lead to obsessive worry. Or they may involve themselves in a manner that stunts the other's growth, babying and overprotecting. "The helping hand strikes again" describes the behavior of an Earth whose life has lost its balance. In their joy at helping others flourish, they may neglect to give enough attention to their own growth. Skilled at helping others integrate lessons and experiences, they may have a harder time integrating their own. Knowing bone-deep that loss is an inevitable part of transition, they may anticipate it and try to prevent it, staying with a bad marriage or an unfulfilling job. So they may turn their strongest suit into a losing hand by interfering with the cycle of necessary change, leading to a life full of regrets. Also, because they do not have a designated season of their own, people living in the rhythm of the solstice and equinox may live with heartrending questions always in the background, such as: "Where is time for me? When will my season come?"

The talk of an Earth has a singsong quality, like a mom making baby talk to her infant. The walk has a relaxed, lyrical manner—a slow, rhythmic side-to-side sway, light-footed as a deer. The characteristic mental state is compassion. The stress emotion is worry. In moving from one season to the next, the two seasons come into a resonance as one transforms into the other. In your own transitions, regardless of your Element, you can activate the Earth Mother archetype within yourself, to support you through endings and new beginnings. The harvest of the season that is passing must be incorporated into the season that is coming. Earths instinctually help others in transition to transform past mistakes into lessons for the future. An Earth's generosity may be martyrish; with maturity, however, exaggerated sympathy ripens into a wise and balanced compassion. Earths can love many, deeply and personally. And theirs is a more intimate love of many than a Fire's passionate, generic love for all.

If You Have an Earth Partner

When your partner is pulled by many people, overly responsive to their needs, hurting for everyone, or immersed in the middle of a conflict (and championing both sides), rather than throwing up your hands in frustration, ask about the quandary inside. As too much compassion for others is a core problem, showering your partner with your own compassion will reach in deeply. Be alert also to when your partner is suffering for you, trying to anticipate needs you are not feeling, or putting you first in ways that throw the relationship out of balance. Reflect this back with the intention of reestablishing balances between you. Draw out what your partner is not saying because of not wanting to hurt you or disappoint you. It is important feedback for your own evolution that you might otherwise miss. Because your partner tends to cater to the real or imagined needs of all who are close, assume extra responsibility for working through your own problems and encourage your partner to have self-compassion. Know, also, that your partner needs ample time to process information and make a decision.

METAL ELEMENT: ENDING

Metal Element carries the rhythm of autumn, the season of completion. Each day turns to night earlier than the last. The warmth fades. Yet autumn embodies the peace of a concluding chapter, the meaning found in attainment, and faith that dying to the old makes way for the new. The leaves fall to earth, fertilizing the next cycle. This rhythm garners the meaning of the cycle that is coming to an end, evaluates what has been useful and what has not, and eliminates all that is not valuable so as to bring about a worthy completion. The energy of a Metal seems to be stretched between the heavens and the earth. Like a tall tree that has lost its leaves, the energies seem restrained yet serene, barren yet dignified. The rhythm glides like a ballet dancer—elongated, still, and graceful.

Metals have the ability to mine truths out of their experiences and apply those truths. Living in the final cycle, there is an urge toward perfection, high achievements, and model results. Metals can see what needs to happen and are highly motivated to bring it into being. Out of this vision of perfection grows a standard of excellence that is concerned with a higher good and is inspiring to others. That which is impure—whether in ideas, behavior, or systems—is eliminated. As the last season of the cycle, autumn carries a sadness, and those whose rhythm vibrates with autumn are simpatico with the world's grief. This affinity with sadness engenders kindness, honesty, and integrity. Metals have a capacity to express themselves clearly, and they receive well the ideas and inspiration of others, for they have a gift for discerning the pure from the impure. They have an urgency to find meaning and serenity in what has been, for theirs is the final cycle. Forgive them their persistence. It is their rhythm.

Metals are vulnerable to becoming overly serious or sinking into depression. Shunning fun and lacking pleasure, they may find their energies becoming restrained and dry, like the tree without leaves. They may appear dreary and aloof. Living always in the energy of the final cycle, they may have difficulty with time, trying to cram more into each day than it can contain. Oriented toward the future, their wisdom about life is tempered by their awareness of death's inevitability, so they may become trapped in depression or in the pressure to reach perfection before the last grains of sand have emptied from the hourglass. Their ability to make pure judgments may be clouded by this despair or perfectionism, and their standards may be tarnished by hopelessness or inflated through unrealistic assessments. Either may paralyze them so that they become unable to let go into change, obsessively evaluating and reevaluating to the point of exhaustion, lacking the capacity to complete a cycle of their lives, again failing to reap the benefits of their strongest suit.

The talk of a Metal has a weeping sound. The walk is tall, straight, and subdued, gliding with head high and gaze forward. The characteristic mental state is reflectiveness. The stress emotion is grief. As the leaves fall and the wildflowers die, loss is in the air. The cycle draws to its close. When you come to the close of a cycle in your own life, there may be sadness for opportunities missed and for what must be left behind. If autumn is your primary rhythm, you are oriented toward completions, toward discerning what has been worthy and meaningful. There is a heaviness in these tasks, and you know the grief of what might have been but was not to be. With maturity, however, a Metal's grief transforms into an identification with the whole cycle, at peace with life, at peace with death.

If You Have a Metal Partner

While you may long for an easier flow of feelings, it is in your partner's rhythm to apply mental solutions to emotional problems. Still, you will serve your partner's evolution by beckoning him or her into the realm of feeling, and you will be more effective if you can begin by meeting on the mental plane. Metals expect others to approach tasks and fulfill their obligations according to their own exaggerated standards. Your partner's perfectionism can lead to beautiful creations, but it can also become a tyrant that makes your partner miserable and, if turned upon you, can be a ferocious assault on your self-esteem. Articulating this vulnerability gives your Metal partner a chance to recognize the arrogance of expecting others to run their lives according to his or her own inner tyrant. Your partner's single-minded focus, an asset for getting the job done, can, however, lead to isolation and detachment, specifically detachment from you. While you may need to accept that your partner does not want to be disturbed while in the creative process, establish agreements about when you will meet and expect them to be honored and honored wholeheartedly. Your partner longs—often at a level deeper than conscious awareness—to resonate with your heart, and the same single-minded focus that goes into a project can be directed to establishing intimacy.

Understanding Your Own and Your Partner's Element Is a Lifelong Process

The above descriptions are a brief guide for understanding your own and your partner's Elements and living from them more effectively. While each of us is a unique energy system with a unique vibration, our vibrations tend to cluster in these five areas. Your vibrational signature will likely be a combination of two or three of these elemental rhythms. It is not all or nothing. David is a Water/Metal combo; Donna is Fire/Earth.

As you come to know your primary Element and its dynamics, you come to understand a great deal about your needs and your blind spots in all areas of your life, and you will also be able to meet other people's behavior with greater insight and compassion. The more that the energies composing your life force are in harmony, the more the strengths of your Element, rather than its liabilities, will express themselves. Beyond understanding the nature of your own and your partner's Elements, another invaluable step you can take is to balance your energies (pp. 83–94) when you or your partner is caught in the downside of your Element.

On to Part 2

Carl Rogers, among the greatest American psychologists of the twentieth century, was, toward the end of his long career, one of David's graduate school professors. David idolized Carl, to Carl's immense annoyance . . . but that's another story. Rogers' work is still commonly cited in psychological literature. One of his most frequently quoted statements is, "The curious paradox is that when I accept myself just as I am, then I can change."[44] He goes on to explain, "We cannot change, we cannot move away from what we are, until we thoroughly *accept* what we are."

In terms of self-initiated change, this "curious paradox" applies to all of us. Up to this point, the instructions in *The Energies of Love* have not tried to change you. Yours and your partner's Element, Energetic Stress Style, biochemistry, and gender are all inherited. What you have been learning is how to become more adept in the way the two of you avoid clashes in your inborn styles while building on your strengths. This begins by understanding and accepting what cannot be changed in your natures. Other core dimensions of how you relate to one another, however, were learned early in your life and may also seem to be fixed and unchangeable. But they are not. Learning to recognize, accept, *and* change them is the topic of Part 2.

PART

2

The Learned Aspects of Love

5

The Energies of Attachment

The Nitty-Gritty of Intimacy

[The infant's] profound attachment to a particular
person is both as strong as, and often as irrational
as, falling in love, and the very similarity of
these two processes suggests strongly that
they may have something in common.

—JOHN BOWLBY[1]

WHILE YOUR ENERGETIC STRESS STYLE IS INHERITED (DONNA CAN SEE IT IN THE energies of a newborn infant), the way you bond to others, called your *attachment style,* is to a large degree a product of learning. Behavioral scientists have studied in-depth the way your early experiences are likely to impact your adult relationships.

How the Infant Brain Gets Wired

At birth, your brain was a book whose story line was yet to be written. The pages, the binding, and overall organization were already apparent in their embryonic forms, but the words had not yet been inscribed. Your genes determined the basic structure of your nervous system and even primal temperamental patterns, but the early experiences that would come to shape the life you are now living would only unfold as a result of your interactions with your environment.

While the mutual influences of nature and nurture are no doubt familiar to you, what you may not know is how *directly* the neural pathways in your developing brain were impacted by the subtle and not-so-subtle ways your primary caregivers responded to you. Life was a stream of sensation. Hunger pangs would intrude into a peaceful rest. You would cry reflexively. If you were met with soothing words, a tender embrace, and the taste of warm milk, all was good again. The neural pathways that would eventually form meaning about hunger pangs would not link to neurons that activate anxiety. Hunger would eventually become associated with positive expectations. If, however, your cries went unheeded, that episode established a different set of pathways. Hunger was not only a temporary pain. It became pain laced with anxiety, uncertainty, and negative anticipations.

→ THE ENERGY DIMENSION ←

Infant Being Nurtured
When an infant's needs are responded to promptly, it is very beautiful. The surrounding aura moves in toward the baby and then gently moves away. This steady rhythm comforts the body like a pulsating warm blanket, keeping all the baby's energies in a tender glow.

Infant Being Neglected
When an infant is crying out of unmet need, the energy reaches out toward the caregiver, but it looks confused. It is disorganized and sometimes jagged. When the baby finally stops crying from exhaustion, the energies are pulled back from the world, the aura looks collapsed and thin, and its natural pulsation seems subdued.

As an infant, you could not soothe your discomforts. While the part of your nervous system that mobilizes action in response to stress and pain (the sympathetic nervous system) was already well developed by the time you were born, the part that would allow you to soothe yourself in the face of distress (the parasympathetic nervous system) was still undeveloped. Nature gave that job to your parents, counting on them to soothe you and to teach you about soothing yourself. When discomfort roused you into action, your repertoire was limited mostly to squirming and crying. When your caregivers held you and cuddled you and cooed soothing sounds, you were not only comforted; you learned about *self-comforting*.

These early learnings shaped your most basic assessments about yourself and your relationships. They told you whether you were worthy of intimacy, confirmed whether or not you could rely on your intimates for support and protection, showed you how to care for and be cared for by those to whom you were closest, and guided you in how to manage your emotional needs.

Early Imprints of How to Be in a Relationship Are Usually Lasting Ones

In the wild, a child's survival depended on establishing a close bond with whoever would provide care. The infant's brain is wired to seek, bond, and communicate with a caregiver, and it is from caregiver relationships that skills for self-nurture and relating intimately with others are, for better or worse, formed. John Bowlby—the British psychiatrist who blazed the trail for our current understanding of the infant's attachment to a primary caregiver and its lifelong impact—provocatively claimed in 1951 that the young child's hunger for the mother's love and presence was as primal a drive as the hunger for food.[2] No survival without food, but also no survival without nurture and protection. And bonding is the route to securing each. The baby is driven by inner forces to seek proximity and contact with the caregiver.

Bowlby's assertion that the child's need to bond is as primal as the need for food was put to a test a few years later in classic experiments by Harry Harlow. Baby rhesus monkeys would bond to and seek comfort from a terry-cloth mother they could cling to, though it provided no food, rather than to a wire mother outfitted with a nipple that provided milk.[3] Infant monkeys placed in an unfamiliar room with their cloth surrogate parent would cling to it until they felt secure enough to explore. If the cloth surrogate was not present, they would crouch and freeze in fear, perhaps also rocking, sucking, crying, or screaming. This behavior was displayed in the absence of the cloth surrogate even if the wire surrogate—which they had suckled but could not physically embrace in a manner that produced bonding—was present. That primal is the infant's drive to bond with a caregiver.

In the infant's impulse for attachment, the sight of the caregiver's face, hands, and hair are triggers for grasping and clinging. The caregiver's voice and caresses initiate smiling and babbling behavior. Communication had to, of course, first be accomplished without words. Facial expressions, eye contact, voice tone, gestures, postures, timing, and intensity showed on the outside what was happening to you on the inside.[4] Before you could talk, this was the primary information available to your caregivers about your moment-to-moment experience. The accuracy with which they read and were able to respond to your needs determined a great deal about your sense of well-being. Their attunement or lack of attunement was your first, deeply imprinted lesson about what to expect in a close relationship.

These early imprints are usually lasting ones. Bowlby compared the sweeping effects of maternal deprivation on psychological development to the impact of poor nutrition on physical growth.[5] His first speculation on the role of early emotional deprivation traced to experiences prior to his psychiatric training when, as a volunteer at a residential school for delinquent and other troubled children, he noticed how some children would show anger and rejection even to those who tried to befriend them. Their self-defeating interpersonal styles seemed to have been established during their troubled home lives.

Fast-forward eighty years. Study after study suggests that early attachment relationships set the foundation for subsequent personality development. Infants who enjoyed a secure attachment relationship with a primary caregiver, as inferred by systematic assessments, grew up to have higher self-esteem than children whose primary attachment relationship was insecure. They also developed closer friendships,

---

→ THE ENERGY DIMENSION ←

Infant in a Secure Moment
The infant's energy moves outward into the world, whether or not an adult is there. It is as if the energy is exploring the environment. Then it comes back in and soothes the infant. Then back out into the surrounding world. Like the breath, the energy moves inward, bringing the infant support and harmony, and then outward, securely contacting the world.

Infant in an Insecure Moment
The energies look confused, disorganized, and chaotic. Because the infant can't make sense of what is happening and can't control it, there is a surrender into powerlessness. The energies do not focus or coalesce, and they become disconnected from the environment.

greater social competence, more fulfilling romantic partnerships, greater capacity to regulate their emotions, more ability to accomplish their goals, greater resilience, enhanced leadership qualities, and less anxiety and depression.[6]

Secure Attachment; Anxious Attachment; Avoidant Attachment

We are wired to bond to only a small group of intimates, with one special person at the top of the hierarchy, and it is during times of threat or separation that this wiring is most strongly activated. However, the *way* we will react when it is activated is shaped by our experiences. The dynamics of "secure" and "insecure" attachment styles have been investigated in hundreds of studies.

Secure Attachment

Secure attachment in childhood sets the stage for greater ease with intimacy as an adult. People with a secure attachment style tend to be optimistic about their primary relationship. They have a strong sense of self-worth, expect closeness, warmth, and comfort in their relationships, and they tend to find it. They are effective in communicating their needs and feelings, and they accurately read and respond to their partner's emotional cues. They are able to soothe as well as self-soothe, and they are capable of moving easily between intimate engagement and independence, leading to the emotional and behavioral *inter*dependence required for a successful relationship.[7]

Insecure Attachment

Insecure attachment in childhood sets the stage for later troubles with intimacy. Children who are insecurely attached did not receive the imprinting from their caregivers that would help them learn to regulate their own nervous systems, making them vulnerable to emotional difficulties throughout life.[8] Insecure attachment generally involves anxious clinging or emotional avoidance in intimate relationships:

ANXIOUS ATTACHMENT

Anxious attachment is typified by a strong need for closeness, worry about and preoccupation with the relationship, and reliance on strategies such as clinging, angry, and controlling responses that attempt to minimize the emotional distance from the partner.[9] People with an anxious attachment style tend to be extremely sensitive to small fluctuations in their partner's moods and behavior, to take them personally, and to be easily upset by any sign of real or imagined distancing. Because they may alternate between clinging when their partner is available and showing anger because of times their partner was not available—or refusing comfort for that reason—this attachment style is sometimes called *anxious-ambivalent*.

AVOIDANT ATTACHMENT

Avoidant attachment is typified by exaggerated self-reliance and strategies that maximize emotional distance from the partner.[10] Adults with an avoidant attachment style tend to be isolated, unaware of their emotional hollowness, and put off by any sug-

---

→ THE ENERGY DIMENSION ←

Secure

The aura is full. It fluctuates easily in response to others, influenced by them but then returning to center. There is also a fullness in the chakra energies, which reach out in front of the person as if to greet others. This fullness in the aura and the chakras is soothing, leaving the person less dependent on others for emotional and energetic support.

Anxious

The energy of an anxious aura is jittery, its patterns unstable. Sometimes it will engulf or cling to the partner's energies. Other times it will repel them or appear to attack them. This makes it difficult for another's energies to connect and dance with those with an anxious-avoidant style.

Avoidant

The energy is pulled back into the avoidant person, or it focuses or fragments in other directions, any direction but toward a person where commitment might be called for. This may be toward projects, acquaintances, casual social situations, entertainment, surfing the net, or intellectual pursuits.

---

gestion that they might have more needs for intimacy than they recognize. They view their emotional detachment as a sign of strength and independence. Research, however, shows that when the relationship is at risk, individuals with an avoidant attachment style are just as distressed on physiological measures (such as the galvanic skin response) as other people. They are simply better at keeping themselves from expressing or even experiencing such thoughts and feelings.[11] Avoidant partners have the same core need for a primary relationship but manage it by attempting to deny it.

MIXED ANXIOUS/AVOIDANT ATTACHMENT

Mixed anxious/avoidant attachment is a combination of both strategies, characterized by seeking closeness and then fearfully avoiding it. A traumatic or abusive relationship with a primary caregiver is often found in the person's history. Borderline personality disorder often corresponds with an anxious/avoidant attachment style (which is sometimes called *disorganized attachment*). Closeness with the partner is longed for as a source of comfort and intimacy, but at the same time, intimacy provokes fear and anxiety. Anxious/avoidant attachment is typified in the quip, "If you won't leave me, I'll find someone who will." This paradoxical style is relatively rare but can be extraordinarily challenging for the partner.

While the descriptions of attachment styles are, by necessity, of "pure types," human beings are rarely *pure* types within any classification. A given individual may be a mix of these qualities or more like one type in a particular situation and more like another in a different situation, and the person's primary attachment style may also shift over time.

The potential for developing a *secure* attachment style is there in your genes. It is what nature intended. But the way this capacity manifests or doesn't manifest is shaped by your experiences. Secure attachment helps individuals, intimate relationships, and human communities thrive. Even though no parent is perfect, nature teams with the family to achieve secure attachment more than half of the time.[12] The rest are divided fairly evenly between the anxious and the avoidant styles, with a minority having the disorganized anxious–avoidant style. However, such classifications don't capture the rich nuance in an individual's ways of relating intimately. Even within the "secure" majority are innumerable traits and habitual patterns that may dampen or strengthen intimacy.

When the attachment bond is strained or threatened by the inevitable hurdles in building any close, creative relationship, primal responses that trace back to early attachment experiences are evoked. Understanding how your style and your partner's style were once upon a time adaptive strategies for less than perfect circumstances allows you, when such primal responses erupt, to proceed with greater compassion for yourself as well as for your partner.

✦ THE ENERGY DIMENSION ✦

When Donna witnesses couples interacting, the choreography of their energies is exactly the way you might imagine it to be:

Secure Relating

When two people engage intimately during a secure moment, the energy interchange Donna observes is smooth and strong. That is exactly what would be predicted by the "smooth, ordered, coherent patterns" that spectral analysis revealed in the electromagnetic field radiated by the heart during moments of love or appreciation.[13]

The Anxious Style in Relationships

The energies around a person with an *anxious attachment style* seeking contact with an intimate partner who is not responding in the moment tend to become disorganized and move somewhat chaotically but forcefully toward the partner.

The Avoidant Style in Relationships

The energies surrounding a person with an *avoidant attachment style* tend to contract so much that they take on what looks to Donna like a shell. These compacted energies then retreat from an intimate partner who is making an emotional demand. In interactions with others, the avoidant partner's energies may be much more fluid and engaging. This corresponds with clinical observations. People who seem well adjusted and at ease in most social situations may still use an avoidant (or an anxious) attachment style in their most intimate relationships.

The Anxious-Avoidant Trap

Combining the above two descriptions provides a vivid picture of what has been the "anxious-avoidant trap," in which one person's energies move toward the other and the other's retreat inward or move away.

Is your attachment style—whether secure, anxious, or avoidant—also reflected in the electromagnetic energies emanating from your body? Of course our answer is yes. One of the most interesting discoveries for David as he learned about Donna's work is that memories, emotions, and behavioral programs are stored not only in the brain but also in the body's energy systems. The secure, anxious, and avoidant ways of responding when feeling distressed are not just products of your mind. They are visible to Donna as patterns of energy.

The Dance of David's and Donna's Attachment Styles

We will once again feature our relationship in discussing how the principles discussed play out, not because it is an ideal model, but because we've had to struggle with and work through so many issues and some of them may resonate with you. Anxious or avoidant strategies—pursuing or retreating—are the two basic ways a child can respond when caregivers are not able to meet the child's needs. For instance, David's mother tried to breast-feed him but was unable to produce the amount of milk his body required. A determined woman, she kept trying for three weeks, as he approached semistarvation, until the doctor insisted that his diet be supplemented. So David's earliest formative experiences, about so basic a drive as chronic hunger, were that no matter how much he cried, he was not going to get what he needed. With consistent physical or emotional deprivation, the infant finally stops seeking the caregiver's attention, dampens internal sensations, and withdraws—avoidant attachment in the making.

For David, this was reinforced because the wisdom of post–World War II child experts was to feed on a schedule and not soothe or reinforce the infant for crying. Family legend has it that Mr. and Mrs. Cohen, an elderly couple who were renting a room in the same Brooklyn tenement where David's parents were staying during David's first year, would cry themselves to sleep each night hearing David's unheeded screams through the thin walls and being powerless to override the child experts of the day and intervene. Children will finally stop screaming and retreat within. Such experiences laid the foundation for David's attachment style. They combined with his being an only child, and one who had no age-matched playmates in the neighborhood, into the development of a boy who was comfortable spending long periods alone, who tended toward self-soothing rather than sharing his vulnerabilities with others, and who was not at ease in the casual emotional give-and-take that seemed natural to his peers.

He grew up proud of his independence and self-sufficiency. He did not view his style as an avoidant attachment disorder, though his failure to form a lasting partnership despite a number of intense romances during his twenties might have been a clue. He couldn't understand why his relationships, which usually started with strong passion, would deteriorate into an emotional roller coaster where his partners felt he was not giving them what they needed. It seemed patently obvious to him that their neediness and emotional volatility were what was pushing him away. This initial attraction between a person with an avoidant attachment style and a person with an anxious/clinging style has been characterized in literature as the "anxious–avoidant trap."[14] If an avoidant person with David's aptitude for the role gets close enough even to a relatively secure partner, however, the partner may still be drawn into this anxious–avoidant dance.

David was thirty when he met Donna. After so many experiences where his paramours became wounded puddles of emotion, and with no inkling of his role in inflicting the wounds, Donna's independence and self-reliance were very attractive to him. She was the middle child of three. While her older sister was still commanding special attention as the firstborn, their little brother came along, eighteen months after Donna, with some special needs, and Donna was in many ways left to fend for herself. In assuring her young second daughter that she would be fine, though she got relatively little parental attention, Donna's mother would say to her, "The Lord protects angels and fools. I'm not sure which you are, but I know you are protected." As you will see in chapter 7, Donna learned self-sufficiency. In her first marriage, her emotionally remote husband would be away for long periods and her self-reliance was all she had for bringing up their young daughters. When we met, we each wanted a lot of space and were happy to give the other a lot of space. But the self-reliance that is an effective way of coping when no one is available can be a liability for forming a lasting intimate relationship. It can also be a bit of a delusion. People identified in scientific studies as being secure in their primary relationships were not only capable of greater intimacy and interdependence, they were more autonomous and independent.[15]

Being with a partner whose strong self-reliance can trump intimacy has been part of the journey for each of us—sometimes propelling one of us or the other into the anxious/clinging polarity of self-reliance as we have traveled together for well more than three decades toward more secure attachment styles. Attachment style is not rigidly fixed, may shift with the context, and may become more secure over time.[16] Our tumultuous ride has transformed us both, so we know what is possible, as well as how challenging the journey can be.

Obviously, however, not all adults have an intimate partner or are in a relationship that is meeting their basic needs for closeness, security, love, and support. Does this mean they drew the short straw and must lead empty, emotionally barren lives? By no means. Some people seem well suited for single life. Particularly if your early attachment experiences provided you with healthy internal models for self-care, you are poised to manage your emotions effectively, to soothe your own sorrows, and to self-validate in the absence of a primary partner. Many single people do indeed find enough of the emotional benefits that might be provided by an intimate relationship to do very well. Nonetheless, there are strong reasons that people who are in fulfilling partnerships tend to live longer, healthier, happier lives than those who are not.[17]

The Influence of Your Energetic Stress Style on Your Relationship Style

The years have proven that Donna, as a kinesthetic, was more readily capable of intimate connection than digital David, but her self-reliance made her so tolerant of emotional distance that David's avoidant style set the tone for both of us. Your Energetic Stress Style—visual, kinesthetic, digital, tonal—is an aspect of your inborn temperament that we believe influences your attachment style throughout your life.

It is not hard to understand how your Energetic Stress Style would interact with your attachment history in forming and maintaining your patterns of intimacy. Donna's kinesthetic orientation *countered* the early experiences that might have produced a person with a more avoidant attachment style. Although she had a high tolerance for distance based on her early experiences, her kinesthetic nature allowed her to also easily resonate with whatever bids for closeness her parents, and later David, managed to express and meet them there. David's digital orientation, on the other hand, *amplified* the early experiences that fed into his avoidant style. Digitals tend to cut off emotionally from themselves and from their partners, so it is a double whammy to be a digital whose early experiences forged an avoidant attachment style. Learning to soothe oneself instead of seeking contact and support (risking feelings of vulnerability and dependence) combines with the digital's more insular ways

The Interaction of Energetic Stress Style and Attachment Style

As we were trying to convey how the digital stress style can amplify an avoidant attachment style, David bravely ventured, "Okay, Donna, let's tell the folks what this looks like in me energetically." Her analysis: "Sometimes you are in a digital bubble. And you show no interest in leaving it to enter my world. If we're having a difficult time and I'm desperately trying to reach you, that bubble looks like a thick, impenetrable wall. Other times it is just where you go when you are involved in a project. The bubble is not so thick, but it is still not easy to penetrate. And when I do penetrate it, it is like I have disturbed you from a dream, like I have literally burst your bubble. You don't transition easily from that space to meet my energies. I've come to understand that this is your nature and to not take it personally that you are such an automaton. And to appreciate that at so many other times, you are fully and readily present."

of relating—which favor mental retreat over emotional engagement. This is a recipe for a seriously avoidant attachment style.

The "motto" that typify each sensory mode (pp. 35–36) provide insight into the way Energetic Stress Style interacts with attachment style. You can see how the kinesthetic's "I don't want you to suffer or feel wrong" reinforced "I don't want to cause trouble" and played into Donna's allowing David's avoidant style to set the tone for the relationship. An overlay of the digital style's "I'm right!" is to not question the role of his or her own behaviors in the lack of intimacy. An overlay of the visual's "You're wrong!" is to blame the partner for the difficulties the relationship encounters. Meanwhile, the tonal's "I'm angry at you for making me feel wrong!" undermines the partner's efforts toward being close. Tonals whose backgrounds led to an anxious attachment style are dealing with another double whammy, quite different from that of the digital. As tonals, they characteristically read between the lines and, when stressed, negatively distort their partner's intentions. If they in childhood also developed an anxious attachment style, they will be overly sensitive to tiny nuances in their partner's mood. With those two filters acting in concert, it is not surprising that they tend to feel emotionally abused and abandoned by their partners. Being aware of the filters you characteristically use when under stress, and those your partner tends to use, will provide a helpful backdrop as you move toward more secure attachment.

What Does All This Mean for Your Relationship?

Does the scientific understanding of attachment mean that in order for you to have emerged from your childhood psychologically unscathed your parents needed to have anticipated your every need, correctly read your every gesture, and soothed your every discomfort? Nature knew better than to set the bar at that level. The concept of the "good-enough" parent recognizes that no one can always interpret a child's signals correctly, avoid separations, or hit the bull's-eye with every attempt to soothe.[18] A child's innate programming to thrive is remarkably robust. Doses of adversity and want build self-reliance even as the neural pathways for secure bonding seem to require a somewhat steady accumulation of positive interactions with the caregiver. Children are naturally resilient, so even imperfect parents, as all parents are, are able to raise healthy kids.

Many people, however, didn't have even minimally "good enough" parenting, or at least there were areas of breakdown, and problems in their adult relationships often trace back to these earlier lapses. Are these patterns indelibly stamped on your psyche? For most people throughout history, the answer was "probably yes." Attachment style during childhood is likely to shift only if significant external changes occur, such as a divorce, the onset of chronic depression in a parent, or the entry of a different primary caregiver.[19] As people develop into adulthood, the tendency is to choose partners and situations that correspond with and reinforce early psychological patterns.[20] In this sense, the past predicts the future. What people receive from their parents sets into motion deep patterns they usually bring to their marriages.

The hopeful and encouraging reason for this section of the book is that the possibility of repairing wounds and compensating for damages tracing to fallible parenting and unfavorable circumstances is now open to anyone willing to invest the time and effort. Even in infancy, programs that improved the quality of interaction between a mother and a child who evidenced early attachment problems resulted in more positive mother-child relationships that included significantly less anger, avoidance, and resistance.[21] For instance, it is well established that babies who are irritable from birth are less likely to create secure bonds at the end of their first year and are

→ THE ENERGY DIMENSION ←

Attunement between Infant and Parent

In one another's presence, the auras of the infant and the parent grow larger, and another field appears that surrounds the pair, ensconcing them in a cocoonlike energy. This is like a third aura, a property of infant and parent as a unit.

Non-Attunement between Infant and Parent

Depending on the quality of the relationship, the shared energy will differ. In general, the two auras will not overlap. If infant and parent are interacting but in a non-attuned manner, the infant's aura sucks further into itself and starts disconnecting from the environment. If the parent is angry or exasperated, a forceful energy that is threatening and confusing will move toward the child, sometimes causing the child to energetically retreat but other times literally entering the child. When the adult's more powerful energy enters the child's, it creates an energetic bridge for the transmission of beliefs as well as emotions. We are all familiar with how children may take on their parents' judgments and worldview as their own. This starts in the energies and can grow out non-attunement as well as out of the attunement in which you would expect it.

more likely to be anxious than infants who are more tranquil. However, early adjustments in parenting style can yield quick and significant results. In a Dutch study, mothers of babies diagnosed as "highly irritable at birth" were given three counseling sessions of two hours each, when their babies were between six and nine months old. By the time they were one year old, 68 percent of these infants were "securely attached." Only 28 percent of a matched control group that did not receive this counseling were "securely attached" by age one.[22]

What occurs in our lives beyond childhood can also have a strong impact on our bonding behavior. Favorable life events, such as successfully moving into the role of parenthood or forming a relationship with a partner whose attachment style is healthy and secure, can help transform an insecure attachment style.[23] So can individual psychotherapy, couple counseling, or other efforts that improve a challenging relationship.[24] It is never too late.

Attaching by Detaching

We will open our discussion of how to retrieve insecure attachment moments and begin to repair deep patterns with one of the simplest methods possible. If you have avoidant attachment tendencies, stay alert for times that you pull away from your partner and invite your partner to join you in this exercise. If you have anxious attachment tendencies, stay alert for times that you become clinging or controlling and do the exercise. In either case, when you realize you are caught in the attachment habits that do not serve your relationship, this simple wordless exercise can quickly interrupt the pattern, help you find your center, and open a path toward developing a more secure attachment moment with your partner. At such times of opportunity (we know—they don't *feel* like opportunities), ask your partner to participate with you. That alone acknowledges your awareness of tendencies in yourself that hurt the relationship and of your intention to overcome them. Your partner will probably find this encouraging in itself and cause for appreciation or at least hope. The exercise begins by coming into yourself and establishing an internal sense of safety. That is, you will, ironically, begin to enhance your capacity for healthy attachment by *detaching*. Then, as you become centered, you can turn back to your partner to energetically establish a stronger connection:

1. **Coming into Yourself.** Sitting directly across from your partner, both of you place your hands on your chest, close your eyes, and keep your focus on your heart for three deep breaths or until you are feeling more calm, safe, and centered.
2. **Softly Reconnecting.** When you are both ready, look at your partner's hands while keeping yours over your chest. Allow yourself to simply be with this connection for three more deep breaths.
3. **The Secure Gentle Gaze.** Lift your eyes and meet your partner's eyes. Feel an energetic bridge between you reconnecting. If this becomes difficult, return to step one and continue through the exercise until you can securely engage one another's gaze.

Simple as it is, this exercise is powerful. Starting when you are caught in the energy of an old and dysfunctional way of relating, it begins to repattern your nervous system. Each time you do the exercise, you are building a stronger energetic foundation for secure attachment.

> → THE ENERGY DIMENSION ←

Deep Breathing

The simple act of taking a deep breath engages a branch of the vagus nerve that slows the cardiovascular and respiratory systems in ways that allow us to relax and be present with one another. Taking a long deep breath when stressed not only slows respiratory and cardiovascular processes, it also smooths the movement of energy in the meridians, chakras, and aura. It counteracts the "rigid-alert" energy configuration of distress.

Heart Connection

When you bring your consciousness to your heart, you evoke feelings that are more positive and loving. The energies of these feelings not only travel to your cells, organs, and through your entire body, your heart's expanded electromagnetic field radiates outwardly and will impact anyone around you.

The Gentle Gaze

When you are open and relaxed and your eyes gently meet your partner's, the energies connect, but not as a straight line. Rather they look like a soft, hazy suspension bridge between your eyes and your partner's. As your eyes stay in contact, the energies in this downward curve begin to loop upward, eventually taking on the form of a figure eight between you. This connects you and actually grows stronger for as long as you remain in comfortable eye contact. When the figure-eight energy has grown quite strong, it will continue to connect you even after your attention has shifted from one another.

How Triple Warmer Maintains Your Attachment Style

An energy system identified by ancient Chinese physicians and given a strange name has an invisible but emphatic impact on your attachment style. It is called Triple Warmer.

The infant needs the caregiver's nurturing and protection in order to survive.

The foundational issue for attachment strategies, deeper even than the need for love and affection, is safety. Safety is the domain of Triple Warmer. It is the energy system in your body that is charged with responding to any threat to your survival. The Triple Warmer energy system—invisible yet as real as your cardiovascular or respiratory systems—supports your survival in three basic ways: It governs your immune system; it orchestrates responses to external threat, such as whether to fight or flee; and it maintains habits that are geared toward keeping you out of danger.

How Triple Warmer Keeps You from Changing

In carrying out these three basic survival strategies, Triple Warmer reveals the remarkable intelligence of the body and its energy systems. Consider, for instance, your immune response. Your body's surveillance energies are continually on alert for invading bacteria and other harmful intruders, and they initiate complex, ingenious strategies to destroy and dispose of them. Anyone who examines the workings of the immune system realizes that immense intelligence is involved. Triple Warmer uses an analogous strategy to that of the immune system for keeping you safe in the outer world. It assesses the information brought in by your senses. When it recognizes a potential threat, it implements preprogrammed behavioral strategies (just as your immune system implements preprogrammed biochemical strategies) that evolved because of their survival value for your ancestors. All this occurs without the need for your intellect or even your conscious awareness.

Triple Warmer approaches its mission of keeping you safe by working in concert with the hypothalamus. While Triple Warmer is an *energy system*, your hypothalamus is a tiny *organ*, an almond-sized gland that governs your autonomic nervous system. The hypothalamus is the highest up on the chain of endocrine glands, regulating the hormones that influence much of your emotional life, from how you bond to what you do in the face of threat.

Both Triple Warmer and the hypothalamus are oriented toward advancing the same ends: your safety and well-being. The way they work together is reminiscent of a computer and its software. As a physical structure, the hypothalamus, like a computer, has relatively fixed wiring. Triple Warmer (or any other energy system) is much more flexible and responsive, more like your word-processing software. You can create a poem, a blog entry, or a thriller novel. The software tells the computer what to do based on the input from the keyboard. Your body's energies, which are responsive to the ever-changing input from the environment and from within, are always at the "keyboard," telling your body what to do. Triple Warmer tells the hypothalamus which hormones and other chemicals to produce and disperse. Your mood, automated thoughts, and behaviors follow.

Triple Warmer evolved during the preponderance of human history when physical threat was part of daily life. When a saber-toothed tiger walked into the cave of your ancestors a hundred thousand years ago, Triple Warmer worked in partnership with the hypothalamus. They diverted bloodflow away from digestive, reproductive, and other systems not involved with immediate survival, and directed it toward systems that support fighting, escaping, or freezing to become less detectable. Triple Warmer also learns. It was continually establishing new survival habits for your ancestors, such as creating an aversion to the kinds of caves frequented by saber-toothed tigers or to the smell of a predator that just moved into their territory. Triple Warmer, in fact, still maintains innumerable survival habits tracing to your ancestors. These operate largely beneath your awareness, and Triple Warmer is quite unyielding about giving up habits or programs that were designed over eons to ensure survival. After all, you are here. It worked!

The challenges and stresses of modern life, however, are far different from those

→ THE ENERGY DIMENSION ←

Triple Warmer at Rest
Even when there is no perceived threat, Triple Warmer is usually still on alert. So Donna rarely sees Triple Warmer at rest. When it really is at rest, it fades into the background and seems to play more of a supportive role. You don't so much see Triple Warmer then, and with the safety that is signaled as Triple Warmer relaxes, the meridians become stronger, the chakras more vital, the radiant circuits activated, and the aura more full. You see the impact of a peaceful Triple Warmer in all the other energy systems.

Triple Warmer in the Face of Threat
When an immediate danger is detected, Triple Warmer orchestrates all of the body's energies to deal with the threat. They become sharp and focused. A cascading en-

ergy from the aura above the head and into the physical body prepares it for fight or flight, activating stress chemicals. If the response is to be flight, the energy leaves the face and upper body and goes into the legs to support their ability to run. The blood flow follows these energies, directing extra blood to the legs. If the response is to be fight, energy goes into the face and pumps up the arms and chest, which is also followed by the flow of blood.

Triple Warmer Maintaining a Habit

Triple Warmer regulates the activities of a spectrum of energy systems that are involved with habits that were formed in an attempt to ensure survival and well-being. For instance, the aura includes a band that holds the energy of established habits and behavioral patterns. When someone is in a situation that evokes a habitual emotion or behavior—whether the habit is an effective one or a dysfunctional one—this band becomes more pronounced. Triple Warmer's role in this orchestration becomes most obvious when the person tries to change the habit. Then Triple Warmer's energies rise to preserve the habit. Triple Warmer is a conservative force that is not oriented toward change. You've survived this long with the habit, so Triple Warmer has no incentive to change it! A similar process occurs at the level of the chakras. Habitual anger may too often scream out from the Third Chakra (solar plexus). Excessive compassion may ooze out from the Heart Chakra. Energy may move up quickly from the Root Chakra when your safety or sense of self is threatened. Triple Warmer is at the foundation of these reflexive responses, and if you try to change them, Triple Warmer's energies become activated in an attempt to retain the status quo.

in the world that existed while Triple Warmer was evolving. So Triple Warmer's brilliant programming is keyed to a world that no longer exists. Beyond its outdated strategies, Triple Warmer does not discriminate particularly well between life-threatening situations and relatively benign events. If you go into threat alert or full fight or flight or freeze mode half a dozen times a day—when your daughter won't obey you, when you are late for an appointment, when your computer isn't cooperating—the cortisol and other stress chemicals that are generated accumulate in your body and become harmful in a multitude of ways. Your risk then increases for anxiety, depression, digestive problems, heart disease, sleep disorders, weight gain, and concentration difficulties—collateral damage of Triple Warmer's survival strategies. In trying to save you, Triple Warmer is powerful enough to leave you with any of the symptoms mentioned above. It is the military-industrial complex of your body. Like the military, its job is to keep you alive and safe, and it is steadfast with that assignment, even if it means a lot of excessive effort, false alarms, inadvertent harm, and unsparing expenditure of precious resources to ensure security.

A peculiarity about Triple Warmer is that it won't support your desire to change a habit, even a harmful habit. Its assessment much of the time, since it is using outdated maps, is that you are in territory that is not safe, and introducing change of any sort exaggerates that perceived danger. So Triple Warmer's default response is to resist change. The habits and programs it maintains have kept you alive to this point, so it endorses every one of them. It is also uninterested in subtleties. It doesn't care if you are happy or unhappy, only that you are surviving and safe. Operating beneath your consciousness and with its own agenda, Triple Warmer can be a formidable enemy of your intentions. Of particular relevance for this book, your attachment style is one of the behavioral systems Triple Warmer crafted to help you adapt to your childhood circumstances, and it does not readily allow it to transform.

Attachment and Triple Warmer

Triple Warmer is particularly reactive about your family and primary relationship. In addition to the attachment style formed during your childhood, your ancestors' survival and propagation depended on their mate and clan, so Triple Warmer is alert for any disturbance in the interpersonal field. When it finds one, it can trigger an emotional tempest that leaves both you and your partner stupefied.

The concept that safety, the domain of Triple Warmer, is a core issue in attachment is revealed by the intensity with which couples argue. Who else would you fight with so passionately about disagreements you cannot recall the next day but the one you love? In fact, mammals have a special pathway in their brain that triggers "primal panic" when an attachment relationship seems endangered.[25] When the love between you turns to tension and your collaborative alliance seems to be on the line, your primal instincts are activated. Your ancestors depended on their bond with a partner to survive and bring the next generation forward. When that bond is threatened—whether your overall attachment style is secure or insecure—you and what matters most to you do not feel safe. Triple Warmer goes into overdrive and your rational mind has little influence over what comes next! The Pact (Chapter 3) can restore the balance, but glitches in your attachment style can keep reigniting conflict and tension.

A way to bring your attachment style closer to the secure side of the secure-insecure spectrum is to keep Triple Warmer calm in situations that might trigger feelings and behaviors that are rooted in painful experiences from childhood. While Triple Warmer does not readily release its grip on its survival strategies, you will be more effective if you recognize that not only are you up against a powerful foe, but this "foe" evolved to be your friend. It is, in fact, still helping you stay alive, though it is confused by the plethora of circumstances that did not exist while it was evolving. A basic step you can take to improve your relationship with your partner is to bring Triple Warmer to a calmer default position. Energy medicine offers techniques for working directly with Triple Warmer to do just that. From this more favorable base-line, Triple Warmer is less likely to go into a threat response or to revert to attachment patterns from childhood that were formed in the face of threat or deprivation.

Retraining Triple Warmer

Triple Warmer can hijack your brain, propelling it into outdated fears and thought habits that are the antithesis of secure attachment. An effective approach for changing such habitual strategies is to communicate to Triple Warmer that you are safe in situations where it tends to initiate false alarms. How do you communicate with Triple Warmer? Triple Warmer's language is energy, not words. The following three techniques realign the energies that impact Triple Warmer, bringing Triple Warmer into a more secure state even while you are actively recalling challenging moments in your relationship. The more Triple Warmer is helped in these ways to recognize that such situations do not constitute mortal danger or the annihilation of a primary relationship, the less likely it will overreact.

The Triple Warmer Smoothie

Triple Warmer has its own energy pathway. You can calm and sedate Triple Warmer by tracing your fingers over part of this pathway in the direction that reduces excess energy:

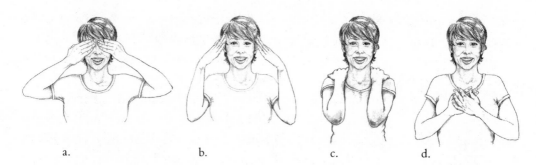

FIGURE 5-1 *The Triple Warmer Smoothie*

1. Bring to mind a situation where you "lost it" with your partner. This can simply be a time that the two of you had a challenging interaction, but even better for this technique if it is an instance of an ongoing pattern.
2. Lay your fingers sideways across your closed eyelids and take a deep in-breath (see Figure 5-1a).
3. As you let your breath out, drag your fingers across your eyes to your temples.
4. With your fingers at your temples, take another deep in-breath and bring your fingers up so they are just above your ears (see Figure 5-1b).
5. As you let your breath out, trace around the back side of your ears with light pressure and go down the side of your neck.
6. Lay your hands over the top of your shoulders and, with an in-breath, push your fingers into the back of your shoulders (see Figure 5-1c).
7. Let your breath out as you pull your fingers hard over your shoulders and drag them down to the middle of your chest (Heart Chakra). Place one hand over the other (see Figure 5-1d).
8. With several deep breaths, softly cradle in your heart the words, "I am safe!"

Triple Warmer Neurovascular Points

You have already learned, with the Stress Release Hold (p. 90), to work with one set of neurovascular points as a way of turning off the fight/flight/freeze response and shifting the neurochemistry of stress. Triple Warmer's neurovascular reflex points are at the temple and can be held along with the points on the forehead to shift outmoded habits of thought:

1. Bring to mind a second situation where you "lost it" with your partner.
2. Lightly place your thumbs on your temples and your fingers on your forehead (see Figure 5-2).
3. Continue to keep the situation in mind during several deep breaths.
4. The energy will begin to shift within a minute or two. End with the words, "I am safe!"

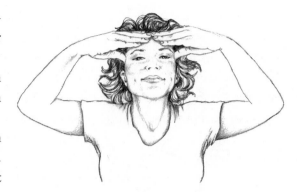

FIGURE 5-2 *Triple Warmer Hold*

Heart Chakra/Triple Warmer Tap

Another part of the Triple Warmer pathway, this one on the back of your hands, can be stimulated to manage anxiety and fear. Holding your hand over your Heart Chakra and tapping Triple Warmer back into balance:

1. Bring to mind yet another situation where you "lost it" with your partner.
2. Put one hand over the middle of your chest (this is your Heart Chakra), and find the V between your ring finger and little finger on the back of that hand.
3. Below the V is a ridge. Tap inside this ridge with the four fingers of your other hand (see Figure 5-3).
4. Finally have both hands resting over your Heart Chakra as you end with the words, "I am safe!"

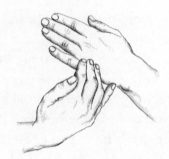

FIGURE 5-3
Heart Chakr/Triple Warmer Tap

Tapping on the ridge of the hand that is over your Heart Chakra can also provide quick emotional first aid *any* time you are feeling anxious or afraid.

These three simple energy techniques, individually (selecting the one that seems to work best for you) or in combination, can be used to desensitize Triple Warmer to interpersonal situations that have tended to hook you.[26] As you shift the energies that maintain fear-based reactions, you are opening a door for changing them. Additional techniques presented in the following two chapters focus on healing the residue of difficult childhood experiences and transforming the emotional and behavioral patterns that arose from them. These techniques involve the stimulation of acupuncture points while bringing specific memories or visualizations to mind, and they can laser into the energies of attachment. You will begin to get a feel for how this is accomplished in the three case histories presented during the following discussion.

Soothing Yourself, Managing Your Emotions, and Repairing Ruptures

While it is beyond the scope of any book to be a *substitute* for psychotherapy or for interactions with a partner that heal childhood attachment wounds, you can do a great deal to enhance your relationship by using techniques that shift the energetic underpinnings of attachment difficulties.

Three basic skill sets that promote secure attachment—soothing yourself, managing your emotions, and repairing ruptures within an intimate partnership—were ideally learned early in life during daily interactions with your primary caregivers. Where you have gaps in these skills, your primary relationships are directly impacted. But it is not like signs are imprinted on our foreheads as we grow up that say "deficits in self-soothing ability" or "poor manager of emotions" or "anxious about intimacy." We develop our skill sets for self-soothing, emotional management, and relating intimately to the extent that we do (or that we don't), and we try to make the best of what we have. What might have been theoretically possible is not on our radar. It is not part of our living reality. Donna's orienting her early life around the theme of not causing trouble made her very good at self-soothing but not as practiced in getting what she needed from her closest relationships, an essential skill for thriving in an intimate partnership. Conscious choice, however, was not involved. If she had a need that would cause any inconvenience for her partner, it did not occur to her to express it and risk being trouble for him.

Can we improve our relationship patterns by further developing and refining these skill sets? For each, we will present some of the basics and describe a person who made a significant positive shift using the energy psychology techniques you will be learning in the following two chapters.

Self-Soothing

Since infants aren't equipped with the ability to soothe themselves when they feel distressed, but only to cry out, they depend on their caregivers to provide comfort. From the responses they receive, they acquire strategies for coping with distressful emotions or difficult experiences. Adults who haven't developed adequate skills for self-soothing tend to become overly reliant on their partner for emotional comfort and resentful when it is not provided.

Skills for improving your mood and bringing calm, nurturing, and pleasure can be learned at any point in your life. They are generally quite basic, relying on your senses. A hot bath is one of Donna's favorites. We both like to take walks in beautiful natural settings. Energy techniques such as those presented on pages 82–94 are always in our tool kit. Music, dance, art, sports, and meditation are other popular forms of self-soothing. Simple enough. Readily available. Often free or almost free. But for people who didn't learn in their formative years that they can make themselves feel better, calmer, or more relaxed, times of distress can lead to an internal panic and often a clutching toward others or an escape into drugs, junk food, or other addictions. It does not occur to them that they can take simple, healthy steps that will help them feel better.

Elizabeth, at thirty-one, frequently felt rebuffed, disregarded, and unloved. While her husband demonstrated his love for her in many ways and was always trying to comfort her, she was, at these times, inconsolable. To make it worse, after these episodes she would withdraw from him further because, despite his sincere efforts, she felt he hadn't been there for her. Self-soothing wasn't even in her repertoire as she would ruminate on how she had been wronged and sank ever deeper into a dark hole of despair. Not only hadn't Elizabeth learned much about self-soothing as a child, you might wonder how she managed to make it into her thirties so unskilled about helping herself feel better during times of emotional distress.

Unfortunately, this type of lapse is not particularly unusual. While many people pick up new skills for self-soothing as they mature, others face internal obstacles that prevent them from learning and using even the most obvious self-soothing skills. So rather than simply trying to teach them techniques for self-soothing, these internal obstacles also need to be addressed.

A theme in Elizabeth's bouts of feeling unloved was that someone else always seemed to be receiving the credit and recognition that she deserved. At another level, however, she felt undeserving of the very recognition she desired and expected. This was particularly evident in her inability to accept compliments even after she had done something extremely well. Rather, she would find flaws in her actions that no one else would even notice and relentlessly beat herself up for them. Obsessing about her own flaws and sinking into her resentment of those who she felt had wronged her consumed her so completely that doing things that might make her feel better simply did not come into her mind.

Derived from the field of energy psychology, the protocol used with Elizabeth (which you will be learning in chapters 6 and 7) includes two basic steps. The first involves giving a zero-to-ten rating on the level of distress or discomfort you feel in relation to an issue you wish to change. The second is to stimulate a set of acupuncture points by tapping on them while keeping the issue active in your mind. This simple combination is proving to be extraordinarily powerful in rewiring the neural pathways that underlie a range of emotional difficulties.

Elizabeth's initial rounds of tapping focused on the fierce judgments she would place on herself, which she had rated as being at a 10 in relation to the amount of distress she felt when thinking about them. What emerged as she continued to tap were childhood memories of longing for her father's approval, which she never received (as she remembered it), yet when her younger brother was born, he got the praise and adoration she so desperately craved. Tapping on her pain about this started a healing process that went very deep. She was eventually able to recognize and tap on the exaggerated authority she was still giving her father to determine her sense of worth. In a subsequent session, she focused on and neutralized her emotional response to specific, recent incidents where she had judged herself harshly and was unable to accept sincere compliments about things others felt she had done well.

By the time she'd made some progress with these issues, the tapping was able to directly address self-soothing. A mental association was made by using energy techniques to link times of feeling despondent with doing activities that consoled her (e.g., "Even though there may still be times that I feel down, I know I will feel better if I sit on the porch and listen to Enya"). Not only did the episodes of struggling with her self-worth become much less intense and less frequent, but it now occurred to her when they did happen that she could take positive steps that would bring her comfort and relief. Finally, she was given instruction in four ways to "put money in the bank" so her reserves would already be stronger at times she needed self-soothing.

These were simple physical or interpersonal actions that were in her control: enough sleep, enough exercise, enough physical touch, and enough emotional contact.

Learning to self-soothe had an enormous impact on Elizabeth's marriage. She no longer would desperately look to her husband to make her feel better or rage at him when he couldn't. By having a way to amp down to a manageable level the intensity when she was feeling bad, she was also able to let her husband help her. Now that his overtures of support could be received when they were needed, what had been a thorny obstacle to their being close to one another became a source of bonding.

Emotional Self-Management

The second skill set that grows out of your early attachment experiences is the ability to manage your emotions. More than a hundred human emotions have been identified,[27] with most of them being combinations of or the social shaping of a few basic emotions found in people of all cultures, such as anger, fear, sadness, disgust, surprise, anticipation, trust, and joy.[28] The English word *emotion* is derived from the Old French *esmovoir*, meaning "to excite." While psychologists define this basic concept in numerous ways, all would agree that emotions involve arousal ("to excite") and that they influence the way we process our thoughts and experiences.

At the most basic level, in the life of an infant, an internal event (such as hunger or feeling cold) or an external event (such as a warm blanket or a loud sound), results in simple appraisals: "this is good" or "this is bad." While this is the prototype for the more nuanced emotions that will come later, this basic assessment of good or bad, Daniel Siegel explains, "prepares the brain and the rest of the body for action."[29]

The parents' responses to the infant's expressions of positively toned or negatively toned arousal lay down the neural pathways that help children learn to regulate their own nervous systems. You figured out how to manage your "states of arousal and inner processing"[30] through those early interactions. If your parents' responses to you were attuned to your internal experiences, you were likely to form a secure foundation for navigating through life with confidence about the validity of your feelings and thoughts. If your early caregivers usually failed to validate your internal experiences in their moment-to-moment exchanges with you, your foundation for trusting your feelings and thoughts as valid guides became shaky. If this lack of attunement is extreme, as in cases of abusive, emotionally disturbed, or severely neglectful parents, children are set on their journey through life with a compass that is fundamentally flawed. They may find themselves regularly pushing down the truth of their emotions and experiences, distorting them, or becoming overwhelmed by them.

Early caregivers not only validate or fail to validate the child's internal experiences, they also model for the child how to respond when others express their emotions. A parent whose internal state is dominated by fear or anger simultaneously evokes fear or anger in the child and also, through reinforcement, teaches the child specific ways of responding to fear or anger. A girl may take it upon herself to give a fearful mother the support she herself really needs from that mother, or try to make herself invisible in the presence of an angry father. These patterns tend to carry over into her adult relationships even when they no longer fit.

Individual childhood experiences involving trauma, severe loss, or other emotionally intense experiences, if they are not adequately processed, can also lead to patterns of emotional response that are not appropriate to the current situation. In *Parenting from the Inside Out*, Siegel and Mary Hartzell identify two basic types of responses to emotionally challenging situations: the "high road" and the "low road."[31] The *high road* is dominated by advanced brain structures that came later in evolution and sit "higher," toward the top of the head, in the cerebral cortex. The *low road* is dominated by brain structures that sit below the cerebral cortex, including the amygdala, and that govern automatic behaviors such as the fight/flight/freeze response. When you are on the "high road," your responses are well considered, flexible, and appropriate to the situation. When you are overly stressed or in a situation that otherwise triggers you into the "low road" state of mind, which includes being trapped in your Energetic Stress Style, you may be flooded by intense emotions such as fear, sadness, or rage, leading to "knee-jerk reactions instead of thoughtful responses."[32]

We have all experienced "low road" behaviors from both sides—we've received them and we've acted them out. Unresolved childhood issues make us more susceptible to these storms of difficult feelings and inappropriate actions. When "low road" responses occur, and particularly when they repeat themselves, notice what triggers them. If you can't identify the triggers, your partner probably can. You can then use the energy psychology approach presented in chapters 6 and 7 to defuse these emotional triggers.

Sometimes, however, this requires more than just focusing on the trigger. You saw how, in order to learn self-soothing, Elizabeth had to first overcome emotional obstacles rooted in earlier experiences. A seminar on self-soothing wasn't going to be very useful to her until these interfering issues had been resolved. Learning how to manage intense emotions also often requires a focus on unresolved issues from the past. Fortunately, as you work with the behaviors you want to change, earlier experiences that are at their root often come into your awareness, making them accessible for healing using the energy psychology protocol you will be learning.

For example, a successful medical technology executive named Raul would become furious when younger associates disagreed with him, even if the disagreements were trivial. While in most situations he had a very sweet disposition, this pattern was also carrying into his marriage and his relationship with his children. It was clear to him that his outbursts were hurtful to everyone, including himself, but he was failing to prevent them despite his resolve to do so. Tapping on recent incidents and imagined situations that might trigger him lowered the intensity he felt to a degree, but it could be no match for these deeply ingrained behaviors until their roots were being addressed.

Raul's father, a physician, was very stern with his three sons and imposed his will on them with criticism and rage. Raul was chagrined to realize that he had, in terms of those traits, become a carbon copy of his father. Imprints from such emotional models do not change easily, but over several energy psychology sessions, significant shifts occurred. The tapping focused on images of his enraged father, the feelings they brought up in him, and the thoughts and conclusions he came to as a result of these experiences. Each childhood experience involving anger that he could recall was addressed using the tapping. With these earlier experiences revisited and emotionally reworked, the triggers in his current life were easily brought down to zero on the zero-to-ten scale, and he found himself able to stay on the "high road" when these same triggers presented themselves. The neural pathways maintaining the old pattern had shifted, and managing his anger was now rarely a problem (yes, we are trying to get you excited for the energy psychology instructions in the following chapter).

Repairing Ruptures

To thrive, we need both intimate contact and alone time. Most ongoing relationships provide ample opportunity for both. They are composed of an unending series of separations and reconnections, part of the ebb and flow of daily life. If your parents gave you space for solitude and were then available when you needed connection again, you are already practiced in the dance of coming and going. More challenging for everyone, however, are separations that are experienced not just as a temporary time apart but as a rupture.

With children as well as adults, the consequences of a rupture depend more on whether, how, and how quickly the rupture is repaired than on its nature. How to repair the unavoidable ruptures that occurred as you were growing up was modeled (and in other ways taught to you) by your parents. In some families, ruptures are ignored as much as possible. You are supposed to "get over it" and just go on. In others, resentments are built and harbored. These strategies tend to echo into the person's adult relationships.

Families that are effective at repairing the inevitable ruptures among their members feel safer, produce children who are happier and more emotionally secure, and meet life's challenges with greater ease and flexibility. To repair a rupture, you first need to bring yourself from the "low road" of mental functioning back to the "high road." Siegel and Hartzell suggest steps that will be familiar to you as elements of your STAR Pact (chapter 3), including a temporary separation (the Pact's "Stop"), physical activity (the Pact's "Tap" and other energy techniques), empathically stepping into the other's experience (the Pact's "Attune"), and finally reengaging (the Pact's "Resolve").[33]

Vern and Gloria rarely argued. Whenever they had differences, Vern would quickly tune into Gloria's position and take it as his own. If this was not possible and a rupture between them did occur, Vern would be disheartened, certain it was his fault, and feel full of shame as he tried to grovel his way back into Gloria's good graces. While having a spouse who is so eager to agree with you might seem desirable, it was Gloria who brought them into therapy. Although the peace and easy flow they enjoyed in their first two years together had been a relief in comparison to her other relationships, by their fourth year it was seeming to her that she was with a caricature of a real person instead of someone who brought his own feelings, thoughts, and opinions into the relationship.

Vern's parents had minimized or made light of their differences rather than acknowledging and resolving conflicts, a workable if not ideal strategy, discussed in Chapter 1 as that of the Avoidant couple. A product of his past, Vern brought this style to his relationship with Gloria. But for Gloria, emotional engagement was a vital aspect of a relationship, and all Vern's agreeableness only left her feeling lonely. True to form, Vern agreed to Gloria's suggestion that they enter therapy to change *his* basic way of relating.

Just as you saw with Elizabeth and Raul, work that began with a stated concern quickly shifted to childhood experiences. Vern recounted the way he was witness to unspoken tension between his parents on a myriad of issues, from dinner choices to which car to buy. With little discussion, his mother's preferences would generally carry the decision, but expressions of his father's resentment and his mother's guilt, which couldn't be concealed, were prominent in Vern's memory.

Vern used the acupuncture point tapping protocol while focusing on those memories, on his shame about not being able to do a thing about the tension in his family, and on his reluctance to introduce any tension into his marriage. While his zero-to-ten rating rapidly went down in relation to his past, it would not go below 5 as he focused on his being more forthcoming with his preferences in the marriage. He was clearly ambivalent about that objective.

As Vern explored his ambivalence, it became clear that he had dire misgivings about what would happen if he ever took a strong stand that challenged Gloria's position on virtually any matter. One big reason for this, it turned out, was that he had no idea of how to repair a relationship rupture since he was so inexperienced with them. He imagined, instead, that it would spread like a wildfire until the marriage had been destroyed. In the safety of the therapy office, he was able to tell Gloria clearly and firmly that he felt she was being much too strict with their adolescent daughter. This triggered Gloria into a strong defensive reaction. She was proud of her parenting skills and thought her husband appreciated and fully supported them. Hearing that he didn't shocked her and flooded her with feelings that brought her onto what we have been calling the "low road." She was deeply hurt, felt betrayed that Vern had given her no clue, and was soon ruminating about all the other areas where he might be secretly judging her. She also let him know, with escalating volume, how absurdly wrong he was in the beliefs about child-rearing he was expressing.

It suddenly seemed as if Vern's fears had been well taken and that if they ever got through this therapy-induced mess, he should keep his opinions to himself forever after. Gloria was completely unaware that she was fulfilling Vern's catastrophic expectations about doing exactly what she was asking him to do. I (David) was, at that moment, reflecting on the dubious wisdom of having chosen a profession that messes with a family's established adaptations. But I also knew that this was an opportunity for them to have the experience of repairing a relationship rupture. I took them through the steps of the Pact. By the end, Gloria was back on the "high road" and we were all laughing about the ironies that had just played out. Vern had had the experience that even one of the worst reactions he could imagine to his having stated a disagreement had been repaired within half an hour.

During the week following the session, they had numerous deep and creative discussions about discipline for their kids and were feeling closer to one another than they had for a long time. In the next session, with Vern now having a sense that ruptures could be repaired instead of being something to be avoided at all costs, additional acupuncture point tapping dissolved his knee-jerk discomfort about stating a disagreement to Gloria. Being able to tolerate ruptures and repair them were essential skills in Vern's ability to take a next step in the evolution of his marriage.

The three skill sets discussed in this section—self-soothing, emotional self-management, and being able to repair ruptures within an intimate partnership—are laid down in our family of origin and early interactions with our caregivers. But they are skills that we can continue to develop and refine throughout our lives. Particularly in the crucible of our intimate partnerships, we discover the shortcomings of the strategies we have brought forth from childhood. The cases described here illustrate breakdowns in these three core relationship skill sets. Each was quite challenging—but not particularly unusual. We hope this discussion has provided a context for recognizing your own strengths with these skills as well as for assessing areas where they may need attention, along with instructive models. Healthier attachment in your most intimate relationships is a reward well worth striving toward.

On to Chapter 6

As you saw with Elizabeth, Raul, and Vern and Gloria, tapping on acupuncture points—the core physical procedure in energy psychology—can be applied to overcoming lapses in your relationship skills while strengthening the foundation of your bond. These focused efforts can also help with many other aspects of your relationship and, not just incidentally, with your own personal evolution as well. Chapter 6 introduces you to the basic steps of a simple but powerful energy psychology protocol.

6

Changing Your Future by Not Repeating Your Past

Tapping Your Way to a New Brain Chemistry

The real voyage of discovery consists not in seeking new landscapes, but in having new eyes.

—MARCEL PROUST[1]

ASED ON OUR THREE DECADES OF TEACHING ENERGIES OF LOVE SEMINARS, OUR editor at Tarcher/Penguin asked us to write this book. We found it an exciting invitation, but we had a somewhat superstitious hesitation. We have known several couples over the years who have written books on couples work whose marriages dissolved shortly after their book was published. We did not want to tempt the relationship gods. Along with the personal catastrophe and awkward embarrassment that would be involved, we were wary about the arrogance of holding ourselves out as a couple who had somehow "figured out" the sweet and not-so-sweet mysteries of love.

And sure enough, as soon as we were earnestly discussing the book with the publisher, our relationship took a serious downhill turn. Our organization happened to be exploding at the time, growing exponentially. We were both under tremendous pressure. Not surprisingly, given the chasms between the ways each of us approaches the world, we weren't seeing eye to eye on many of the critical decisions we were making that would shape the future of our organization and our life's work. To make it worse, the sensory systems that are our defaults when under stress (chapter 1) seemed to be getting so exaggerated that misunderstandings were amassing. Donna, as a kinesthetic, is highly expressive emotionally while David, as a digital, wants to crawl into his interior cave and regroup at times of distress. So Donna would feel unmet and discounted, and this would of course escalate her sense of distress. Feeling pressed to not retreat, David tried to center himself for each hot topic we would encounter, but he began to respond in a way that "I could hardly believe was me."

With unrelenting stress between us, and both of us locked into our threat response styles, David would be pushed over the edge of his calm defenses. He would begin to scream at Donna, swear at her, and generally escalate a situation that was already too escalated. Yes, even a die-hard digital can lose it. Your Energetic Stress Style is a way of processing information, but pushed far enough by the one you love and your reasoning abilities can regress to roughly the equivalent of a four-year-old during a tantrum. That your partner can send you down the rabbit hole into another encounter with your rough edges seems part of nature's grand plan to help you evolve.

After each incident, David would will himself to not get triggered the next time. He would use all the techniques he knew. He could bring to mind the last fight and use tricks to decrease his emotional response while recalling it, and that seemed to help. He would then enter the next encounter centered, clear, and confident, but within five minutes find himself screaming again and slamming doors. What ominous portents for writing our magnum opus on relationships! One day after it had happened for about the fifteenth time in three months, he went out to the hot tub of the condominium where we were staying. Fortunately, no one else was there. He decided to try a mindfulness practice to go deeper into his understanding of what was happening. Here is his account of what occurred:

> I set my intention on noticing the texture of my experience at the time of these explosions and right before them. With that in place, I simply followed my breathing and noticed what emerged. At first there was a lot of inner chatter, self-justifications, self-judgments, anger at Donna, seeing Donna's sweet countenance having turned fierce in frustration and anger, fear of being discovered to be a fraud, images of the headline in our energy e-letter announcing the divorce of the self-proclaimed relationship virtuosos. I just noticed each and let it go. Back to the breath. Then a very vague image emerged. But I was able to place it. It was the bus stop where I was left off every day after

school during first grade. Another boy and I were the only two left off there. Unfortunately for me, he was the class bully, a wiry but very strong boy who for some reason was called Pudgy. I remember that his father was a police officer and that he was the toughest kid and the best fighter in our class. I, on the other hand, was tall, skinny, highly uncoordinated, painfully shy, and socially awkward—the perfect target for bullies of far less stature than Pudgy. So it wasn't a big rush for him to beat me up, and I usually got away with just a punch to the stomach or jaw, just enough to make me cry. Once he was satisfied that he had done enough damage to reaffirm his dominance, he would turn away and walk home.

But on the day that came up in my vision, something ominous had happened in school. The teacher was angry at the class for being particularly unruly. She kept us in instead of letting us go as usual to the playground for recess. But she had to deal with us needing a bathroom break, so she had all the boys line up in one line, all the girls in another, and marched us to the boys' and girls' lavatories. But first she gave a warning that if even one of us spoke, the entire class would have to put their heads down for thirty minutes afterward, a most unwelcome punishment for children with growing, restless bodies. If we retained perfect silence during the bathroom break, she would instead read us a story we were all eager to hear. After I finished at the urinal, I walked up to the sink to wash my hands and another boy walked up to it at the same time. I stepped back and invited him to go first. At that unfortunate moment, the teacher happened to glance into the boys' bathroom, saw my mouth moving, and that was that. The whole class spent the next interminable half hour with our collective little heads on our folded little arms on our uncomfortable little desks. The teacher did not announce the name of the culprit, but she said it was someone she never would have suspected. Of course, by the end of the school day, everyone knew it was me. I could not have been more humiliated or felt more ostracized.

It also gave occasion for Pudgy to give me an extra-vigorous beating that day. And that was the scene that emerged out of the initial vague image of the bus stop. I was surprised it came up right then, in part because I had decades earlier dealt with my relationship with Pudgy ad nauseam in psychodynamic talk therapy. I felt done with it, processed, complete. I particularly didn't, at first, see any relationship between this memory and my arguments with

Donna. But even as I kept bringing my awareness back to my breath, I had opened a portal that kept presenting different aspects of the memory and then connections to my current problem. While no one would ever see Donna as a bully, with the pressures on us, the complex demands of the organization, and the curse of having agreed to hold our relationship up as a model, we became about as acrimonious as we'd ever been in our thirty-three years together at that point. I felt I was giving my heart and soul to the organization, and Donna's disagreement and judgment of my best efforts felt as unfair as becoming the class villain for having simply indicated to another boy that he could use the sink first.

The sense of unfairness and injustice was the invisible link between what I was playing out with Donna and what still was unhealed in my psyche. My sense of feeling bullied became the psychological context of our interchanges. I would simply be in a discussion with Donna about a sensitive issue and suddenly and uncharacteristically find myself screaming at her as if my life depended on it. I was desperate as each unresolved encounter was not only damaging our relationship; the unsolved problems were hurting our organization in ways that were making our lives more difficult. By "acupoint tapping" [the technique you will learn in this chapter] on the memory and on the theme of being bullied, the triggers lost their power, and my reactions to more recent altercations could be neutralized as well. I've not been hooked in one of those discussions since. This had a positive domino effect. Now Donna could express her frustrations and be heard rather than fought, allowing genuine problem solving to occur, and we were soon back on track with one another. I have a large bag of clinical tricks, but acupoint tapping was what popped me through the doorway that eliminated this explosive trip wire from our marriage.

The steps David took when life had thrust him beyond his usual coping strategies began with identifying a childhood experience that was at the root of a current difficulty. This is where many transformational approaches, from Freud's psychoanalysis onward, begin. The difficulties we run into with our partners often have an analog in our past, our attachment history. What is *new* is a deepened appreciation of the role of the body in matters of the mind. A powerful new order of psychological healing is emerging with psychotherapies that work with soma (body) as well as psyche. After all, we are, fundamentally, "embodied psyches." The entire body—not just the brain—carries our memories, our conflicts, our life lessons, even the latency of the next stage in our evolution, and it does so in its energy systems.[2] From the body and its energies emerges a whole new order of transformative healing, unavailable when psychotherapy was limited to *psychological* treatment. Bringing the viscera into the process of emotional healing opens a body-mind dynamic that has not previously been integrated, raising a whole new spiral of possibility.

How a Little Knowledge about Acupuncture Points Can Do a Lot of Good

The organs of emotion—such as the heart, stomach, kidneys, and liver—are energetically connected to points on the skin known as acupuncture points (acupoints). Simplistic as you may find it to be, tapping on acupoints while focusing on a problem is the most direct and potent route we know for involving the body in the psychotherapeutic process. It initiates a reprocessing of unresolved emotional experiences, allowing current patterns to rapidly shift, and it is one of the main interventions used in energy psychology.

Acupoints are gateways into the body's energy system, acting like switches that can increase or decrease the flow of energy to specific areas of the body. The traditional use of acupuncture needles is not necessary. Energy psychology teaches you how to tap on or massage about a dozen points that influence your emotions while you think about specific scenes that are associated with a problem or a goal. The process shifts not only the *psychological atmosphere* that surrounds the situation being focused upon—reducing anxiety, increasing confidence, healing old wounds, and generally enhancing your freedom to move through the situation more effectively and more joyfully—it also changes your *brain chemistry.*[3] With acupoint tapping, you can eliminate outdated emotional patterns by altering the neural pathways that maintain them.

Energy psychology practitioners, in fact, often comment on the way a client believes a particular issue was resolved in previous psychotherapy, only to discover that the old thoughts, feelings, and behavior are still intruding. After addressing the problem at the body level, in this case with acupoint tapping, the pattern is transformed at its neurological core. David had previously talked to therapists "ad nauseam" about the bullying he had experienced, and this did increase his insight and under-

> **→ THE ENERGY DIMENSION ←**
>
> **Acupuncture Points**
>
> More than three hundred points on the surface of the body, known as acupuncture points, fall along the meridians—energy pathways that were identified by ancient Chinese physicians thousands of years ago. The acupuncture points are vital spots on the surface of the body that have lower electrical resistance and greater sensitivity than other areas of the skin. They are situated on meridian lines that have been verified by modern scientists as corresponding with the body's connective tissue.[4]

standing. However, his visceral response during situations that brought up emotions tracing to his having been bullied was still occurring. The good news for us, and for you, is that by combining simple acupoint tapping techniques with current understanding about how the brain works, energy psychology is making available, to anyone, straightforward procedures for bringing about deep change. We can quickly and decisively shift long-standing patterns that limit us and our relationships.

The way it works may seem simple, yet *embodying* psychological change via a body-based intervention such as tapping is a profound advance within psychotherapy. You bring to mind an emotional memory or trigger, tap on a sequence of acupoints, and a shift occurs in your brain, your energies, and your psyche. Old wounds heal. Destructive patterns lose their grip. New possibilities open. Improbable as this sounds, the science and clinical research showing how this is possible, why energy psychology is effective, are laid out in a journal article that was originally written for this chapter. It became too long and academic, but it is available as a free download from www.tapping.innersource.net.

My Beloved, You Are the Catalyst for My Growth—Thanks a Lot!

Psyches become intertwined in deep relationships. "Neural feedback loops" get formed that are so potent that two brains begin, in some ways, to function as one, as a single *collective nervous system*.[5] The partners' energies respond to one another before a word has been spoken. Attachment at work! One spouse begins to feel an emotional need, energetic signals are transmitted, and the other's brain is activated in response to it. Sweet . . . assuming that your partner's brain is inclined toward loving, attuned, and validating thoughts.

We do not, however, come into our relationship with a clean slate emotionally. Many of the psychological difficulties people have in their relationships trace to difficult emotional experiences from the past. These result in entrenched learnings that are at the core of emotional responses, behavioral patterns, and beliefs about ourselves and our world that can undermine our best intentions. They are the leopard's spots of the human psyche, notoriously difficult to change. David's closing down or striking out when a situation felt unfair traced back to his being unjustly blamed and bullied more than fifty years earlier. Such internal scenarios are often at the root of destructive patterns that follow people throughout their lives. David's unprocessed experience regarding the bullying incident and the impact it was having on our marriage is a drama that repeats itself in untold varieties for all couples.

Your relationship has, in fact, an astounding capacity to re-create whatever issues are unresolved within you. Many couples suffer with the intrusion of the same persistent issues day after day and year after year. To protect themselves, they may—consciously or unconsciously—structure their interactions to try to avoid these painful areas. Our dear friend Peg Elliott Mayo, who was David's first clinical supervisor in 1968, refers to this strategy as "wallpapering over the cockroaches." Such "no-fly" zones may work to some degree, but when you draw lines beyond which you or your partner may not venture, your spontaneity and intimacy suffer as well. This limiting arrangement may descend beneath the surface and become embedded in the foundation of your relationship. A woman's oversensitivity to criticism results in her husband withholding information that is vital for an intimate flow between them. A man's hair-trigger anger causes his wife to hatch down her spontaneity with him. This decreases the frequency of his outbursts but does not eliminate them, and she is systematically dampening her spirit every day.

What was nature up to in arranging things so those we love most bring out the parts of us that are most difficult to love? The impulse is strong for our emotional wounds to be played out again and again in our deepest relationships. Perhaps this strange twist of Love's plan is designed to make us catalysts for one another's growth and healing? Old patterns repeat themselves—again and again—until they are brought to a new resolution.

While this new resolution is not automatic or guaranteed, healing old wounds that are at the basis of ongoing difficulties opens new vistas. Painful as it may be to enter this territory—even when mindful and armed with tools for healing—the outcome can transform you as well as your relationship in many-splendored ways. Your partnership provides not only the *context* in which old wounds play out; it can also be a *container* for healing them.

What Tapping Can Do for You and Your Relationship

Some of the most potent tools for bringing about such healings involve working with your energies. Energetic patterns that trace to childhood carry into new situations. Think of how a magnet under a piece of paper on which iron filings have been placed will create a pattern. You can replace the iron filings with a totally different set of iron filings and you will still see the same pattern. Childhood experiences are coded in your body's energies, and these energies act as templates that impose the same essential patterns—again and again—on the unfolding panorama of your life, even as the characters and circumstances change. Articulating the way this works was Freud's landmark contribution, but the talk therapy he developed for transforming persistent themes tracing to earlier times was often not powerful enough to produce deep, lasting change. It turns out that energy fields, by organizing the brain's neural pathways, provide the glue that keeps old patterns in place, and also hold the key for changing them.[6]

Energy psychology addresses problems at this level, impacting the energy fields that maintain outdated psychological habits. When you bring to mind an emotional problem—such as a situation with your partner that triggers irrational hurt or anger—you activate the energy field involved with that problem. Simultaneously, tapping on selected acupoints that produce calm shifts the internal landscape around the problem.

Can tapping really make that much difference? David's reactions to Donna, tracing to his childhood experiences of having been the victim of bullying, were transformed in a single evening. Numerous studies have established the effectiveness of acupoint tapping in resolving a range of psychological difficulties quickly and permanently.[7] Here are seven ways energy psychology can help improve your relationship:

1. Navigate through emotional intensity without escalating.
2. Change how you respond to triggers that had evoked anger, hurt, or resentment.
3. Trace emotional challenges to formative attachment experiences.
4. Heal emotional wounds that emerged from those experiences.
5. Transform the patterns that grew out of those wounds.
6. Complete any other "unfinished business," including "baggage" from earlier relationships or from an earlier time in your current relationship.
7. Establish a strong mental vision of how you want yourself or your relationship to change and rewire your brain to support that vision.

Extraordinary promises? Yes! We discuss limitations and caveats shortly, but we can say that over the course of our long careers, energy psychology is the most powerful single tool we've found for helping couples change unwanted patterns in their interactions. We invite you to set aside your probable disbelief if you've never seen it in action and give it a try.

Important Guidelines and Responsibilities to Review before You Begin

Energy psychology is a simple but powerful tool. Like any powerful tool, it should be used with care and a consciousness about its limitations as well as its strengths. We will be showing you how to apply it on a self-administered, self-help basis. At the time of this writing, more than half a million people have participated in *each* of the last four annual online World Tapping Summits, and over two million people have downloaded a manual that provides the basics of using energy psychology on a self-help basis. These are unprecedented numbers for any self-help approach. People are finding that it works for them. Studies of clinical outcomes when administered by psychotherapists have uncovered virtually no reports of harm being caused by the protocol,[8] though no research has, to date, investigated its safety as a self-help technique. Thus the following cautions.

Learning a method like this from a book has all the limitations of any one-way teaching process. Beyond that, mastering the basics of energy psychology won't make you a therapist if you aren't already one. The human psyche is the most complex terrain in the known universe, and it can be delicate. From our workshops, however, and from seeing the work of others who teach energy methods, we believe that virtually anyone can use energy psychology in ways that will benefit them. Just as deep breathing can relax your cardiovascular system, tapping on selected acupoints can reduce dysfunction, anger, jealousy, anxiety, fear, and other unwanted emotions. This is a straightforward mechanical process. You bring a problematic emotional response to mind and then you create an internal energetic context that is not compatible with that emotional response. After showing you how to do the mechanics, we will guide you in applying it in ways that are designed to benefit your relationship.

How far you can take this depends on a variety of factors. First of all, there are some circumstances where you should proceed *only* with a well-trained, licensed psychotherapist or marriage counselor. If you have a history of severe trauma in your background, a serious mental health condition, or if your relationship is deeply troubled, if it involves emotional or physical abuse, drugs, alcohol, gambling, or other serious addictions, or if it is on the brink of separation, your needs are beyond the scope of an unguided application of the techniques presented in this and the following chapter. The chapters may inspire you to use acupoint tapping, but you should not use it except with professional guidance.

If the above cautions do not apply and you are using the approach taught here on a self-help basis, your success with the methods will depend in part on your motivation. The chapters in this section teach you a skill that requires practice and application. You can read about them and acquire a good deal of information without applying them, but for the benefits listed above, you need to dig in and give it a try. When you do, you will almost certainly find the tools empowering, but you may also run into some obstacles. The first is that we all have blind spots, particularly in areas where old learnings and unprocessed experiences are interfering with our current responses and understanding. You may simply not be able to navigate your way through this territory in a manner that brings you to the healings and empowerment that is nonetheless available. If you get stuck in your own self-help efforts, asking your partner for assistance may bring in another set of eyes, ears, perspective, and understanding that helps you get to the other side. But it may require someone with professional training or at least someone who is not intimately involved in the situation.

Counselors who use energy psychology can be found in virtually any major city.[9] Some are licensed mental health professionals. Some operate as life coaches, as peak performance consultants, or with similar designations. Many athletes and entertainers, for instance, find energy psychology extraordinarily useful in enhancing their performance. Business and community leaders find that it provides invaluable tools for building on their strengths and overcoming their foibles. The line between being able to benefit from self-help methods and needing professional assistance can be blurry and deserves careful and responsible examination.[10]

In addition to the circumstances mentioned earlier, brain health is another consideration. Particularly for people who have suffered brain injuries, severe emotional trauma, exposure to toxic substances, abuse of alcohol or drugs, ongoing sleep deprivation, or chronic poor nutrition, the impact on your brain may be limiting your relationship. Fortunately, much can be done to overcome these limitations. In his book *The Brain in Love*, psychiatrist Daniel Amen provides information on how to identify deficiencies in specific brain areas and how to address those deficiencies with mental or physical exercises, diet, nutritional supplements, or medication when necessary.[11]

We also want you to be aware that tapping on an issue *can* increase the intensity of your emotions and distress about it *before* it reduces them. This is not what usually happens, nor is the tapping itself actually increasing the distress. Rather, as the tapping begins to reduce your distress, it may open a way for you to more fully engage the situation emotionally, and repressed feelings may flood in. New layers may also emerge, such as memories of similar situations from your past that were never fully resolved. Continuing with the protocol presented here will usually get you through these seeming setbacks, but if you are feeling overwhelmed, go directly to the instructions in "If the Program Becomes Unsettling" at the end of this chapter. You can return to the issue later alone or with the support of your partner, another person with a facility in using energy psychology techniques, or a psychotherapist. When an issue gets worse before it gets better, the good news is that you are on to something significant and have the possibility of moving blocked energies out of you. This is freeing not just psychologically but physically as well.

One more important caveat. Please don't use the tools offered here as a weapon against your partner! If your partner is angry or otherwise upset with you, that is *not* the time to say, "Just tap it away, dear!" It is a time to listen. If listening and responding from your heart doesn't resolve the issues, then it is time to apply your Pact

(Chapter 3). Acupoint tapping may be one of the tools you use to center yourself and bring balance to your own energies (Part 2 of the Pact), but it is not a method for either partner to try to impose on the other. The line between *suggest* and *impose* can, however, be deceptively thin.

The "Basic Recipe": A Simple, Effective Energy Psychology Protocol

We must admit that for all the reasons just discussed, we were reluctant to present these methods here. We could have simply advised you to take a class together in Emotional Freedom Techniques (EFT), Thought Field Therapy (TFT), Tapas Acupressure Technique (TAT), Be Set Free Fast (BSFF), or one of the other popular forms of energy psychology. Such classes are increasingly available in local communities and regularly taught at seminar retreat centers such as Esalen Institute, the Omega Institute, and Kripalu. Reports from individuals who have used the procedures safely and effectively on a self-help basis have, however, been accumulating. We have heard them not only from our colleagues and students. Thousands of case reports describing positive outcomes have been posted on websites, blogs, and other electronic media.[12] While still anecdotal, the positive results being described have given us confidence that—after offering the above precautions and the additional guidelines you will find at the end of this chapter—we can offer the method to you responsibly and with optimism.

The best way to learn the techniques of energy psychology from a book is to experiment with them on yourself.[13] Again, as with any powerful tool, there are some skills to master and some inherent dangers. While tapping itself is as safe a self-help intervention as exists, opening yourself to past wounds or traumatic memories can evoke unpleasant emotions that may be challenging, particularly for people who are going through a highly stressful time or are already emotionally unstable. Thus the above words of caution that if you are concerned that using these methods on a self-help basis may be too unsettling for you, please discuss them first with someone whose perspective you trust—friend, spouse, family member, therapist, spiritual counselor. If you are dealing with the aftermath of severe trauma or a diagnosable psychiatric condition, please use these techniques only in consultation with a qualified mental health professional. You can also simply read or skip these chapters for now, go on to Part 3, and decide at a later point whether and how to experiment with the guided instructions.

But if you are ready and interested in learning an important skill that can serve you and your relationship for the rest of your lives, take the time to use the following instructions as a tutorial. They will teach you a skill that can be of enormous value in bringing the energies of love into full bloom. Begin by going through these steps individually, even if you are working with your partner. The text will tell you when to start working together.

PREVIEW: A BARE-BONES
→ ENERGY PSYCHOLOGY PROTOCOL—THE "BASIC RECIPE" ←

Preliminaries
Select a memory or problem, rate your distress from zero to ten, center yourself with energy balancing, and formulate an Acceptance Statement and a Reminder Phrase.

Part 1: Rub the Central Meridian points (see Figure 6-1) while saying, "Even though [name problem]" (Reminder Phrase) and then place your hands over the center of your chest while saying, "I deeply love and accept myself" (Acceptance Statement). Repeat three times.

Part 2: Tap the points (see Figure 6-3) while saying your Reminder Phrase out loud.

Part 3: Do the Integration Sequence: Tap the ridge beneath the V where your ring finger and little finger meet on the back of either hand as you (1) close your eyes, (2) open your eyes, (3) look down to the right, (4) look down to the left, (5) circle your eyes, (6) circle your eyes in the opposite direction, (7) hum a bar of a song, (8) count to five, and (9) hum again. Optionally, end by sweeping your eyes from the floor to the ceiling, sending energy through them.

Part 4: Repeat Part 2.

Repeat this sequence (Parts 1 through 4) as needed, until your rating for the memory or problem is down to zero or near zero. Challenge the results by trying to invoke the disturbing feeling.

Select a Memory

To get right into the Basic Recipe, begin by bringing to mind a memory, preferably from childhood, that has a negative charge for you. Later you will learn to apply the same techniques to unwanted emotional responses that emerge in current situations as well as to other challenges, but for this initial run-through, we suggest you begin with a memory. Most memories that evoke a strong negative feeling have not been fully processed. The experience may have been horrible, and psychologically processing it cannot erase that, but it can alter the brain pathways that cause the memory to evoke the kinds of emotions and physical sensations that were part of the original experience. When this has been accomplished, the memory can be integrated in new ways that make it a resource and source of emotional resilience rather than an area of vulnerability.

For the purposes of this exercise, the memory should not be of an event that involved physical injury or any type of abuse, but it can be one that carries a strong emotional charge, such as the loss of a loved one; the moment you learned your parents were getting divorced; a move from a comfortable home to a neighborhood of strangers; getting lost in what seemed like the wilderness; a pet dying; a betrayal; an embarrassing incident in which your peers, team, or whole class were laughing at you or were upset with you; or a situation where you hurt someone you cared about. We all have them, and while we may not think of them frequently, such memories, until they are fully resolved emotionally, carry an energy that drains us just a bit from our full vitality. They also narrow our world a little because at some level we restrict ourselves from behaviors or choices that might create a similar circumstance. And as we saw in David's "heads on desk" memory, they can bleed through and distort our current experiences.

The memory should be of a specific scene. For example, if the memory is about your family moving and you having a difficult time adjusting, rather than focusing on the challenges you faced in a general way, identify a *specific* memory that epitomizes the difficulties you faced (e.g., "I got lost walking home on the first day of school and thought I'd never find my parents again"). Once you have your memory, write it down. If you are working alongside your partner or with a friend, you can describe your memories to one another at this point instead of writing about them. One of the great strengths of energy psychology for couples is that not only can the procedures be successfully applied on a self-help basis, you can be a tremendous support to your partner by simply being a witness through the process.

Give the Memory a Subjective Units of Distress (SUD) Rating

Once you have selected the scene you wish to work with, the next step of the Basic Recipe is to give it a SUD (subjective units of distress) score. Rate the memory on a scale of zero (no distress) to 10 (extreme distress), based on the amount of discomfort you experience in your body and/or mind when you think about the memory or, as we are about to suggest, as you vividly re-create the memory in your mind.

It is, however, neither necessary nor desirable to do this so vividly that you risk retraumatizing yourself. You can have a successful outcome using energy techniques by just touching into the incident lightly. If the issue you are focusing on is particularly intense, a variety of techniques can be used to keep the memory or feeling "at a distance." You could, for instance, give the scene a rating by "viewing" it through a long tunnel or through the wrong end of binoculars. Or you could simply think about what it *would be like* to think about the issue. In this method, referred to by Gary Craig, the founder of EFT (the most widely used form of energy psychology), as the "tearless trauma" technique,[14] you simply *guess* at what the emotional intensity would be (on a scale of zero to ten) *if* you were to vividly imagine the unpleasant incident.

If, on the other hand, you find yourself having difficulty keeping focused on the memory or accessing your feelings about it, rather than *viewing* the scene, you might use your imagination to help you *enter* the scene. Imagine as vividly as you can what you *might have* seen, heard, smelled, tasted, felt, and/or thought during the incident. This can bring you more deeply into the memory if it is seeming too distant to you, but, again, it is not necessary to immerse yourself in an emotionally traumatizing incident from your past—only that you touch into it. That is enough so it will be neurologically active as you are doing the tapping.

The Movie Technique

While you can simply bring the memory to mind and give it a rating, the technique we suggest for most people, at least initially, is called the "movie technique."[15] You create a short mental movie clip of the scene, play it in your mind, hit pause at the point of maximum intensity (the "crescendo" moment), give that a rating, and then complete the movie. Inner movies are experienced differently from one person to the next. Some people see sharp internal images. For others, imagination is based more on feelings or words or somehow just "knowing." Whatever way your mind creates the "movie" is the right way for you. You will still be able to rate the scene and use energy techniques to work with it. Another alternative for rating the memory is to tell it (again, focusing only on a brief snippet that includes the moment when it reached an emotional crescendo) as a story and giving a rating to the crescendo moment.

If your memory has several climactic points, focus on only one of them. The other crescendos may need to be treated one at a time as separate aspects of the event. If the memory is, for instance, of an automobile accident where you escaped injury, the crescendo points might include hearing the tires skidding, realizing an accident is about to happen, hearing the crash, wondering if you were hurt, and seeing others on the ground. You would treat each as a separate memory, but you will find that once you have neutralized your physiological response to a few of them, the rest will probably fall away quite readily. If your memory has several crescendos, select only one for now.

When you give the zero-to-ten rating on the discomfort or distress you feel while activating the scene, you are rating the intensity the memory evokes in you *right now*, as you tune into it (as contrasted with what you *think* you would feel if you were in the situation again). Once you have rated the scene and finished the movie, you may wish to release any pent-up energy that was stirred. An energy technique such as the Blow-Out (p. 86) can be effective for this.

Memorizing the SUD

Next, share with your partner, write down, or fix in your mind the precise scene you went to and the zero-to-ten SUD rating you gave to it. For some people, children in particular, a more concrete way of rating may be preferred, such as indicating the amount of distress by extending both hands with palms facing to indicate "this much." You will be using the rating as a gauge of your progress as you go through the various procedures.

Center Yourself

Tapping on acupoints is effective for a wide range of situations, but it will tend to be more powerful if you can remove the "static" from your energy system. A way of quickly accomplishing this is to use one or more of the centering techniques on pages 82–94. While this step is not always necessary, it will always bring some benefits, and it can make a great deal of difference if your energies were already scrambled before beginning the energy psychology protocol.

Select a Reminder Phrase

Memories, thoughts, or circumstances that elicit negative emotions cause disruptions not only in the brain but also in the body's energy system. To address a problem by stimulating acupoints, the energy disruption must be mentally activated. For instance, if the memory is of your mother crying because of her disappointment in you, the emotional weight you carry from the incident is not activated or available for healing while you are thinking about what to have for dinner. Tapping the points shown in Figure 6-3, while thinking about the problem, will not only balance the energy system in the moment; it will also retrain your body to be able to hold the memory (or to be able to be in a similar circumstance) without the energy disturbance, and therefore, without the unwanted emotional response.

You may, however, find it a bit difficult to consciously think about the problem while you are doing the tapping. By continually repeating a Reminder Phrase as you tap, you are able to keep yourself psychologically attuned to the situation that has been triggering the disruption in your energy system. The Reminder Phrase is a word or short phrase describing the problem or memory—for instance, "the time my pants ripped during the high school play." A statement like this can activate the problem enough to create a reaction in both your energy system and your brain. Abbreviated versions of the statement, such as "humiliation from the play," or simply "ripped pants," will also suffice as long as their full meaning is clear to you.

You will use your Reminder Phrase in both the Acceptance Statement and the Tapping Sequence. Choose your Reminder Phrase now, a few words that bring the memory to mind, and write it on a piece of paper, in a journal, or electronically.

The Acceptance Statement

The Acceptance Statement is a way of establishing a psychological and energetic receptiveness for changing an emotional response or behavioral pattern. It is simple, mechanical, and effective. It is structured around your Reminder Phrase and uses the following format:

"Even though [Reminder Phrase or slight variation], I deeply love and accept myself."

While many people are accustomed to stating affirmations only in the positive, in this method you describe the difficult memory or undesired response exactly as you experience it. So if your Reminder Phrase is "the time my pants ripped during the high school play," the Acceptance Statement might be:

"Even though I still carry humiliation about my pants having ripped during the play, I deeply love and accept myself."

or shortened, as in:

"Even though I was humiliated during the play, I deeply love and accept myself."

The affirmation is best stated out loud, with feeling and emphasis. Other examples:

- Even though I still feel terrorized about the robbery, I deeply love and accept myself.
- Even though my heart rips in two when I think of Mary rejecting me, I deeply love and accept myself.
- Even though I feel overwhelming guilt about the awful thing I did to Bobby, I deeply love and accept myself.
- Even though I resent the hell out of my mother, I deeply love and accept myself.
- Even though I tend to get headaches at work, I deeply love and accept myself.
- Even though I feel resentment about not getting the promotion, I deeply love and accept myself.
- Even though I am obsessed about my son's grades, I deeply love and accept myself.
- Even though I can't stop smoking, I deeply love and accept myself.

Various alternative wordings could serve the same purpose, which is to accept the problem while at the same time affirming your worthiness despite the existence of the problem. Other wordings are discussed later in the chapter, but the format shown in these examples is easy to memorize and has been used widely with good success. So, in the same place you recorded your Reminder Phrase, write your Acceptance Statement in the form of "Even though I [your emotional reaction about the memory], I deeply love and accept myself." This wording is usually effective for energetically preparing yourself for the next steps, whether or not you fully believe the words!

The Acceptance Statement is different from any other affirmation format you have likely ever before encountered. It begins by summarizing the problem. Most affirmations don't state a negative. In fact, some people who have been trained in the use of hypnosis or self-suggestion are puzzled that a phrase that activates the *unwanted* feeling or response is used in energy psychology. The Acceptance Statement, however, is worded to acknowledge and accept the condition you want to change, such as resolving the lingering embarrassment that traces back to the high school play. It then pairs the statement of what you want to change with a positive affirmation such as "I deeply love and accept myself." If the problematic situation comes into your mind at a later point, you will have already begun to accept the problem and associate it with the positive affirmation.

While the second part of the sentence, "I deeply love and accept myself," may seem a simplistic and overly pat self-affirmation, it seems to somehow interact with the acknowledgment of the problem in a way that eliminates the energy disruption. Any deep suggestion that fosters self-acceptance, despite the unwanted pattern, made with focus and intent, also seems to help people address the problem without the interference of the energy disturbance. "I deeply love and accept myself" is usually effective. If you feel incongruent with this wording, most people can at least say, "I am *learning* to love and accept myself" or "Deep down I know I am a good and worthy human being." Any positive, affirming statement—such as "I know I am doing my best" or "I know Mary loves me"—can have the needed effect. The association between the problem and the positive affirmation can be strengthened by using a pair of energy techniques—involving the Central Meridian and the Heart Chakra—while saying your Acceptance Statement. A caveat is that if *any* positive statement about yourself feels shameful or seems arrogant, you have entered territory where outside help is needed.

Stimulating the Central Meridian

This first technique optimizes the movement of energy in what is called the Central Meridian. The Central Meridian helps govern the energy flow in the central nervous system. For most people, certain points associated with the Central Meridian become sore simply as they go through a normal day. Energy becomes clogged there, particularly at the points on the side of the chest, where the arms attach to the body (see Figure 6-1).

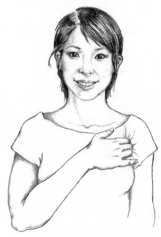

FIGURE 6-1
Stimulating the Central Meridian

To boost the energy moving through the Central Meridian, press in deeply on your left arm attachment points with the thumb or fingers of your right hand. Simultaneously do the same on the right side with your left thumb or fingers. Breathe deeply as you proceed. Massage up and down the lines where your arms meet your body. You will probably find that some of these points are tender. This usually simply means that energy has become clogged there. Massaging it can free the clogged energy and give a boost to your central nervous system. You can press in deeply, but never so much as to cause more than a little discomfort. If painful, decrease the pressure. Also, if you have had an injury in that area or if there is another medical reason not to massage these spots, or if you cannot find a spot that is sore, see if another spot in the general area of your chest is sore and use it. Massage these points as you say the first part of your Acceptance Statement: "Even though I still carry humiliation about my pants having ripped during the play . . ."

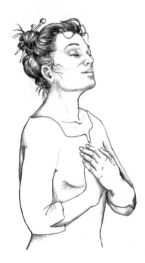

FIGURE 6-2
Activating Your Heart Chakra

Activating Your Heart Chakra

Next place either hand on the center of your chest, your Heart Chakra, and your other hand over the first hand (see Figure 6-2). Hold this position as you say the second part of your Acceptance Statement, "I deeply love and accept myself." Repeat the affirmation three times, alternating between massaging your Central Meridian points on the first phrase and holding your hands over your Heart Chakra on the second phrase.

The Tapping Sequence: The First Part of the Sandwich

The core of the Basic Recipe is called the Sandwich. It includes a tapping sequence, a set of simple physical procedures, and another, identical tapping sequence. Use the eight points or pairs of points shown in Figure 6-3. State the Reminder Phrase while tapping each point. Tapping can be done with either hand or both hands simultaneously. You can tap with the fingertips of your index finger and middle finger, or make a three-finger cluster by including your thumb. Tap each point as you say the Reminder Phrase. Tap solidly but never so hard as to hurt or risk bruising yourself.

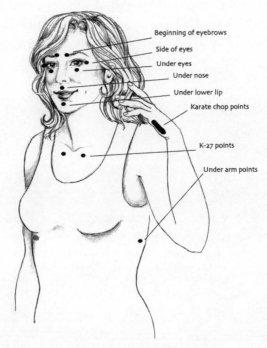

Beginning of eyebrows
Side of eyes
Under eyes
Under nose
Under lower lip
Karate chop points
K-27 points
Under arm points

FIGURE 6-3 *The Tapping Points. Note: You stimulate the "karate chop" points by hitting the edges of your hands against one another. Two additional optional points are (1) the "Tarzan point" at the center of your chest (tap them right after the K-27 points) and (2) the points on the outside of your legs, midway between your hips and knees (tap them right after the under arm points).*

Most of the tapping points are matched on both sides of the body and can be tapped simultaneously. Take a tour now through the eight tapping points or pairs of points, tapping each as you state your Reminder Phrase. Tap about three beats per second for as long as it takes you to say the Reminder Phrase. Breathe freely as you tap.

The Integration Sequence

Introduced as the Nine Gamut Procedure by psychologist Roger Callahan, the founder of Thought Field Therapy,[16] the Integration Sequence stimulates specific areas of the brain to help it process emotional material more effectively. It is one of the more strange-looking procedures within energy psychology—or any form of psychology, for that matter—with tapping, eye movements, humming, and counting all designed to activate parts of the brain that are involved in processing information.

The Integration Sequence does not use a Reminder Phrase and does not even focus on the memory or problem directly. The eye movements and sounds are done simultaneously with tapping. Use the four fingers of one hand to tap on the back of the other hand in the ridge beneath the V where your ring finger and little finger

---

➡ THE INTEGRATION SEQUENCE ⬅

While tapping on the back of your hand (see Figure 5-3), perform the following nine actions:

1. Close your eyes.
2. Open your eyes.
3. Move your eyes down and to the right.
4. Move your eyes down and to the left.
5. Circle your eyes, rotating them 360 degrees in one direction.
6. Circle your eyes in the other direction.
7. Hum the first few bars of a familiar tune (e.g., "Row, Row Your Boat," "Zip-A-Dee-Doo-Dah," "Mary Had a Little Lamb").
8. Count slowly and deliberately from 1 to 5.
9. Hum again.

---

meet (see Figure 5-3). Tap firmly but not aggressively, again at about three taps per second as you carry out the nine simple steps. Alternate which hand is being tapped as often as you wish.

Sometimes the Integration Sequence ends with an Eye Roll, which is believed to increase the potency of the entire tapping protocol. Begin the Eye Roll with your face straight ahead. Then bring your eyes down to the floor. Next, slowly and deliberately, move your eyes across the floor, up the wall, up to the ceiling, and across the ceiling back toward you. During the entire Eye Roll, forcefully and deliberately send energy out your eyes. Project the "old" energy out into the distance as your eyes move up the arc.

Go ahead now and do the Integration Sequence. It can also be done on its own, independent of the other parts of the Basic Recipe. It is a good "brain balancer" in its own right.

Completing the Sandwich

Next is a second tapping sequence. Do another round of tapping exactly as you did it earlier. You can think of the three ingredients after the Acceptance Statement as making a sandwich:

1. The Tapping Sequence (with the Reminder Phrase)
2. The Integration Sequence
3. The Tapping Sequence (with the Reminder Phrase)

Reassessing

When you have completed the second sequence of tapping, again assess the intensity of the memory. Close your eyes, bring the original memory to mind or play it as a movie, and give a zero-to-ten SUD rating on the moment of greatest distress. Again, you are giving the rating to the amount of distress you are feeling in your body and/or mind *right now*, not what you *think* it would be if you were again in the earlier situation.

If you can get no trace whatsoever of your previous emotional intensity, a final step is to challenge the results (discussed shortly). If, on the other hand, you go down to, let's say a 4, you would perform subsequent rounds until, ideally, zero is reached (see "Mission Accomplished?"). You may recognize that the event being recalled was still as bad as it ever was, but you are now able to bring it up without a physiological distress response being activated. This is a tremendous shift. It almost invariably means that the unprocessed emotion will no longer invade its way into current situations, as evidenced in the way that David stopped projecting feelings about being unfairly attacked onto Donna.

Working with a Partner

If you are learning these techniques at the same time as your partner or with a friend, review with one another your experiences to this point. Then proceed with "After the First Round of the Basic Recipe" (below), working together rather than independently. Your partner will be a witness as you go through the steps. Say what you are doing out loud as your partner listens. Your partner can also consult the book and coach you on the mechanics, at your request, but should in no way impose his or her agenda on your work. Once you have taken the process as far as you can with the issue you are focusing on, switch roles.

After the First Round of the Basic Recipe

Continue with additional rounds until you reach zero or until you have done three rounds with the rating no longer decreasing. Following each round, do a new zero-to-ten assessment of the distress you feel when you tune into the original memory or problem. While the instructions had you focusing on a memory the first time through, the same procedures are applied when focusing on a problem—usually an unwanted emotional response, core belief, or behavior pattern—so you can return to these instructions throughout the book, and beyond, for working not only with memories but also emotional triggers, outdated beliefs, or behavior patterns that don't serve you.

Sometimes a problem is resolved or a memory is fully processed after a single round of treatment. More often, only partial resolution is obtained and additional rounds are necessary. Two simple adjustments need to be made for these subsequent rounds:

Adjusting the Acceptance Statement

The Acceptance Statement is a self-suggestion targeted to the subconscious mind. The subconscious mind tends to be quite literal. After the subjective distress rating has gone down, the Acceptance Statement needs to change to reflect the internal shift. A slight adjustment—the addition of two or three words—accomplishes this. The adjusted format for the Acceptance Statement is:

Even though I still have some of this _____, I deeply love and accept myself.

The words *still* and *some* or *some of* shift the emphasis of the affirmation toward a focus on the remainder of the problem. The adjustment is easy to make. The revised wording for the humiliation experience described earlier might be: Even though I *still* have *some of* my humiliation about the split-pants scene, I deeply love and accept myself.

Adjusting the Reminder Phrase

Simply place the word *remaining* in front of the original Reminder Phrase. For the humiliation example, the new Reminder Phrase would be:

"*remaining* humiliation about the split-pants scene" (or simply "*remaining* humiliation")

Do another round now with your disturbing memory, repeating the Acceptance Statement while using the words *still* and *some of* as appropriate, and inserting the word *remaining* into your Reminder Phrase as appropriate (sometimes other wording needs to be slightly revised as well—this will be apparent when it is required). Again bring the memory to mind and rate it from zero to ten. If you are still able to activate disturbing feelings in relationship to the memory or problem, continue to repeat the Acceptance Statement and the Sandwich until you are unable to feel distress in relationship to the issue, or until you have been unable to lower the degree of distress after three rounds (see "Overcoming Obstacles to Resolving the Problem").

Mission Accomplished?

How do you know you have really overcome the problem in a way that will last? Does a SUD rating of zero ensure that the unwanted feeling will not return? There is one more step.

Challenging Your Results

Once you do get the subjective distress rating down to zero, a final step is to *challenge* it. Try to recall or visualize the situation in a manner that evokes the earlier sense of distress. Find a way to intensify the scene. If the disturbed energy pattern and neurological sequence have been corrected—that is, if the earlier memory, thought, or situation does not produce a disturbed response in your brain and energy system— you will not be able to activate your earlier feelings. The speed with which this can often be accomplished is among the most striking benefits of energy psychology. A difficult situation from your past will still be recognized for its inherent dangers, injuries, or injustices, but the stress response in your autonomic nervous system that had been paired with that memory will no longer be triggered.

If you are unable to reproduce any trace of the initial emotional response, the probability is strong that your autonomic response to the memory has been deactivated. If you were working with an emotional trigger such as your wife's tone of voice when she feels sad or a memory that intrudes into your current life, chances are that the internal changes will translate into new situations. If the internal changes do not translate into daily life, or if there is some slippage, you can do another round or two of tapping as the situation is occurring. This often is all that is needed to anchor the changes into your life. If in spite of this follow-up the desired changes still seem tenuous, it may mean that an aspect of the problem still needs attention, as discussed below.

Claiming Victory Even if the SUD Did Not Get down to Zero

We should mention that sometimes the rating will get down to a 2 or a 1 but will not go down any further. This is not necessarily a bad outcome. For some problems, you may not be able to conceive of the rating going down to zero, and a 1 or a 2 is essentially a "cure" in your subjective world. In some circumstances, such as taking a test, or giving a performance, a small measure of anxiety increases your ability to function. So while zero might be thought of as the ideal, and it is the outcome that is most frequently obtained, it is not always realistic or necessary.

Overcoming Obstacles to Resolving the Problem

If after three rounds the rating has not budged, you may need to shift your focus or wording, or you may have identified a problem where you need outside assistance. There are many possible reasons that improvement can become stalled. A small proportion of people do not respond to tapping on acupoints (if you suspect you are one of them, try massaging the points or simply touching each point while breathing deeply). Sometimes the problem needs to be formulated with more specific or altogether different wording.

A more frequent reason the process may get stuck is that an aspect of the problem that has not been addressed requires your attention for progress to continue. Another is that internal conflict about resolving the problem may need greater exploration. A third is that the energy fields in your body may have become so disorganized that they need to be balanced before tapping on an emotional issue can be fully effective.

Addressing Unresolved Aspects of the Problem

In the hands of a relatively proficient newcomer, the Basic Recipe seems, in our experience, to produce effective results 70 to 80 percent of the time when applied to reducing the emotional charge on a specific negatively charged memory. The tapping sends signals that reduce arousal in the threat response centers of the brain. It is that simple. While by many standards this is an extremely favorable success rate, a better percentage is possible when you know how to handle potential blocks to progress.

The most common reason the distress rating would not have gone down to zero or close to zero if you followed the instructions precisely is that another aspect of the problem is involved that was not focused upon during the energy tapping. In addition, the most frequent reason an apparently successful treatment, where the distress rating *did go down to zero*, won't translate into the actual situation is that a new aspect of the problem came up in the real-life situation that wasn't there when you were just thinking about the problem and wording your Reminder Phrase. While many problems are straightforward and do not have multiple aspects, some have a number of physical or psychological aspects that each require attention if the problem is to be fully resolved.

Physical Aspects

The *physical* aspects of a problem include the look, sound, smell, taste, or feel of the situation. A thirty-eight-year-old account executive emerged from a serious car accident with no physical injuries, but he subsequently felt extremely anxious whenever he drove. He was told it would go away, but after six months, it had only become worse. In his first energy psychology session, he tapped on the words "when my Volvo was totaled." His zero-to-ten distress rating began as a 9 and fairly quickly went down to a 6, but it would not go down further. When asked what came into his mind when he was rating the scene, he said that what bothered him the most was recalling "the sound of the screeching tires followed by the loud crash." After tapping on "the sound of the screeching tires" and "the loud crash," his rating went down to a 3. Reflecting then on what kept it at a 3, he described the feeling of helplessness as the car went into a skid. After tapping on that, he was able to vividly recall the accident, scene by scene, with no stress reaction, and he was again able to drive without anxiety.

Unresolved physical aspects of a problem are not always obvious, but you can usually identify them by noting what is prominent in your mind when you focus on the remaining distress you feel, or by examining how your experience in the actual situation differs from the scene you imagined during the tapping. Consider, for instance, a fear of spiders. Usually the energy disruptions that occur when someone with this fear is thinking about a spider are very similar to those that occur upon actually seeing a spider. After the response to the thought or image of a spider has been brought down to a zero, the response to seeing a real spider will usually be zero as well. But not always.

Perhaps during the tapping, the person was thinking about a stationary spider. The imagined spider was not moving. If movement is an important aspect of the fear, and if it was not addressed in the original rounds of tapping, then a moving spider can still trigger fear. So you would apply the Basic Recipe to this additional aspect ("*moving* spider") until the emotional response gets down to zero. Once all aspects have been resolved, the phobic response to spiders will have been eliminated. The person will be able to stay calm in the presence of a spider. The physical aspects of a traumatic event, such as an accident or an abusive situation (the *taste* of the mud in my mouth after I hit the ground, the *smell* of his breath, the *look* in her eyes) may remain in play until you recognize that they require attention. At that point, they can usually be neutralized quite readily by tapping while keeping them active in your mind.

Psychological Aspects

Many issues also carry psychological associations that go beyond the obvious stresses connected to the problem being addressed. If your fear of spiders started when your brother dropped a spider down the back of your blouse at the carnival when you were eight and you ran screaming through the crowds, simply tapping on the image of a spider to overcome your spider phobia isn't likely to do it. The terror, shock, embarrassment, and sense of betrayal tracing to the earlier incident may all need tapping. Or if the account executive with the fear of driving had, as a child, witnessed a terrible automobile accident that had been repressed from his memory, the emotional residue from that experience may have been activated by the recent car crash and his anxiety may not be fully eradicated until the earlier trauma has been addressed. Early experiences of this nature may have been forgotten or totally repressed, but analogous experiences can reactivate them.

Suppose, for instance, that you were bitten by a dog when you were seven. This memory has long been forgotten. But then you hear of a neighbor receiving a dog bite and you instantly develop a fear of dogs, rated at 9 or 10. This level of fear and physiological arousal suggests more is at play than just having heard a report of a single incident. Applying the Basic Recipe to "fear of dogs" may reduce your fear a bit, but it is not likely to be effective until the childhood incident has been addressed. Having been bitten as a child is an important aspect of "fear of dogs," and it probably will need attention before the fear of dogs that recently appeared can be successfully resolved. Fortunately, when you use tapping to reduce the charge on a recent event or current problem, earlier experiences that have become psychologically entangled with the current problem tend to reveal themselves and will also be responsive to tapping.

Any recent trauma or loss can unearth a network of earlier unresolved traumas or losses. In focusing on the first memory that reveals itself, you may find that it also has a number of aspects. Neutralizing each physical and psychological aspect that emerges brings you deeper into the heart of long-standing emotional issues, like peeling the layers off an onion. Haunting physical aspects of the memory may be at the outer layers. You may vividly recall the feeling of your blood rolling down your leg or the icy terror in your chest when you saw the dog baring its teeth and about to attack. These may, in turn, tie into psychological aspects of the problem, such as other situations where you felt helpless. Your subconscious mind knows what you are working on and tends to present whatever requires attention. By neutralizing the emotional charge on such memories, you are not only making it possible to fully resolve the original problem, you are also healing early emotional wounds that were limiting you. That is why the most popular form of energy psychology is called Emotional Freedom Techniques (EFT).

When focusing on the aspects of a problem, be as specific as possible. Not just "fear of dogs," but specific memories—recent or past—that feed that fear. Recall, rate (zero to ten), and work with them one at a time. This is a good guideline for addressing any problem, but it is particularly important for emotional responses that occur in multiple contexts, such as free-floating anxiety or incessant feelings of shame. In these instances, it is useful to work with your earliest memories of the feeling. For instance, rather than tapping on "this shame I feel," you could focus on the earliest experiences of shame you can recall, tapping on each until it has been neutralized. Then, when you return to more recent incidents, the underlying sense of shame will have been cleared away and the current concern is likely to be resolved quite readily.

It is not necessary, however, to clear related incidents in any particular chronological order; nor do you need to remember and treat every aspect that was involved with a problem in order to overcome it. This is particularly important to understand in working with a history of ongoing abuse, the aftermath of warfare, or when other kinds of traumas have been experienced repeatedly. Fortunately, a "generalization effect" kicks in. After you have resolved a few related incidents, the effects start to generalize to the broader issue. For instance, someone who has thirty traumatic memories of having been beaten will find that after neutralizing five or ten of them (this would be done in the context of psychotherapy), the others will begin to lose their emotional charge as well.

In summary, our experiences working with a wide range of individuals suggest that when they patiently apply the Basic Recipe to neutralize the physical and psychological aspects of the problems they present, self-limiting psychological difficulties can often be fully and permanently resolved.

"Psychological Reversals": Internal Conflicts about Overcoming a Problem

Another reason—besides an unrecognized aspect of the problem—that the SUD rating would not have gone down to zero or close to zero is that a "psychological reversal" is involved in the problem you are trying to resolve. In a psychological reversal, unconscious resistance is blocking the consciously desired outcome. A woman wanted to get over her phobia of being on airplanes, but when her distress while thinking about flying wouldn't get below a 5, she explored what was in the way of further progress. She came to realize that if she did overcome her flying phobia, then she would have to "go on those dreadful business trips" with her husband.

In a psychological reversal, a part of you seems to want the reverse of what you consciously desire. Or it simply plays out that you consistently *do* the reverse of what you intend. Remember the toy straw tubes where you place your forefingers into each end and when you try to pull them out, the tube tightens so you can't free your fingers. That's how a psychological reversal feels. The harder you try, the more powerful the resistance that emerges to counter you. Your efforts produce the opposite of the result you intend. All effective therapies address psychological reversals in one way or another, using a variety of terms, from *unconscious resistance* to *self-sabotage*. Until these are resolved, other therapeutic interventions are less likely to have a deep or lasting effect.

When Roger Callahan was formulating Thought Field Therapy, he recognized an energetic dimension to such conflicts about a treatment goal. The psychological resistance was being compounded by a disruption in the body's energy system whenever the person brought the goal to mind. Addressing a psychological reversal at the energetic level can cut through the need for the long, complex analysis that is typical for many therapeutic approaches.

If the tapping is not decreasing your internal distress when bringing the problem to mind, and you have worked through all the aspects you can identify, looking inward for possible conflicts about overcoming the problem may show you where you are caught. Psychological reversals are often subconscious, but they will usually reveal themselves after a bit of reflection. For instance, you may at some level be concerned about certain possible consequences of overcoming the problem, such as, "If I truly learn to relax and not push myself so hard, I won't achieve as much" or "If I get an A in math, boys will stay away from me." The possibilities are endless.

Keeping a problem may be a way of lowering people's expectations about you. It may even be a way of punishing someone: "If I am no longer devastated about the affair, he gets off scot-free!" Another form of psychological reversal is when a person is deriving "secondary gains" for having an emotional problem—from gaining sympathy to receiving disability insurance.

Some psychological reversals are specific to a particular aspect of the problem or goal. They may have to do with:

- conflicted *desire* about reaching the goal
- a sense of *not deserving* to reach the goal
- a feeling that it is *not safe* or *not possible* to reach the goal
- a feeling that reaching the goal is not compatible with the person's *identity*

For instance, a person who wants to lose weight may have no energy disruption with the thought, "I *want* to lose weight." But an energy disruption may appear with the related thought, "I *deserve* to lose weight," or "It is *safe* to lose weight," or "It is *possible* for me to lose weight," or "I will do what's necessary to lose weight," or "I would no longer *be me* if I lost weight," or "If I lose weight, men will start hitting on me." Useful themes to explore when identifying whether a psychological reversal is at play include:

I want to [name the goal].
I deserve to [name the goal].
It is safe for me or my relationship if I [name the goal].
It is possible for me to [name the goal].
I will feel deprived if I [name the goal].
I will do what's necessary to [name the goal].
I would still be me if I [name the goal].

An approach to working with psychological reversals that we find effective is similar to the technique you have already learned of using an Acceptance Statement combined with the simple physical procedures of massaging points on your torso and placing your hands over your heart (pp. 198–199).

In the Acceptance Statement, you formulated a phrase that acknowledges that the problem you want to change exists (e.g., "Even though I have this unwanted weight") and at the same time affirms that you accept yourself even though you have that problem (e.g., "I deeply love and accept myself"). While making this statement, you work with points that move energy through your body (pp. 199–201). Recall the statement, "Even though I still carry humiliation about my pants having ripped during the play [rubbing sore spots on the chest], I deeply love and accept myself [with hands over center of chest]."

Resistance to any psychological or behavioral problem or goal—from attempting to overcome a self-defeating habit to eliminating irrational anger toward your spouse—can be translated into this format. Once such inner conflicts are discovered, the same strategy applies. Find a statement that acknowledges the problem, such as "Even though I don't deserve to lose weight," and then, while doing the energy interventions, pair it with a statement of self-acceptance, such as "I deeply love and accept myself." So if you were to discover that any of the above themes were at play, the wordings might be:

Even though I don't want to [name the goal], I deeply love and accept myself.
Even though I don't deserve to [name the goal], I deeply love and accept myself.
Even though it's not safe to [name the goal], I deeply love and accept myself.
Even though it's not possible for me to [name the goal], I deeply love and accept myself.
Even though I will feel deprived if I [name the goal], I deeply love and accept myself.
Even though I won't do what's necessary to [name the goal], I deeply love and accept myself.
Even though I wouldn't still be me if I [name the goal], I deeply love and accept myself.

Again, the points where your arms meet your torso are massaged during the first phrase (or other acupoints are stimulated, as discussed earlier) and your hands are held over your heart as you say "I deeply love and accept myself."

The Choices Method

An alternative format for the second phrase in the Acceptance Statement, as well as for addressing psychological reversals, is called the Choices Method.[17] It emphasizes choice and opportunity. "Even though I still obsess about my son's grades, I choose to know that I deeply love and accept him" or "Even though I neglect my body, I choose to know that I deserve to have time for regular, enjoyable exercise." Regardless of the wording, the strategy is to stimulate acupoints that help pair a negative self-evaluation with a positive thought or with the recognition of an opportunity. This causes the negative thought to become a *trigger* for a positive choice.

The Choices Method can be tailored to any situation, even those that are bleak or overwhelming. A depressed client in his first psychotherapy session developed the affirmation, "Even though my life is hopeless, I choose to find unexpected help in this therapy." Writing to her colleagues the day after 9/11 on how to assist people dealing with the psychological aftermath of the attack, psychologist Patricia Carrington, who developed the Choices Method, suggested using it with phrasings such as, "Even though I am stunned and bewildered by this terrible happening, I choose to be a still point amid all the chaos," or "Even though I am stunned and bewildered, I choose to learn something absolutely essential for my own life from this event," or "Even though I am stunned and bewildered, I choose to have this dreadful event open my heart." Additional examples:

Even though I was rejected, I choose to remember how many people love me.
Even though I feel deprived if I don't have that extra helping, I choose to know my body is fully nourished.
Even though I'm completely driven by my work, I choose to know that my worth as a person is not about my accomplishments.

In summary, if tapping is not decreasing your emotional distress about the problem or increasing your confidence about overcoming it, be alert for the possibility of an inner conflict about your goal. If you identify such conflict, you can formulate an Acceptance Statement or use the Choices Method to resolve it.

→ THE BASIC RECIPE IN A NUTSHELL ←

Identify and Rate a Problem That Is Suitable for Energy Interventions
Identify an emotional response, physical reaction, thought pattern, or behavioral pattern you would like to change, state it as a Reminder Phrase, and rate it from zero to ten according to the amount of distress you feel when you bring it to mind (p. 193).

Establish a Psychological Receptiveness for Change
Say the Acceptance Statement (p. 196) three times in the format of: *Even though I have this* [Reminder Phrase], *I deeply love and accept myself.* Simultaneously rub your chest sore spots on the first statement and hold your hands over the center of your chest on the second.

Initial Round of Treatment ("The Sandwich")
1. Tap the energy points shown in Figure 6-3 while stating the Reminder Phrase at each point.
2. The Integration Sequence (p. 200): While tapping on the back of your hand (see Figure 5-3), close your eyes, open them, move them down to the right, move them down to the left, circle them clockwise, circle them counterclockwise, hum, count, hum.
3. Again tap the energy points shown in Figure 6-3.

Subsequent Rounds of the Sandwich
Add *still* and *some* to the Acceptance Statement; add *remaining* to the Reminder Phrase. Repeat until down to zero or adjust based on aspects, psychological reversals, or scrambled energies.

Challenge the Results
After the distress level is at zero or near zero, try to bring up the initial emotion. If you cannot, you are done. If you can, do another round of the Basic Recipe. If progress becomes stuck, identify and address any hidden aspects, psychological reversals, or scrambled energies.

"Scrambled" Energy

A third possible impediment to progress is that sometimes a person's energies become so disorganized when bringing the problem to mind that tapping a set of acupuncture points is too subtle an intervention to be able to take hold amid all the static. In such cases, it is necessary to shift your focus to the energy disruptions. The methods presented in Part 2 of the Pact (pp. 82–94) can be extremely useful. Taking a few minutes to balance your body's energies before bringing your attention back to the psychological issue may be an essential step.

In brief, if applying the Basic Recipe is not going as planned, an analysis almost always points to one of the following being active: hidden aspects of the problem, psychological reversals, or scrambled energies, as discussed earlier. A fourth possibility is an overwhelming emotional response. Emotional responses that become unsettling are addressed next.

If the Program Becomes Unsettling

A delicate issue in presenting the potent methods offered in this chapter is that any useful psychological tool can stir strong emotions or uncover dormant psychological problems. The methods you are learning here will not create new emotional problems, but it is possible that they may bring to the surface underlying emotional turmoil. One of our colleagues[18] was doing a demonstration in front of a large group with a woman who wanted help regarding spells of extreme shyness and a tendency to go silent in certain social situations. Just standing in front of the group, her shoulders slumped, as if trying to make herself take up less space, and her voice became tiny. With the tapping treatment, her stress rating went from an initial 8 down to 6, but it stayed at 6 for the next two rounds. Then a childhood memory surfaced of her and her mother walking into their home while a burglary was in progress. Her mother started to scream and the intruder began to viciously beat her mother. The girl ran and hid behind some curtains. She was sure the burglar was searching for her and managed to silence her own tears and screams of terror. While she had totally repressed her memory of this incident (she was able to later confirm it with her mother, who had been reluctant to revive the memory), whenever she felt any stress in front of other people, she would have to fight against herself to be able to speak.

Now with the memory rushing back in vivid detail, she went through the same kinds of physiological reactions as when the incident occurred: shaking heavily, face blanched, heart pounding, hardly breathing. Of course at this point our colleague saw the symptoms but did not yet know the story. He offered reassuring words while unwaveringly instructing her to continue tapping. By the second trip through the tapping sequence, her breathing had returned to normal and she had stopped shaking. A couple more rounds of tapping (no Acceptance Statement, no Integration Sequence, just the emotional first aid of stimulating the acupoints involved with the stress response), and she was able to describe what had occurred. Then her work was able to proceed by focusing on various aspects of the memory, neutralizing them one by one. Finally, to test the degree to which she had overcome her shyness, she described her experience to the group in full-bodied posture and voice.

While tapping itself reduces rather than increases distress, touching into traumatic memories can be destabilizing. Activating a past trauma may make it feel like the problem is getting worse. Simply bringing to mind a difficult emotional issue or disturbing memory can shake one's confidence, open an old wound, or stir up overwhelming feelings. Any potent experience can, in fact, bring to the surface underlying issues that have not been resolved. If repressed emotions are on the verge of breaking through one's psychological defenses, a reaction might be triggered by seeing a powerful film, helping one's child through a difficult time, having an argument with a loved one, experiencing a volley of criticism from a friend, entering psychotherapy, opening oneself to the deeper recesses of one's psyche while working with one's dreams, participating in an intensive "personal growth" workshop, or using techniques such as the ones presented in this book. The following pages offer steps you can take if working through this program becomes unsettling.

Before offering procedures that will calm and steady you if this happens, we want to emphasize that intense emotional reactions are not a setback. Critical, however, is that when they occur, you find the support and resources so you are able to resolve them and come out stronger rather than with an additional unresolved trauma that leaves you feeling more fragile or more defended. Energy work can, like any other psychological approach as well as many other life experiences, bring old emotional wounds to the surface. Although this may be challenging, emotional problems that lie beneath the surface often drain a person's vitality and foster defensive thought and behavioral patterns. By bringing them into your awareness, doorways open for healing them. With that healing, the energies that had been defending against the old wound can be directed toward a more dynamic response to life.

We have made every effort to present the techniques in this book so you can adjust them to your own needs, readiness, and pace. If, however, you should feel disturbed or unsettled as you apply the procedures, and if those feelings persist after you have used the suggestions given next, we strongly encourage you to elicit support from family and friends or seek professional assistance.

For a first course of action if the program becomes upsetting, you can take any of the following "psychological first aid" measures. In most cases, one or more of these will suffice. But do not forget that prolonged upset can also be an opportunity, an opening for a highly beneficial course of healing and growth facilitated by focused effort, psychotherapy, a spiritual discipline, or other healing resource. Immediate steps you can take if you find yourself becoming upset include:

Tap on the Reaction You Are Having

Acupoint tapping is a powerful way to calm yourself. If focusing on your personal issues leads to emotional discomfort, take a step back and apply the tapping to the emotional discomfort itself. Since you are in the midst of the emotion, begin by simply doing the tapping sequence. It is not necessary to create a Reminder Phrase since you are already tuned into the feeling. With intense emotional reactions, you may need to go through several rounds of the tapping sequence. During the period that the feelings are intense, it is not necessary to stop for the Acceptance Statement or the Integration Sequence.

Do the Stress Release Hold

This procedure (p. 90) can have a similar effect to tapping, relaxing your body and calming your emotions. A stress reaction sends blood away from your brain and into your arms, legs, chest, and other organs involved in the fight/flight/freeze response. Holding these points counters the stress reaction by directing blood back to your brain. Simply place the palm of one hand over your forehead and the palm of your other hand over the back of your head just above your neckline. Hold comfortably for two to three minutes, breathing in through your nose and out through your mouth. This can be done standing, sitting, or lying down.

BALANCE YOUR ENERGIES

Do an energy "emotional first aid" sequence consisting of some or all of the following: the Hook-Up (p. 88), the Crossover Shoulder Pull (p. 89), the Wayne Cook Posture (p. 91), the Triple Warmer Smoothie (p. 167), the Blow-Out (p. 86), and Connecting Heaven and Earth (p. 92).

SHIFT TO A CALMING ACTIVITY

Listen to music, work in your garden, phone a supportive friend, take a walk in nature, meditate, watch an entertaining video, do yoga or stretching exercises, breathe deeply.

REST YOUR BODY

Take a break. Take a bath. Take a nap. Take a vacation. Rest your body. Rest your spirit.

STIMULATE YOUR BODY

Involve yourself in an invigorating physical activity, such as swimming, running, dancing, jumping on a mini-trampoline, cleaning your house, or waxing your car. Regularly discharging pent-up or stagnant energies is an excellent form of emotional self-care.

USE YOUR IMAGINATION

Experiment with imagery that takes you to a protected, beautiful, sacred place—an old oak tree, a mountain stream, a childhood hideaway. Later, cultivate your ability to go there in your mind whenever you feel the need for safety, sustenance, or renewal.

REACH INTO YOUR INNER GUIDANCE

Archetypes are elements of your psyche that bridge to powerful forces beyond your conscious mind. An archetype that connects you to greater wisdom can be accessed by going inward and imagining an inner guide who is able to nurture and advise you. This inner guide may appear as a wise man or woman, a spiritual or religious figure, or someone you looked up to as a child. Imagine this person vividly, perhaps in the beautiful, sacred setting suggested above. Ask for the guidance you need. Listen carefully to the response. Cultivate a relationship with this inner guide.

FIND SUPPORT FROM ANOTHER PERSON

Share intimately with someone who cares about you. Use this person as a sounding board and a source of support.

BE PATIENT WITH YOURSELF

In applying energy psychology to your own life and issues, you are affirming your ability to change and evolve. Appreciate yourself for your intention and efforts, *and* use the Basic Recipe to counter your self-judgments and to increase your ability to accept yourself *just the way you are.*

DEVELOP A SELF-AFFIRMING PERSPECTIVE FOR YOUR TRIALS AND TRIBULATIONS

When deep changes occur, old and familiar ways of perceiving, thinking, and behaving all transform. This by its nature is disorienting and can be destabilizing. Give yourself time and support for adjusting to new understanding and new ways of being. Use the Basic Recipe to foster optimism, welcome a new perspective, call on your creativity, and find the humor, ironies, and lessons in the process.

BRING IN NEW SOURCES OF INSPIRATION

From inspirational reading to great movies to sacred ceremonies to worship services to prayer to meditation, we are all fed by experiences that expand our understanding of the invisible patterns behind the visible world, that remind us of the courage and vastness of the human spirit, and that call us into a keener relationship with ourselves and our surroundings. Dedicate time to such activities.

Healing the Aftermath of a Catastrophe

While we have just been focusing on the possible hazards of self-guided exploration, we want to close with another story that demonstrates the powerful benefits that can result from working directly with the energies that are at the foundation of your habits, thoughts, and feelings. When June was twenty-four, her high school sweetheart and then-husband was killed in a traffic accident, the victim of a drunk driver. The loss was horrendous. She was depressed and almost inconsolable for the next two years. Eventually, however, she returned to school, started a new career, and was able to rebuild a meaningful life.

At age thirty-one, she met Ralph and, after dealing with her sense of being dis-loyal to her first husband, she allowed herself to fall deeply in love with him. They married and had two sons. June's worry about their well-being became problematic. If Ralph was late coming home from work, she would be a bundle of frayed nerves by the time he arrived. It was very difficult for her to allow either of their sons to part from her sight, and their going to school was agony for her. She would ruminate about all the terrible things that might happen. Earlier in their relationship, Ralph had been very patient with June when her worry was primarily about him. He un-derstood the loss she had suffered. But now her worry was stifling the boys as they became more independent, and he insisted that they attend therapy.

After a thorough history was taken in the first session, it became clear to David that while June had received grief counseling following her husband's death and had healed in many important ways, the shock of learning of his death still reverber-ated within her in nightmarish proportions. As difficult as it might be, the treatment had to revisit that moment. Fortunately, with acupoint tapping, it is not necessary to vividly relive a trauma. A technique that our colleague Gary Craig calls "sneaking up on the problem" uses general terms rather than the highly specific language that is usually suggested. When working with a devastating memory, you don't need to relive it, only to activate it slightly. So June's first round of tapping simply used the words "that horrible day." Her SUD rating went from a 10 to a 7 after a few rounds, but then other losses came into her mind, specifically of her grandmother when she was eight and her dog, Smithers, when she was in her teens. We focused on each until the emotional charge had dissipated and the memory of the joys each had brought into her life could be fully experienced without intrusion by unprocessed pain about their subsequent loss.

In the next session, we returned to the moment June learned of her first husband's death. It had come back up to a 9 and was quickly lowered to a 6 after a bit of tap-ping, again using the Reminder Phrase "that horrible day." At this point, the ap-proach was refined. First June was asked to describe what she was doing just prior to learning of her husband's death and to tell the story of that day. She had already done enough work that she was able to manage this, not without tears, but without being overwhelmed. Then we took the account she had just presented in stages, using lan-guage that was more specific than had been used in the earlier tapping.

We began with her shopping in a grocery store prior to receiving the call on her cell phone. That was not hard to neutralize. Then hearing the cell phone ring and taking it out of her purse. She could recall exactly what aisle she was in. The distress triggered by this memory was neutralized within a couple of rounds of tapping. Then hearing the doctor identify himself and say the awful words, "I'm afraid your husband has been in an accident." Everything that followed was addressed in segments, from the anxious drive to the hospital to learning he had died to insisting on seeing his disfigured body to the long and terrible night of being home alone after it was all over.

Because overwhelming emotion is not compatible with the signals sent to the brain during tapping, the signals turn off the emotion without distorting the memory. The memory becomes manageable and stops intruding into other areas of one's life. This emotional processing and healing changes the person's psychic landscape. From there, it was relatively easy to identify several of the most recent times that June had been obsessively worried about Ralph or one of the boys and to tap each down to zero. Finally, we worked with some situations that had not yet happened but that she imagined might be challenging. From that point on, she was able to send her men off to work or school with a smile on her face and a heart that was at peace.

You do not need to have had a tragedy like June's to fall prey to a self-defeating thought or emotional pattern that is hurting your relationship. If you are prone to excessive worry, judgments, comparisons, avoidance, or a sense of threat, your tapping can focus on the last time the pattern occurred. Freeing yourself from these echoes from your past using the energy psychology protocol taught in this and the following chapter can be a large step toward clearing the way for a relationship that is blessed by increasingly secure attachment.

7

Recurring Patterns, Triggers, and Other Inconveniences

Reprogramming Responses
That Hurt Your Relationship

Love is *everything it's cracked up to be. . . .*
It really is *worth fighting for, worth being brave for,*
risking everything for. And the trouble is, if you
don't risk anything, you risk even more.

—ERICA JONG[1]

J EREMY WAS THIRTY-SIX WHEN HE MARRIED MELISSA. HE WAS EAGER TO HELP RAISE her sons, ages seven and nine. He had gotten to know them quite well during the year prior to the marriage; he had brought them to baseball games, zoos, parks, and other local attractions, and he had participated in their hobbies. The boys liked their stepdad and the attention he was giving them, and the new family was blossoming within an atmosphere of affection and promise. Melissa's ex-husband, Steve, the boys' biological father, had not been particularly eager to spend time with his sons during the marriage, but he also loved them. He had moved to another town several hours away after the divorce but had been reliable in taking the boys for the afternoon every other Sunday.

During his courtship with Melissa, Jeremy had never met Steve. But now that Jeremy had moved in with the family, the twice-monthly visits became a fixture in his life. He was civil enough toward his new wife's ex, but he avoided having much contact with him when the boys were being picked up or dropped off. During the first Christmas vacation after the marriage, Steve arranged to take the boys for a week, and the three of them flew to Orlando for a Disney marathon. The boys were so excited about it that they seemed to talk of little else for the week before and the week after the trip. When Steve came for the next Sunday visitation, Jeremy could hardly look at him. He began to criticize Steve's parenting style to Melissa, point out his culpability in the divorce, and generally paint an ugly picture of the man who had fathered her children. At first Melissa acknowledged the truth in some of the observations, but over time Jeremy became increasingly vehement in his criticisms. This grew into a loaded theme in their interactions on the weekends that Steve would be arriving, and Jeremy began questioning the boys about their visits with their father, as if looking for more fodder for his rants. He was eventually unable to hide from the boys his disdain toward their father.

Jeremy's jealousy toward Steve continued to escalate, and the acrimony was seeping into other areas of the family. As Steve's visits approached, tension would descend on the household. The boys were confused. Melissa began to judge Jeremy harshly. She had more than once called him a "spoiled brat." This was the state of things when they scheduled a couple counseling session with David. Jeremy knew at some level that his reactions were not rational, but this knowledge could not compete with the strength of his emotions. When Jeremy was triggered, Steve was an evil man sabotaging all of Jeremy's fine efforts with the boys and the family, and there was no other reality to consider.

After hearing both of their renditions of the problem, David spoke to the part of Jeremy that knew his reactions to Steve were extreme. David explained that when intense emotions are triggered, they are very real, whether rational or irrational. He suggested tapping to take the edge off the intensity of Jeremy's responses to Steve. Neither Jeremy nor Melissa had any experience with energy psychology, but the couple who referred them had worked with David and described the method, so they were game for anything that could help, however strange it might look. While Jeremy was not open to considering that his assessment of Steve might be wrong, he was interested in feeling less consumed by his reactions.

They proceeded, following essentially the same steps you learned as the Basic Recipe in the previous chapter. The scene that Jeremy chose for his subjective units of distress (SUD) rating was from the previous Sunday, watching as Steve's car pulled into the driveway. It was a 10 on the zero-to-ten scale. After four rounds of tapping, it had gone down to a 7, but even after further tapping it seemed to be stuck there. David asked, "How do you know it is a seven?" Jeremy said that he felt pressure in his chest and a tightness in his throat. David asked him to explore the feelings in his throat. Jeremy said it was almost as if he were trying to hold back tears. David asked if he could recall one of the first times he had that feeling. Jeremy immediately recalled being ten when his parents brought a foster boy into the family. It was to be a temporary arrangement until a permanent placement could be found, a favor for a relative of the boy, but it changed everything for Jeremy.

As an only child, Jeremy had enjoyed his parents' full attention and affection. Suddenly that was history. The foster boy had many problems, both of Jeremy's parents held full-time jobs, and the limited time and resources they had available shifted from Jeremy to the new boy. Jeremy, at ten, did not have words or concepts that could help him come to grips with the loss. He felt emotionally abandoned by both of his parents, he could not fathom why they had brought this troublesome person into their home, and he hated the foster boy. He began starting fights and creating acrimony wherever he could. This strategy seemed to eventually work. After about a year, the agency found a permanent placement for the boy and Jeremy never saw him again. All of this was buried in the recesses of Jeremy's psyche. He hadn't thought about it for years, and no other circumstance in his adult life had triggered his unprocessed feelings around that chapter from his childhood. He had never thought to mention it to Melissa, but the parallels between the foster boy and the situation with Steve became immediately obvious to all three of us.

We tapped on every aspect of the memory we could identify, staying with each until it was down to a zero: Jeremy's loss of his parents' attention; his many times having held back his tears when he felt lonely and abandoned; his confusion and puzzlement about what he had done wrong to deserve having all the attention withdrawn from him; the invasion into his family; his hatred for the new boy; the fights they had; his being punished for starting them and feeling like a bad boy after ten years of being a good boy; and even his confusion when the new boy suddenly disappeared.

Fortunately, each round of tapping takes only a couple of minutes, so all of this was accomplished within that first session (David generally schedules two hours for initial sessions with couples). Jeremy was by then able to talk lucidly and calmly about the foster boy and the boy's invasion into his young life. And he could reflect on how Steve's visits with the boys were bringing up feelings that traced to his experiences with the foster boy. He was entertaining the possibility that his sense of

Steve purposefully trying to destroy the family Jeremy was building had something to do with this earlier scenario. Focusing again on watching Steve's car pulling into the driveway, Jeremy gave it a SUD rating of 3. A couple more rounds of tapping and it was down to a zero. We then briefly focused on Melissa's horror and sense of betrayal about Jeremy's shift over the recent months from an apparently ideal stepfather to an angry, jealous, irrational force in her home. Witnessing Jeremy's work had already put all of this into a welcome new light, and by the end of the session, she was able to review the strange course of their young marriage with no emotional charge.

On a follow-up session two weeks later, the issue had vanished. Jeremy was not triggered by Steve's next visit, the strong relationship Jeremy had established with the boys and with Melissa was back on track, and David had lost customers who could have easily spent a year or two in counseling. Such are the risks a therapist takes when bringing an energy approach into the consulting room.

Can You Try This at Home?

How effectively you can use the techniques taught here to change patterns that really matter to you and to your relationship depends on many factors, but we can tell you that innumerable individuals and couples have gained strong benefits from using energy psychology techniques on a self-help basis. If they don't work, then you will have wasted a bit of time and effort and perhaps gotten frustrated—but you will know you gave it your best shot and it may help you determine that professional assistance is warranted to optimize what you have together. If they do work, you have not only solved the problem at hand, but you have also been building tools for navigating through whatever emotional challenges you may face in the future.

Chapter 6 presented basic energy psychology procedures that can bring about deep transformation. It listed seven areas of relationships where these procedures can be particularly effective in helping couples: (1) moving through emotional intensity without escalating; (2) shifting the way you respond to behaviors in your partner that had been triggers for anger, hurt, or resentment; (3) tracing emotional challenges that play themselves out again and again in your relationship to formative childhood experiences; (4) healing those emotional wounds; (5) transforming the patterns that grew out of those wounds; (6) completing any other "unfinished business" in your emotional life, including "baggage" from earlier relationships or from an earlier time in your current relationship; and (7) establishing a strong mental vision of how you want yourself or your relationship to change and rewiring your brain to support that vision.

In this chapter, we will describe how energy psychology can be applied in each of these areas. We wanted an example to illustrate each topic. While we could have drawn from couples we've worked with, we decided to keep it alive and at our own personal edges. The following describes our personal use of the techniques you are learning, conducted specifically with this chapter in mind. The commentary instructs you on how to work with the theme being explored, and it also includes fresh discussion of the dilemmas in working with one's partner as they emerged for us during our little experiment. David's bullying issue was a theme in the previous chapter. In this chapter, we turn the spotlight on Donna.

The theme you will see Donna focusing on throughout the remainder of this chapter traces to a core decision she made early in her childhood that she would not cause trouble for anyone. Her sister and her brother required a great deal of attention from their parents, and Donna took on the family role of being the one who wasn't a source of difficulty. It is not like she had never before been aware of this issue or worked on it. Rather, as we evolve and reach higher levels of consciousness, certain basic themes may reemerge to be resolved in new ways. We are each a work in progress.

Personal development has, in fact, sometimes been likened to an upward spiral where you revisit the same issues, again and again, but because it is an *upward* spiral, you meet them from a higher vantage point, a new level of personal evolution.[2] The more effectively you deal with the issue during the current round of the spiral, the more the issue becomes a source of experience and wisdom rather than limitation, at least until its number is up again on your life's journey. Donna's theme of not causing trouble had gone through several rounds of the spiral during her life, and it seemed to be up again, just in time for the writing of this chapter.

I. Moving through Emotional Intensity without Escalating

The first step of the Pact (chapter 3) is to STOP your discussion the moment the emotional intensity between you is beginning to escalate. Tapping on the points shown in Figure 6-3 gives you a preventive tool that may keep it from escalating beyond the first emotional bumps. Our close colleague and friend Dawson Church gives this advice to couples:

> The moment you feel a rise in emotional intensity with someone you love, immediately start tapping. [This] instantly tells your body that there's no need to go into the fight/flight/freeze response, that the current situation is not a threat to your physical survival, and that you're not traveling along the same dysfunctional neurological highway you've constructed in the past.[3]

Dawson is suggesting that you both tap while continuing the discussion. He explains that for many couples, well-traveled pathways in the brain are so deeply established that the couple gets "sucked into the same old lose-lose situation"[4] even when they know they are going to crash if they travel along that path. Tapping intervenes at the level of your brain chemistry. It signals safety, slows emotional reactivity, and allows you to take a breath and, in that moment, to look at your partner through fresh eyes and actively listen rather than just react in old ways.

The first time we tried this with this chapter in mind, it worked beautifully. Donna was in a situation where, due to unforeseen circumstances, she had to change some plans without consulting with David. She knew this had caused "trouble" (inconvenience) for him, and she was already on edge when they talked about what had occurred. Part of her "no trouble" pattern was that when she did cause "trouble," she expected the other person to be hurt, angry, or upset. Besides this anticipation in itself having a self-fulfilling quality, it was so rare that Donna did inconvenience the people closest to her that they tended to feel surprised and hurt if she didn't meet their expectations. So, as she began the conversation with David, she already felt upset that he was (presumably) irritated, as if there could never be any room for her to make her own decisions when they might inconvenience someone else. This of course has the effect of bringing out a defensive emotional response in the partner.

Hearing the tone in Donna's voice, David said, "Whoa! This is the moment we've been waiting for. I'm going to start tapping [on the points shown in Figure 6-3], and I hope you will too." David was indeed a bit put out by the inconvenience of the change in plans, but he hadn't gone into the reaction Donna was anticipating. Her essentially accusing him of having gone there did not, at least this time, hook him. He of course doesn't know what would have happened if he weren't tapping, but he later reflected that listening while tapping seemed to help him receive Donna's emotional charge without taking it personally. As Donna tapped while explaining the circumstances, as well as when listening to David's response, she recognized that he was taking her in deeply and understood what occurred, and we were both quickly done with it.

The next time we entered a situation that had an emotional charge and used this "tap while you talk, tap while you listen" method, however, we found that there is a strong caveat. It made things much worse! An effect of tapping while telling a story is that it helps you go more deeply into the story, uncovering emotions to which you did not have access. If the incident you are tapping on touches into a theme that has a great deal of unresolved emotion, you may simply escalate the situation, uncovering layer after layer without resolving a thing before the next unresolved emotion or memory has surfaced. Then the next, and then the next. If you find that continuing the conversation while tapping is escalating the negative emotions or starting to spin out of control, it is time to change strategies. Immediately!

Here is how that played out for us. One of the dynamics in Donna's theme of causing no one any trouble is that her needs, desires, and preferences are not always made obvious, so she often feels dismissed by David, the one who is closest to her. At the time of this writing (we are at this moment no further along in writing the chapter than you are in reading it), there is some heated disagreement between the two of us about this. How much is it the issue that David actually dismisses what Donna has conveyed to him and how much is it that Donna feels dismissed though she never really expressed her thoughts or needs? When David presents his side of this particular argument, Donna of course feels dismissed even further. We can't wait to see how this one gets resolved! Anyway, we have been planning a teaching tour in Europe to correspond with the release of one of our books. Donna felt that David had put the plans into motion without having adequately gone over the details with her, and she was upset about it. When she received the actual itinerary, she was hit particularly hard. The conversation began something like this:

DONNA: "This wasn't my plan. This isn't what I want to do. I thought I was
   so clear about what I wanted. I thought you heard me" (voice escalating).
DAVID: "Another opportunity for tapping, I see" (as he starts to tap).
DONNA (now tapping as well): "I feel so betrayed. You didn't hear me at all.
   You sold me out here! I feel invisible and dismissed. It's just like when . . ."

This led to an intensifying list of unpleasant incidents, each of which we remember quite differently, and we were both getting hooked. David finally said, with due sarcasm about the process we were planning to write about: "Isn't this going well! What was it that we were trying to demonstrate? That we can be as petty as the next couple?" We both agreed it was time to shift out of the nosedive. So we invoked our standby, the Pact (chapter 3), and got beyond the acrimony. Feeling tuned in again to our collaborative alliance, we made a date to return to the issue using the Basic Recipe rather than random tapping.

So the caveat for the "tap while you talk" technique is this: If you both start tapping at the moment one of you feels an emotional bump and the emotional charge seems to be escalating rather than de-escalating, shift to your Pact—Stop, Tap, Attune, Resolve (STAR).

Often enough, however, simply adding tapping to the discussion will keep you calm, centered, and supportive of one another, rather than allow you to be taken over by your emotions.

2. Shifting the Way You Respond to Behaviors in Your Partner That Had Been Triggers for Anger, Hurt, or Resentment

Beyond not escalating an argument, you can use tapping to shift the patterns that trigger emotional upset between you. After using our Pact to clear the air, we returned to the travel arrangements that had originally hooked us.

To get her SUD rating, Donna brought to mind the moment she read the itinerary, how dismissed she immediately felt, and how she then felt like she was talking to a blank wall when she told David about her feelings. Playing this scene as a movie in her mind, she gave a rating of 8 to the emotional intensity at the most distressful moment. Looking for a Reminder Phrase (p. 195)—a few words that capture the scene—Donna thought of a number of phrases: "I'm invisible to you"; "I get discounted when I talk to you"; "I've been betrayed"; "I'm uncared for by you." She then reflected: "*Uncared for* is the wrong word. I know you care for me. What I felt at that moment is 'I'm making trouble for you. That's all you can think of. You've already made your plan.' So what I want doesn't matter." She settled on "I still can't cause trouble for you despite your having betrayed me" as her initial Reminder Phrase.

A difference between a professionally guided session and a self-guided session involves lesser or greater reliance on the Reminder Phrase. In this situation, David is assisting Donna as her husband, but he also brings his professional background and skills in formulating the wordings. Chapter 6 instructed you to keep coming back to the initial Reminder Phrase, adjusting it later as additional aspects (p. 203) of the problem revealed themselves. In the following transcription of our session, you will see that David did not stay with the initial Reminder Phrase but immediately addressed various aspects of the situation. The advantages of this as a teaching tool are that you get to see how flexible the technique is and are given a model of its effective use. The disadvantage would be if you, as a beginner, feel you need to be equally adept at formulating advanced wordings. You don't. Staying with the initial Reminder Phrase and gradually adjusting it as new aspects reveal themselves can be very effective. Always remember that this is more about shifting the energies than anything else, and the tapping is doing that for you.

We did begin with the initial Reminder Phrase in formulating the Acceptance Statement: "Even though I still can't cause trouble for you despite your having betrayed me, I deeply love and accept myself" (stated three times, along with the physical techniques described on p. 198). Then we started the tapping, with our iPad recording it all.

David would offer the phrase that Donna would use as she tapped (she would tap on a point for as long as it took to say the phrase and then go to the next point and phrase, following the sequence of points shown in Figure 6-3). David tapped along with Donna and repeated the phrase with her. That is the format we used throughout the session, and we suggest you experiment with it as well if one of you is guiding the other's work. David suggested the wording except for phrases where the transcript indicates that Donna initiated it. Some phrases were repeated several times while tapping different points and only the first use of the phrase is in the transcript:

I still can't cause trouble for you despite your having betrayed me.
You betrayed me.
We talked about the itinerary, but you ignored me.
I feel betrayed.
Now I'm stuck because I can't make trouble for these people. They've put their time and effort into making this itinerary [wording initiated by Donna].
They will be hurt if I make trouble here.

They will feel deserted, let down, like there is no net beneath them.

They will feel as if I don't care about them.

I could have made trouble, but instead I will be hurt. I didn't speak up. I just had to swallow how betrayed I felt [Donna's wording].

I had to swallow how I let *myself* down because I couldn't let *them* down.

I let myself down again because I couldn't let them down.

At this point, we did the Integration Sequence (p. 200). Then back to tapping:

Feeling betrayed.

I can't make trouble.

I have to go along.

They will probably never trust anyone again if I back out of this [Donna's wording].

People's lives will be destroyed if I make trouble [laughter—overstating an underlying assumption can bring humor and lightness while continuing to address a heavy issue].

They won't survive.

Feeling so trapped.

I'm always trapped.

This time I expected David to make sure I wasn't trapped [Donna's wording].

I expected David to take care of me.

David didn't take care of me.

Now I have to move forward with that same old upset with myself that I have let myself down [Donna's wording].

At this point, David asked Donna to take a deep breath and go back to the scene with the itinerary and give it a SUD rating. She said it was a 4½, down from an 8. He asked her how she knew there was remaining distress. She said, "I still have pain in my heart, though I'm more calm. But even though I'm not as upset, there is still this very painful, kinesthetic wound." This provided the wording for the next Acceptance Statement: "Even though I still have this pain in my heart, I deeply love and accept myself" (repeated, along with the physical procedures). The last time, rather than "I deeply love and accept myself," David had Donna substitute a more specific positive affirmation (see "The Choices Method," pp. 211–212), which was,

"I choose to recognize that I am changing this right now—a four and a half is very different from an eight." Then another round of tapping:

This wound in my heart.

This pain in my heart.

This pain in my heart from all the times I couldn't make trouble.

Nobody ever saw me. I would protect everyone else from having to face trouble, but nobody protected me [Donna's wording].

They were so happy I wasn't trouble [Donna's wording].

What a relief that Donna isn't trouble.

Nobody saw me.

And that's what it felt like when I spoke to David about the itinerary [Donna's wording].

He doesn't hear me, he doesn't know me. He doesn't care. It's okay with him that I'm going to be sacrificed [Donna's wording; David at this moment is glad he is also tapping and staying relatively centered].

It's okay with him if I'm sacrificed for the good of the organization. He didn't step in and rescue me. So I'm just left holding the bag again [Donna's wording].

I'm worried by how much I'm pushing myself. And I'm scared. I feel alone in that fear [Donna's wording].

Nobody is going to worry about me. And it's even worse if I'm trouble [Donna's wording].

They just ignore my needs. If I don't make trouble, nobody ever knows I have a need [Donna's wording].

They don't see me if I don't make trouble. Nobody sees me whether I make trouble or I don't make trouble [Donna's wording].

If I don't make trouble, I'm invisible. If I make trouble, they want me gone.

What a disappointment she turned out to be [Donna's wording].

If I make trouble, they want me gone. If I make trouble, there are awful consequences. If I don't make trouble, I'm invisible. My needs don't get met [Donna's wording].

I want to do this right this time. It's time to do it right. It's time to shift this energy [Donna's wording].

It's time to shift the energy that keeps me trapped in this pattern.

And I can do it differently. And I have [referring to a recent positive interaction with David where Donna had shown her anger. At this point, when much of the charge has been removed, the person is able to consider experiences that counter a deep, long-standing belief].

Yes, I have had some real successful moments. I've been trouble, and I've been loved anyway [Donna's wording].

I've had some successful moments where I've been trouble and I've been loved anyway [David asks Donna to describe one].

Even though you were quick to judge me yesterday, when I told you my side of the story, you switched on a dime. That was love [Donna's wording].

When I felt sick on our last trip, you were there one hundred percent. I was causing you a lot of trouble, and you didn't make me feel guilty.

At this point, Donna went back to the itinerary scene and rated it at a 3. We had skipped the Integration Sequence, but we did it here, bringing the rating down slightly, to 2½. David suggested that the next Acceptance Statement be: "Even though it's still two and a half, I feel power welling up in me." Donna snapped back: "No, I don't feel power. I feel like I will really be betrayed if I let this go. I will never be safe again if I let this go because you will never see yourself. I'm scared to make this go down to zero. I'm scared to make this go away. I'll never be safe then. You'll just go on in your own merry way treating me in the same way. If I let this go, then I'll really be betrayed. I might gain something by getting over being unable to be trouble, but I'm scared that if I get over this, you'll say, 'See, it was your fault all the time,' and you will just keep dismissing me."

This is a point that could derail the process. If David defended himself, *that* would have been a betrayal since Donna was laying herself wide open and had now hit on a psychological reversal (p. 209). While her hope was to no longer feel distress about the situation, she believed David would ignore his side of the problem if she succeeded. If you are guiding your partner in a tapping session, you need to be deeply committed to putting your side of the story aside for the time being so you are taking in and even being an advocate for your partner's reality. David demonstrated that he was doing this by suggesting this Acceptance Statement: "Even though I'm scared that if I get over this I will be even more invisible to David, I deeply accept this dilemma." This worked for Donna, so we proceeded with another round of tapping, this time looking for ways to affirm Donna's power in the situation (note, this was not likely to have been effective before most of the emotional charge had been neutralized):

I'm scared that if I change, David will stay stuck [formulating statements such as this also brought David into deeper empathy for Donna's dilemma].

I don't trust David to do his part.

David won't admit that he discounts me, and if I resolve my part of the issue, he'll never own his part of it.

This is about my power [David now shifts to what he feels is the self-limiting piece in Donna's position].

This is about my being able to say my truth.

This is about my being able to say my truth in a way that no one could ignore.

Not even David.

Even though I'm scared of getting over this completely, I'm getting to be a force to be reckoned with [Donna says, "No, I'm not! Not yet"].

You were yesterday [referring to the earlier incident].

Okay, I'm getting to be a force to be reckoned with [Donna's wording].

Even though I'm scared to get over this, I don't need this anymore [Donna's wording].

I will stay with my power. I will speak my truth. I will speak my truth even if it causes trouble [Donna's wording].

That's what this is about.

Yes, I will speak my truth even if it causes trouble [Donna's wording].

Even though I'm scared to get over this, I will speak my truth. Even if it causes trouble for David, or for the organization, I will speak my truth [Donna's wording].

That's the solution here.

I can speak my truth.

Whatever people's reaction is, that's their issue.

I know I'm basically kind and fair.

I have nothing to be ashamed or guilty about.

I was clear [referring to the situation from the day before.]

I was clear. I was glad for David's reaction.

At this point, Donna's SUD rating had gone down to 1½. When asked how she knows there is still residue, Donna said: "When I look at the scene, I can still feel stress. It is nothing like it was, but I can still feel stress." Going deeper into her feelings, she said, "I still don't believe this will make our marriage stronger because you will get smug and never *get* what you do. You will never get it. I know my part, but I want you to look at yourself. If I get over this issue, you will feel forgiven and I will be forgotten." Again, positioning himself as Donna's guide and advocate and checking his own defensiveness, David suggested this Acceptance Statement: "Even though I want David to look at himself, I don't need to wait for him" and then these tapping statements:

I am becoming such a force that I can't be ignored.

I will be trouble.

I will be trouble if I have to.

Even though I'd like David to "get it," I'm not throwing away my trouble card [Donna is laughing as she repeats this].

Even though I'd like David to "get it," I'm not throwing away my trouble card.

This is giving me permission to use my trouble card.

I claim my trouble card.

I can use it freely.

No guilt.

No shame.

No overcompassion.

I know I'm fair and good.

I can pull out that card any time the situation calls for it.

I can be trouble.

Yea!

Okay, I'm pulling out the card [Donna laughing].

I can be trouble.

You can evolve or not evolve, but I'm pulling out my trouble card whenever I want [Donna laughing].

Get used to it, David.

I'm pulling it out whenever I want.

You're actually very brave to be leading me through this, David [Donna laughs as she repeats David's self-flattering statement].

I can be trouble on my own terms [Donna is laughing].

Returning to the itinerary scene, Donna said, with delight in her voice, "It doesn't have a charge anymore!" Throughout the week, numerous instances came up with David and with others where Donna found herself speaking up even when she knew that what she was saying was different from what the person wanted to hear.

Reflecting on the above transcript, notice how only the initial rounds of tapping focused on Donna's feelings of betrayal and being trapped that were associated with the theme of not being able to cause trouble for anyone. After the first shift in Donna's SUD rating, the focus went to the sensations in her heart and chest. Only after all this was reduced did David's suggested wordings begin to focus on evidence that countered her beliefs regarding not causing trouble (such as when she caused "trouble" by being sick and was nonetheless fully supported). This led to a fear that if she overcame her part of the pattern, David would still persist with his part and continue to dismiss her. This was addressed by embracing her power in the situation, recognizing that she can evolve even if David doesn't, that she can speak her truth and be a force to be reckoned with no matter what David does or doesn't do.

But Donna also knew there was more. She'd not gone into the childhood events that created the "no trouble" pattern or healed the emotional wounds that trace to them. Conveniently, these are the next two interrelated topics we wanted to illustrate.

3. Tracing Emotional Challenges That Play Themselves Out Again and Again in Your Relationship to Formative Childhood Experiences

Tying the "can't make trouble" theme back to an early memory, Donna recalled a family outing when she was about four. They had gone to a forested area in the mountains. Donna had wandered off and become lost. As it grew dark, she was unable to find her way back. With no one having found her either, she was coming to terms with her belief that they had all gone home without her. This seemed natural to her. "Of course they wouldn't wait for me. I could imagine Mama saying in the front seat of the car, 'We loved Donna so much. Wasn't she wonderful! It is so sad that we have to leave her, but what are we going to do? It's getting dark and we have to go.' And I understood completely."

Asked to describe what it is like now to think back on that little girl who understood this completely, she reported feeling "really sad." She reflected that "even though I comforted myself by saying I knew my Mama loved me, I also believed Mama's love would fade into the background if I made trouble. And, in this case, it would be trouble for the family to have to look for me." Donna gave her feelings of sadness about this an 8 on the zero-to-ten SUD scale.

4. Healing These Lingering Emotional Wounds

The Acceptance Statement Donna used while massaging her Central Meridian points was, "Even though I couldn't make trouble, I deeply love and accept myself." Here were the words she used, sometimes suggested by David, but more often now provided by Donna:

Can't make them have to look for me.
I can't be the cause of making them uncomfortable.
It's dark after all. They've got to go home.
I understand.
Of course I'll be left here in the dark.
I'll be left here in the dark.
I hope the wolves will find me and raise me.
But I don't see the wolves yet.
I can't find the wolves.
I really don't know where I am.
I wonder what's going to happen to me.
I knew they had to abandon me because now I was trouble.
I broke the rules.
I became trouble.
I didn't hold up my part of the bargain.
And now I'm all alone.
I'm only four.
I'm out in the wilderness.
The best I can hope for is that the wolves will now raise me.
I had my fantasy world. That made it less awful.
But deep down I knew they had to leave me because I had caused trouble.
My brother and sister caused enough trouble. I wasn't going to create more.
Mama had just come home from the hospital, and I wasn't going to create trouble for her.
But I got lost.

And I would have been trouble if they hadn't gone on home.

But I see Daddy coming around a winding bend on the side of the mountain.

Daddy looked for me. Wow!

He saw me and he started laughing.

His arms opened wide running toward me.

It's making me cry [crying].

I was so surprised!

They fooled me.

I was shocked that they would look for me.

Daddy found me!

Even though I was trouble, they looked for me.

I got back in the car and found out that Mama never said that.

She never said, ". . . it's getting dark, so we have to leave."

They never left.

They stayed for me.

Registering this very deeply now.

I was able to be trouble when I was four.

I got one chance.

Maybe it was okay to be trouble.

Of course, I got over that [laughter at David's lampoon].

It didn't change the contract.

I still had these rules that I couldn't cause trouble.

I couldn't be trouble.

There was already enough trouble.

I'm not gonna be trouble.

I'm gonna make it SO easy for them to have me around.

They won't ever be sorry I'm there.

I won't have any needs [crying].

I'll just make it easy for them.

They'll never know what my needs are.

They'll never know if I get sick or unhappy.

That was my basic rule.

In all my relationships, no one would ever regret that I was around because I
    didn't make trouble.

I didn't make trouble.

It was okay for them to make trouble. They hadn't grown to the place where
they didn't have to make trouble.
But I had.
Whatever people needed to make their lives easier, I would do for them.
They were vulnerable, so I didn't make trouble.

The SUD rating at this point on Donna's sadness in realizing what it really meant
for that little girl that they were not coming back for her had gone down from an 8
to a 5. The next Acceptance Statement was, "Even though she didn't realize that she
was loved enough to be able to make trouble and to be inconvenient, I feel so much
compassion and love for that little girl and feel such sympathy for her." The next
round of tapping included these wordings:

My role in life was to be easy for them.
If I added to the trouble, Mama would get sick again.
If I added to the trouble, Daddy would get all stressed.
They have so much to handle!
I can't make more. I just can't make trouble.
So I don't experience my needs.
I go into fantasy.
The wolves were going to raise me.
Fantasy worked.
I got very good at not causing trouble.
I was happy.
Real happy!
So it worked.
It didn't work all my life, but it worked in my family.
They appreciated it without realizing.
It was okay for me to not be seen.
I had a really wonderful fantasy life.
I came out smelling like a rose.
I didn't cause trouble.

We were both surprised by the next SUD rating: "It's up to a 9! I guess because
I'm having to feel it. I've never felt it." Sometimes coming out of denial is its own

stressor. Donna observed, "I've always kind of laughed about it, how cute that was, but now I just feel sad." This is not unusual for feelings that have been buried in order to support a coping style, and it is not the time to become discouraged or give up. On the contrary, you know you are on the trail of emotionally significant material. The next Acceptance Statement put what had occurred into a constructive context: "Even though I'm really in it and feeling it deeply now, I choose to know that this is how I will heal." Wordings in the next round of tapping included:

That poor little girl.
She was only four.
I had to carry the burden of the family.
And not complain.
And not be trouble for anyone.
I was only four.
It's really sad when I think about it.
But thank God for my rich imagination.
Thank God for my spirit feeding me so well.
Even though it's really sad, I came out of it really well.
Ignorance is bliss.
Denial really served me well.
There's a deep realization here.
It is very healing.
Even though I'm getting in touch with a lot of things, there's a healing going on.
Even though it's sad, I welcome this awareness.
That poor little girl wasn't really so poor.
She had so much going for her that she was able to take this burden within her family.
And she pulled it off.
She came out of it fairly unscathed.
Of course her relationship skills sucked [laughter at another playful dig from David].
But beyond that, she came out of it pretty whole.
So while I'm feeling compassion for her, I'm also feeling some awe for her.
How richly resourced she was.
What a blessing.

She did so well carrying that burden for her family.
She did so well carrying everyone's sadness and being the witness!
She did so well. She did her job well.

This brief round, examining the larger context of the situation with compassion for her four-year-old self, quickly brought Donna's SUD rating down from a 9 to a 2. However, her focus now went to other situations from later in her life that had the same theme. She focused on one of them from her first marriage. She had a miscarriage and got an infection while in the hospital. But she signed herself out against doctor's orders, left the hospital, and stayed with a girlfriend so that she wouldn't cause a financial burden for her husband. When she did see him, although she was in deep grief, she gave no indication that she had signed herself out of the hospital against medical advice and was silently pleased about having spared him any inconvenience or expense. The Acceptance Statement she used for this new aspect of the theme was, "Even though I had that terrible loss that I didn't let him feel, I deeply love and accept myself." She continued, tapping, using these wordings:

That pattern of not being trouble, which was so adaptive in my childhood, caused me to choose a partner who had no tolerance for trouble.
It was a perfect match [laughter].
He couldn't tolerate trouble. I could hide all my needs.
So it played out, again and again and again, throughout that whole marriage.
I couldn't show my needs. I couldn't be trouble. And the pattern just got deeper and deeper.
I couldn't be trouble.
The only thing I could do was to finally leave.
We were like pieces of a puzzle locked together.
He could not tolerate trouble. I couldn't be trouble. That was our bond.
So even though I'm feeling really sad, I'm seeing the pattern.
Even though I'm feeling really sad, I'm having a really empowering insight.
Even though I'm feeling really sad, I choose to recognize that I've come a long way on this.

By this point, her SUD rating on her sadness for the little girl was down to zero, but it was still a 4 for the young woman in the hospital. In exploring what was keeping it at a 4, Donna realized she had a lot of shame about not speaking up. Her next Acceptance Statement was, "Even though I feel ashamed that I was willing to risk my life rather than inconvenience my husband, I deeply love and accept myself." Wordings during the tapping included:

> Feeling ashamed that I checked myself out of the hospital so I wouldn't cause trouble for my husband.
> I wouldn't cause trouble.
> Remembering that it was heroic when I was four to carry the family burden.
> That four-year-old girl wanted to make everyone in the family happy.
> She was able to muster the spirit to carry the family burden.
> She played out what she learned when she was four to keep her mother healthy.
> She just didn't update the program.
> She just kept playing out her family role.
> And she found the right partner to do it with.
> I was doing what I learned.
> It's really hard to see my part in his cruelty.

As her judgment toward the woman in the hospital receded, she was left with humiliation about having been such a doormat. See how the "layers of the onion" unfold? You simply work with whatever emerges. After resolving the humiliation, a few other incidents with the same theme, also from her adult life, were able to be resolved quite readily. The resolution of each specific issue builds on all that had been emotionally resolved before it. Complex as this sounds, the recording shows that the session lasted only forty-seven minutes. Nonetheless, Donna was exhausted. Exhausted but feeling triumphant!

5. Transform the Patterns That Grew Out of Early Emotional Wounds

Even after significant emotional healing, as illustrated in the above transcript, the patterns that become embedded in one's lifestyle or relationships do not automatically shift. But they are ripe at that point for an intervention that does shift them. The theme that Donna wanted to change involved the way she would still hold back from exerting her will if it was going to disappoint or inconvenience someone. This often came up with David in work situations. Couples who work together face a unique set of challenges, and we are not exempt.

Donna selected a situation involving our organization where it was going to be difficult to get what she wanted, and she imagined herself expressing her intentions clearly and with strong resolve. Called the Outcome Projection Procedure,[5] this technique is designed for establishing a new behavior or emotional response. It begins with envisioning a hoped-for outcome rather than a symptom or troubling situation. It also uses a zero-to-ten rating, but it rates the believability of the *hoped-for outcome*, with zero being that it is impossible and 10 being that it absolutely could happen. Except for these differences, it applies the same Basic Recipe you have been learning.

Because David is the CEO of our organization, he periodically finds himself standing with the other key administrators in enforcing a policy with which Donna disagrees, sometimes vehemently. This is not a recipe for family harmony. Donna not only feels outnumbered and powerless, she feels betrayed that her husband is siding with the others instead of her, even though the work they are promoting, Eden Energy Medicine, is her formulation and is in her name. David, on the other hand, feels compelled by considerations that are not even on Donna's radar (state statutes, HR regulations, budgetary concerns, etc.) to keep the operation healthy and running smoothly, so when he digs in, he believes it is ultimately for Donna's good even if she doesn't recognize it.

In Donna's hoped-for outcome, she saw herself standing firm against David and two of our top administrators in asking for an exception to standard procedures that would be quite troublesome for them to implement. It was a theme they had wrestled with innumerable times over the years. The job of David and our administrators is to build a structure that can accommodate the hundreds of people who are involved with the organization as teachers and practitioners and the tens of thousands they serve. But as things played out, people learned that if they wanted to be an exception to a rule, the way to get around the administration was to figure out how to get Donna's ear and plead their case. Her heart would open and she would go to bat for them. This was driving the administration crazy, including her loyal husband, and she eventually became much more discerning about such requests. However, sometimes a case was so compelling that she would open another round of conflict with the people she'd been working with for years in order to advocate for someone she hardly knew.

In the situation that was the focus of the session, a student who had studied with

Donna long ago wanted to get credit toward completing our certification program for courses taken years earlier. Our administration had allowed this during the first couple of years of our program, but as the program evolved and became more sophisticated, we recognized that training from a decade earlier was not equivalent to what we are teaching now. A firm rule was eventually made that giving credit for our early courses could no longer be done. Donna had agreed to this rule, but now she was faced with a person who so represented what she liked in an energy medicine practitioner that she decided to buck the system once more. Our administration is committed to maintaining high standards, and the complex and laborious job of evaluating whether the person had mastered the myriad of principles and procedures that certification represents was going to fall on their laps. Donna felt scared to request the exception, and her aversion to making trouble for others did not make this any easier. She visualized herself presenting the request with confidence and without guilt. On the zero-to-ten scale, with 10 being that it was totally believable that she could do this successfully, she gave it a rating of 4. It was somewhat plausible to her that she could make the request with confidence, but it did not feel very likely.

Her Acceptance Statement was, "Even though I'm not very confident that I can pull this off, I deeply love and accept myself." On her tapping points, she also imagined herself in the situation presenting the request effortlessly as she tapped and used phrases including:

Feeling sure of myself and grounded.
This is the right thing to do.
And it *will* inconvenience them.
And I choose to have this happen.
This is for the greater good.
I'm so sorry it will inconvenience them.
One more time they're going to see me as wishy-washy.
And as a pushover to anyone who brings their problem to me.
But I'm serving a higher truth.
That's how it is.
And I'm going to make it their truth.
I'm sure of myself on this.
I'm using good judgment!

Here she did the Integration Sequence and then returned to the tapping:

I can do this.
It's correct that I do this.
It's right. It's smart. It's ethical.
Even if it makes me feel guilty.
Even if it makes me feel like I'm being unreasonable.
Even if it makes me feel like it's not fair that I am causing them so much extra
    work.
I see myself being so positive that they come over to my side.
I see them willingly go through the trouble!
I'm exuding the rightness of this.
I don't have to cower and be afraid to talk with them.
I see them coming over to my side.

After all of this, Donna went back into the vision of successfully bringing her request to David and the two others and rated its believability: "It's still a four; maybe it's gone up just a bit, to a four and a half. It's so hard not to feel guilty, and that's where I get caught." Her next Acceptance Statement was, "Even though I feel guilty about it, I deeply accept what I am trying to do." Phrases she used in the next round of tapping included:

Exuding the rightness of what I am doing.
Feeling so confident and positive.
Feeling so confident and positive that my guilt just dissolves.
Even they are surprised that I'm not apologizing, saying, "I'm so sorry that I'm
    making trouble!"
This is the higher road.
I'm exuding the rightness of what I'm doing, and it's contagious.
There they are, experiencing me in a new way.
I love standing there just doing what I'm feeling deep down. No apologies.
    No guilt.

After this round, her believability level that she could stand in front of the three administrators and gracefully hold her position had gone up to a 7. She reported, "I feel much more confident and empowered and excited about not apologizing. I still don't feel like I can pull it off, but I'm feeling confidence." For her next Acceptance Statement, David suggested, "Even though I still don't believe I can pull this off, I choose to recognize that I can approach this with new confidence." After trying this, Donna said, "But it gets complicated because my husband is standing there with them, and I want him to choose me over the business." So the Acceptance Statement became, "Even though it feels like David is siding with them against me, I choose to know that if I stand firm and feel positive and exude that positive feeling, I am moving toward a positive outcome." She then returned to the vision of standing in this positive space in front of the others and tapped using statements that included:

No guilt.
I'm seeing myself being very effective.
I'm standing so firm that all four of us are harmonizing.
I'm one of them! They've never seen me as one of them.
I have some power here.
I have some positive power here.
I'm standing up for what is right.
I'm moving the organization in a positive direction.
I'm seeing myself do this.
I'm seeing myself being very effective.

Her believability score had now gone up "from a shaky seven to a very solid eight—feels like a big jump." She reported, "I'm believing the vision that I'm one of them. It isn't me *against* them or them *against* me. We're together as long as I stand firm; I don't have to grovel and cry." Even though additional rounds of tapping are not usually necessary once the believability score reaches 8—the vision will usually translate into the person's life quite readily—Donna didn't want to stop there. She explained, "I think the most important thing I've gotten is that I have finally resigned myself to the idea that the needs of the administration trump what I think is important for the program. You guys run the show, and I don't, and that's all there is to it. Because my name is on the program, you'll sometimes go along with what I want, but you guys represent the business side of things and feel it's your job to convince me I'm wrong. When I stood in that place of holding firm, then it became very different. That's what I want to keep feeling. So I want to take this all the way."

Donna's next Acceptance Statement was, "Even though they haven't respected my opinion on these administrative decisions, I'm taking a stance that they will respect." Returning to the tapping, her statements included:

My perspective matters.
I don't have to grovel.
It feels really, really good to hold my space.
I am taking a stand.
I have my voice. I have my truth.
I am respecting my truth, my stance, my equality with them, and my harmony with them. This feels so positive!
I'm taking this stance.
I am really pulling this off.
I am holding firm.
They know it and I know it.
Even though I'm not an administrator, I carry the spirit of the organization.
I carry the name of the organization. My spirit must be heard. My values must be heard.
I own that and I carry that.

Donna then commented, "What is making it hard for me to get above eight is that I am still looking at you, David. That group is a block of people. You are my husband, yet you will be part of the block against me. I'm looking at you, and I'm hungering for you not to dismiss me." This led to the Acceptance Statement, "Even though David is with the other administrators facing me and it feels like a betrayal and a dismissal, regardless of what David does, I'm standing firm. Regardless of what David does, I'm standing firm." Tapping statements included:

I am exuding the truth of this situation.
I've found my voice.
I am standing tall and firm.
And if David doesn't get it, it's his loss.
If he can't connect with me here, it's his loss.
Because I'm exuding the truth of the situation, I see him coming over to my side.

We're all equals here.

And we all respect one another.

At this point Donna rated the believability of the scene and it was a tad over 9. She reflected that while it seemed very plausible, "It also feels too good to be true. I'm going to have to really practice getting to that state. It's not my default. But I love having done this." Over the next few days, she did raise the issue, she was met with strong resistance, she did hold firm, and over the course of about a week she moved the administrative team to the point where they, with some enthusiasm, took on the challenge of creating a special arrangement for the student in question.

6. Complete Any Other "Unfinished Business" in Your Emotional Life, Including "Baggage" from Earlier Relationships or from an Earlier Time in Your Current Relationship

In the sessions described above, you have seen how a conflict with David was a springboard for Donna to use tapping to:

- resolve the immediate issue
- identify how her side of the conflict was part of a broader theme that traced to her childhood
- heal some of the emotional wounds that kept that theme active in her life
- build a new and more effective way of responding in current situations that call forth the same theme

We will now allow Donna to return from this naked display of her emotional conflicts, necessary when being used as a demonstration case, to the relative privacy of being an author.

Unhealed emotional wounds from an earlier time in your current relationship or from a previous relationship may be an invisible force that is keeping your marriage from moving forward. This chapter opened by describing the way Jeremy and Melissa's marriage took a downhill turn involving Jeremy's irrational anger and jealousy toward Melissa's ex-husband. After Jeremy completed his work, Melissa was the next one to be on the hot seat. The progression, or should we say regression, from their initial marital happiness to the tense, volatile atmosphere in the home had been a nightmare for Melissa. Her first marriage had gone through a similar trajectory and she was questioning whether she was capable of sustaining a satisfying marriage.

The last third of the two-hour initial session focused on her shock about what had occurred with Jeremy and her concern that this was simply what happens for her in a marriage. Watching the transformation in Jeremy during the first part of the session was certainly reassuring. But she had still gone through the nightmarish experience of having what seemed so good become so bad. Acceptance Statements such as "Even though I was shocked by Jeremy's jealousy and wondered if the marriage was over . . ." and "Even though I was deeply wounded by the disaster of my first marriage . . ." led to tapping rounds that worked through the emotional residue of both experiences and oriented her to a recognition that the pattern did not have to repeat itself. At the two-week follow-up session, Melissa and Jeremy both reported that their intimacy was stronger than it had ever been. This is not to suggest that single-session "cures" are typical for most marital problems, but it does illustrate how isolated issues that are interfering in a relationship can readily be resolved.

In any case, it is good to know that painful experiences from earlier relationships or from an earlier time in your current relationship can be processed so that old wounds don't continue to fester or limit the possibilities for your future together. While such wounds are a source of vulnerability if they are not adequately addressed, they can become a source of greater strength and resilience after being processed and healed. Energy psychology is a powerful tool for healing them. In situations where abuse, betrayal, affairs, the death of a partner, or other severe shocks were involved, the assistance of a counselor who is adept in energy psychology can be invaluable and the payoff immense.

7. Establish a Strong Mental Vision of How You Want Yourself or Your Relationship to Change and Rewire Your Brain to Support that Vision

Matt and Jessica had met twenty-two years earlier and married after four years of a stormy courtship. It was the first marriage for each of them. Matt, who was largely an introvert and a loner, was uneasy about committing himself to Jessica. The one context where a more exuberant side of him would come out was in the pursuit of a new woman, and he agreed to Jessica's pleas that they marry, but only under Matt's condition that they have an "open relationship." Open relationships, involving sexual dalliances outside the marriage, were in style when they met in the late 1960s, and Jessica reluctantly agreed, feeling sure in her heart that Matt would settle down and focus solely on her. He did, but it took another decade during which she suffered immeasurable anguish.

THE BACKGROUND

Matt was a workaholic. Before he met Jessica, his pattern was to work intensively for sixty to seventy hours per week and then, every month or so, to take off for three or four days with whomever he was dating at the time for a wild fling. His stored passion from the weeks of intense work would release in a euphoric orgy of sex, food, wine, deep conversation, and other intimate pleasures. Then back to work, with the woman usually wondering why he disappeared after one of the most intensely intimate encounters she'd ever had.

Early in their relationship, this met Jessica's needs quite nicely. They didn't see one another as often as she would have liked between their odysseys, but the intense times together were so fulfilling that they held her over during the times between. About six months after Matt and Jessica started dating, Jessica's roommate moved, so Jessica needed to find a new roommate or give up her apartment. Instead, she persuaded Matt to let her move in with him. His terms were stern but clear. He could still see other women, though he wouldn't bring them to their home. His uncertainty about committing to her was playing out in this ambivalent arrangement. Jessica was happy for the chance to get to see Matt every day and capitulated to his demand. Over time, however, the long weekends were increasingly with other women while the duller routines of daily life were shared with her. Matt started to blame Jessica for not being much fun anymore. All this got old very quickly, and when Matt would return from his trysts, Jessica would be furious, they would fight and then eventually make up, and things would seem smooth until the next time. Meanwhile, about two years into the relationship now, Matt was growing more deeply bonded to Jessica despite the other women and the emotionally heated battles he would periodically have with her. On her side, Jessica believed that they had a "soul connection" and that if they got married, the public/spiritual ritual would seal their deeper bond.

It didn't. After the marriage, the push-pull of Matt becoming closer and then undoing the growing intimacy by going off with another woman did not change. As a result, once their daughter was born, parenting and special projects became Jessica's primary areas of focus, with Matt's cordial but marginal involvement. While Matt's intense, brief affairs became less frequent over the years, Jessica reached a point where she told Matt she would leave him if he had another one. He felt she was reneging on the agreement that got him to marry her in the first place and defiantly made a point of being away at an undisclosed location the following weekend. Jessica had taken their daughter and moved out before he returned home. The only place she was willing to continue to see Matt was in the office of a therapist.

Matt was very confused. He had grown to love Jessica far more deeply than he had ever loved anyone before, but his trysts were the place he would truly feel free, excited, fully alive. Over time, however, even his excursions into new romance were losing their thrill. It was also harder to keep them from getting complicated—in part because the eighties didn't support the sexual freedom of the sixties—but also in part because as he evolved, he wasn't able to be intimate with new women without engaging them at a deeper level. He wasn't able to compartmentalize so wantonly. So by now, he was more ready to hear Jessica's complaints and to consider changing their arrangement. As he registered the amount of pain he had caused Jessica, his whole take on what he was up to shifted. In the past, he had been able to discount her pain since he was only doing what they had agreed on. As he let himself feel how deeply he was hurting this woman whom he had come to love, he found himself agreeing to stop seeing other women. True to his word, Matt didn't have another fling from that day on.

ENTERING THERAPY TWENTY-TWO YEARS INTO THEIR RELATIONSHIP

Fast-forward eight years. Matt and Jessica are again seeking couple counseling. Matt had been the innocent victim of a gunshot during a robbery. He saw the gun point at him, felt the bullet enter his chest, and lay in his own blood, conscious but sure his life was ending. As it turned out, the bullet had entered and exited his body without damaging any organs. After prompt, competent medical attention, he was soon out of the hospital and back into his usual routines. But one thing was plaguing him: "I've just had my life spared. A bit to any side and I could well be dead. But I'm not. I'm alive and well. Why am I not feeling more joy?" Indeed, he was still the same serious, somber, digital kind of guy he had been before his encounter with mortality.

While he and Jessica had been carrying out a very amiable relationship after Jessica had moved back in more than two decades earlier, it had little passion. They rarely made love. Matt was more fully committed to his work than ever, and he was just too busy for much intimate time. His brush with death had brought into stark relief how gray his life had become since he stopped having his affairs. It was as if encountering a new woman had provided the context that brought out his passion, intense joy, and ability to have fun. Without that, he wasn't able to find anything else that stimulated his spirit in that same delicious way. His marriage was comfortable and meant the world to him, but over the years he watched with quiet desperation the withering of his more spirited side.

After Matt's recovery from the gunshot wound, he and Jessica had some of the most penetrating discussions of their relationship. Not only did Matt not feel joy about having survived, he realized that he rarely felt fully alive anymore. He no longer blamed this on Jessica, but he recognized that he had slowly closed his heart over the years. He joked about how the bullet had entered his chest "but fortunately there was nothing there." Jessica was a spirited woman, but she had taken her fervor elsewhere—their daughter, other family, a project with orphaned infants—after years of trying to engage Matt at a more passionate level. Matt's recognition and sadness about how much he had closed himself was welcome news for her, and this led to their decision to once more seek therapy. A friend referred them to David.

They came into therapy with Matt's concerns as the primary focus and with Jessica there to support him. After a thorough history and several "cleanup" sessions where tapping was used to address unresolved issues from their marriage as well as from their childhoods, Matt and Jessica were feeling the closest to one another they had since the charm of their earliest days together. But Matt didn't want to stop there. He wanted to recover the spirit he had once relegated to his trysts and had then lost altogether.

In a poignant session that started with a focus on how lost Matt felt in regard to moving forward with more joy, Jessica recognized at a deeper level than she ever had before the sacrifice Matt had made by stopping his flings. Their focus, going back to the previous therapy, had always been on her pain and his betrayal and blundering insensitivity. Matt had done a great deal to help Jessica heal back then, and he had been faithful now for the past eight years. In this particular session, Jessica had a reverie of appreciation and was able to feed Matt tapping statements such as "I turned away from freedom"; "I exchanged fun and excitement to stop hurting Jessica"; "I gave up my passion, just like my dad"; "I closed the door on the most direct route I had to joy." Besides helping Matt begin to deal with the emptiness he felt, Jessica's empathy for him had a profound effect. They were in this together, Matt's lingering guilt about his flings stopped blocking his creativity about the situation, and he was more motivated than ever to bring his spirited side into their marriage.

While Matt pleaded for our understanding that "there are some limits to the degree to which a man can change his personality," he spoke poignantly about how deeply he longed for a more joyful disposition. David was able to help him identify numerous influences in his life that reinforced his somber side and others that crushed his more joyful and spirited side. After some discussion of these influences, tapping was used to address and change the ways his somber side was being reinforced and his joyful side inhibited.

ESTABLISHING A MENTAL IMAGE OF THE CHANGE

By this point in their work together, David felt that a way of supporting the type of global change Matt was hoping for was to have him create a vivid vision that symbolized his life with that change already having occurred and then to "tap it in." Matt and Jessica's long story is being presented in this section on the seventh way couples can use acupoint tapping to illustrate the approach Matt used at this juncture. It began with a simple instruction that you may want to experiment with as well:

Relax deeply. Feel how life will be once the inner change you hope for has been achieved. Allow a vision that symbolizes this change to emerge. Write it down or share it with your partner.

Again, the word *vision* is used very loosely. You may see images, but it may instead be a word description or simply an understanding. Your vision may be concrete or more symbolic. It could, for instance, be a mental picture of yourself tending a rose garden or it could be a deer running through a meadow. It might be highly detailed or a mere glimpse of a distant scene.

If you are working the exercises as you read the book, choose a personal goal that is important to you and construct a mental image of how your life will be when it is in place. If you are focusing on your relationship, you might, for instance, see yourself and your partner in ecstasy or having just triumphed together during a challenging task. Play with this image. Refine it until it is a vision you are strongly drawn to pursue. If nothing emerges that stirs you, wait until a goal that really matters is up for you. Matt had long recognized that one of the reasons his spirit gets squeezed out of him was the pace he was keeping. The image that came to him was a calendar. His first thought was, "Hey, I can find something more inspiring than a calendar! How about leaning against a redwood and listening to the wind in an old-growth forest? Or seeing myself with Jessica climbing the Eiffel Tower?" But his mind kept returning to the damn calendar, so we decided to go with it.

After settling on an image, he began to examine it. Matt's life was structured so that his vision would have to somehow accommodate his complex career as a software engineer. As an independent contractor, he was always trying to find a balance among the needs of the various clients who had come to rely on him, and he was always feeling stretched. The work was, nonetheless, deeply satisfying and it kept him at his creative edge. But he saw that he had to carve out more time if he was going to give his desire to reawaken his passion any chance of succeeding. He approached the problem like a software engineer trying to make a program more elegant. He saw some routines he could easily cut out and other passion-limiting patterns that would be more challenging to shift. He also knew how readily new projects come in when there is space, so he wanted to envision a new pace, not just a few responsibilities taken off the list.

What better symbol for thinking about this, actually, than a calendar, the very image that had been pursuing him! A one-month wall calendar came into his mind and he had a flash of how he could structure his time very differently. Longer breaks, days off, more sleep, more dedicated time for intimacy and inner work—while obvious—could have substantial impact on his quality of life. While he didn't exactly map it out to the level of "at 8:15 A.M. I'll do this, and then at 9:00, I'll do that," he did have an image of a month and how his time was laid out and he envisioned restructuring it so there was more space, more intimate time, and more sacred time. He wanted to go deeper with Jessica and to share his more joyful side with her. The revised calendar became the symbol of his commitment to have that unfold.

A RATING OF BELIEVABILITY

The next step is to give a rating of how believable the vision is to you. On a scale of zero to ten, how possible does it seem to you? Matt's initial rating was 2, not very likely at all that the calendar was going to support the changes he longed to see. That's how steeped we get in lifelong patterns, but that inertia is exactly what this technique addresses.

PSYCHOLOGICAL REVERSALS

Any heartfelt goal for personal change is meeting some kind of resistance or the change would already have occurred. Some of that resistance may take the form of a psychological reversal, an internal objection or doubt about achieving the goal (p. 209). As Matt tried to embrace the vision of a calendar that supported greater passion in his life, two internal objections immediately occurred to him. The first was that he had made similar resolutions before, but little had changed. As you saw in the previous chapter, a way of addressing such psychological reversals is to begin with an Acceptance Statement in the form of: "Even though" and then briefly describe the old pattern [while rubbing on chest sore spots] and then stating a new and affirming choice [placing both hands over the Heart Chakra]. The wording Matt used to address the first psychological reversal was, "Even though I think this is going to be another disappointment, I choose to recognize that I'm more motivated than I've ever been before." The other concern grew out of his recognition that life can't just be planned out like a calendar on a wall. Situations inevitably come up to disrupt the plans. His Acceptance Statement for this was, "Even though disruptions will occur, I choose to flow with them and then get back into this new rhythm."

THE TAPPING

Matt's tapping (same points as shown in Figure 6-3) at first used statements that addressed his doubts, such as "I can never pull this off" and "I have so much responsibility!" As the tapping neutralized Matt's charge regarding these thoughts, he noticed that the calendar he had seen actually had many empty spaces where rest and renewal could be possible. Beyond sleep, there were sixteen hours every day that were in his control. That eased him, and he tapped in this awareness along with a recognition of how much better his life could be if he carved out more time for intimacy and reflection. Then he tapped on increasing his confidence that he could indeed pull it off and a sense that this new rhythm was his new natural. This part of the work was relatively complex. It involved a review of Matt's entire lifestyle and extended over several weeks, with homework between sessions to incorporate some of the changes in his time management that had been tapped on during the sessions.

A NEW VISION EMERGES

By the time the believability of the new, kinder calendar was up to a 5, Matt's internal picture of the calendar changed. Rather than the entire calendar appearing to him, it was as if he had zeroed in on a single day. What then emerged within that day was a picture of him and Jessica holding hands with intense joy on each of their faces. This became the image for the next round of tapping. There had been no room for it in the old calendar, but after clearing space, this was what his psyche presented.

Tapping on this image was certainly more appealing to him than tapping on the calendar, but the believability rating got stuck at around 6. Two issues that received attention at that point included Matt's intense self-judgment about anything he attempted and the ways his expectations kept him from appreciating what was already good in his life. He tapped on these, as well as seeing Jessica through more appreciative eyes, finding opportunities for affectionate mini-encounters, and making more time for intimacy to occur. Believability was up to a 9 by the end of the session. Phrases he tapped on at home were simple reminders, such as "Even though I'm afraid it's no longer possible, my spirit wants to have more passion." While Matt's energetic structure lent itself more to gradual change than dramatic breakthroughs, over the next several months, he and Jessica reported having more fun with one another than they'd had since their early days.

YOUR TURN

This mental image technique is usually used after the obstacles to reaching your goal have been addressed, which is why we presented it in the context of Matt and Jessica's much longer story. In other words, you would generally identify and work through hindrances and negative emotions about your goal before rating the believability about an image of the goal having already been achieved. Still, it is a powerful technique and certainly does not have to be preceded by twenty-two years of life changes to be effective. You can start with your goal, turn it into a vision, and work backward if other issues emerge that need to be addressed before the goal can be attained. If the believability does not increase, the obstacles usually reveal themselves when reflecting on what is keeping the believability from increasing, and they can be worked on one at a time.

So when you have a clear goal, translate it into a vision or image as instructed above, give its believability a zero-to-ten rating (with 10 being completely believable), identify and address any psychological reversals, and hold the vision while tapping, using the basic protocol taught in the previous chapter (tapping with statements about the goal, Integration Sequence, more tapping, new rating, next round of tapping). Always be prepared to adjust the routine as new developments emerge, such as when Matt's vision morphed from a calendar to a vision of sharing a moment of joy with Jessica.

On to Part 3

In this chapter you have learned seven ways in which acupoint tapping combined with phrases related to your challenges and goals can be used to strengthen your relationship. We are aware that while some readers will be able to put this into immediate use, others will find the technique a little too strange or cumbersome or that there is so much confusion in their relationship that it is hard to know where to start. At a minimum, we hope you will sense that it is possible to identify forces within yourself and in your relationship that may need to be transformed for the two of you to grow into greater intimacy and happiness and that it is possible to transform them. While you may sometimes want a skilled practitioner to help you use these techniques to navigate through difficult territory, acupoint tapping is always available to make things better in the moment, and it can often facilitate changes in long-standing patterns.[6]

Part 2, "The Learned Aspects of Love," has focused on habits of thought and patterns of behavior that you can change. We opened by exploring the way early experiences with your caregivers set the patterns that reverberate into your adult relationships. The attachment style you bring into a relationship may be more or less secure or insecure, and while that is a product of your past, there is much you can do to craft a future supported by increasingly secure attachment. Skills laid down in childhood for soothing yourself, managing your emotions, and living with the ebbs and flows of intimacy are essential for secure attachment, and they become more refined and robust as your partnership matures. You can cultivate each of these skills, and also address many other aspects of your relationship and your personal evolution, by using techniques from energy psychology. Energy psychology works primarily at the individual level, even when it is focusing on relationship issues. You tap your own acupoints. Now you are about to enter the book's final section: Part 3, "The Mutually Created Aspects of Love," where it is your shared journey itself that brings you into ever deeper levels of intimacy.

PART

3

The Mutually Created Aspects of Love

8

Sex Is Nature's Energy Medicine for Couples

Invoking the Passion

Our mothers couldn't tell us and our fathers
didn't know the secrets of great sex.

—JOHN GRAY[1]

THE BEST THING TO HAPPEN TO OUR SEX LIFE IN THE PAST DECADE HAS BEEN TO work on this chapter. It has been *so much* fun! Neither of us is trained as a sex therapist, but we've been reading and listening to the best of them and trying out their methods, as well as innovating our own energy techniques, like kids in a candy store after opening the piggy bank.

One of the first audio talks we came upon was by Alison Armstrong, who suggests that most couples, after the initial passion wears off, go about their sex lives backward.[2] They wait till they *want* sex before they *say yes* to it. She impishly advises the opposite: Say "Yes!" first, and often. Then go about creating the wanting. While some couples remain *passionately* interested in one another's bodies year after year without consciously cultivating that passion, most do not. A *New York Times* article summarizing the findings of more than a hundred scientific studies concluded what everyone knows except those in the middle of it: The passion of new love has a "short shelf life."[3] An NBC *Dateline* survey of 27,500 people showed that two-thirds reported dissatisfaction with their sex lives.[4]

For us, with so much pressure (and pleasure) from our work and so little free time, we were finding that we would choose sleep over physical intimacy, if you can imagine such a choice, or relaxing into a good movie, or buckling under the pressure to squander possibilities for intimate time by returning to the relentless push of unanswered e-mails and uncompleted projects. As we approached the point where we were going to begin writing this chapter, we were wondering, "How are we going to pull this one off without feeling like total hypocrites?"

We did have one advantage over most couples. We could now set aside time for sex as part of our research for the book. So we had the "yes" part in the bag. And after being together for more than three decades, with both of us well into our sixties, getting to an enthusiastic "yes" was not something to take for granted, so this was good. On the other hand, making sex a part of our job descriptions didn't do much for enhancing the intrigue or passion.

Saying Yes and *Then* Creating the Desire That Will Fuel That Yes

Couples can raise the passion in one another in many ways. Activities that get you into your bodies—from dancing to massage to mock wrestling—can be aphrodisiacs. Knowing special words or ways of touching your partner can be turn-ons. Armstrong talks about the "jump-start":

> You get a dead battery and you hook it up, and all of a sudden, "Vroom!" It jumps, it just roars to life! So this is really, really important information to share with your partner. "If you touch me like this in this place, in this way, my battery, vroom, jumps to life." Many men have learned that some women's breasts have a sensitivity that can create a jump-start, but not all women's breasts are that way. For some women it's the palm of her hand . . . rubbing the palm of their hand with a thumb in just this slow way while just looking deep in her eyes. . . . vrooom, she's jump-started! For many women it's words. I know a woman where, if her boyfriend says to her "Oh, honey, we don't have to do anything." . . . vrooooom! She's jump-started. Everybody's different. For another woman, *anything* said *breathlessly*, that's all he's gotta do . . . or kiss her on the back of the neck. Every woman has her own jump-start. And it's really important that her partner knows what they are.[5]

When David puts on soft romantic music, removes Donna's shoes, and massages her feet, he often scores a "vroooom." An important exception is in what Armstrong calls the "pumpkin hours." The pumpkin hours are "when Cinderella's coach turns back into a pumpkin and can't give anyone a ride!" Men and women have different kinds of pumpkin hours: "When a man is extremely focused on a project, a request for sex will be terribly irritating to him. For women, if it's going to cost us sleep—our sleep is so important to us and critical to all our capacities—a request for sex after we're going down and falling off to sleep . . . that's cruel."[6]

Sexual Desire Problems Are Part of a Healthy Marriage

Waning sexual desire is not only common, it is natural. But it is also stigmatized. People don't like to admit it, particularly to their partner, and they don't know what to do about it. If the spontaneous passion and the euphoric cocktail of brain chemicals that often accompany new love are inherently time-limited, how are passion and desire sustained? Passion and desire are sustained by the way you relate to one another in all dimensions—from how you handle differences to how you play to how you grow with one another. Most young people do not enter marriage with the realization that keeping things hot in the bedroom depends on what happens outside the bedroom. David Schnarch, a highly respected psychologist and sex therapist, titled the opening chapter of his best-selling book *Passionate Marriage*, "Nobody's Ready for Marriage—Marriage Makes You Ready for Marriage."[7] He teaches that being with the same sexual partner for years and then decades can stay interesting because "what makes human sexual desire *human* is your brain's unique capacity to bring meaning to sex."[8]

Schnarch surprises couples who have encountered sexual desire problems by telling them, "everything's happening as it should!"[9] He sees sexual desire problems as a normal and healthy part of long-term intimacy, propelling us to grow and to take the next step with each other in the relationship. If we embrace rather than resist them, sexual desire "problems" can help us find a better balance between "two basic life forces: the drive for individuality and the drive for togetherness."[10] Becoming isolated in your own story or so deeply enmeshed with your partner that you lose contact with your own truths are two common imbalances that work against sexual aliveness within your relationship. Sexual desire problems are a warning light indicating that it is time to rebalance the drives for individuality and intimacy. Re-achieving this balance "lets you expand your sexual relationship and rekindle desire and passion in marriages that have grown cold." Schnarch goes on to suggest that maintaining a dynamic balance between these forces "is the pathway to the hottest and most loving sex you'll ever have with your spouse."[11]

We recently received a letter from a friend confiding that while she and her husband are compatible in many, many ways, the sexual charge is not there and they have been thinking of separating, despite their mutual affection for one another and their profound love for their two beautiful daughters. Our reply: "You must know

---

➔ THE ENERGY DIMENSION ✦

How does sexual energy look in the following three states of relationship?

A New Relationship

A single aura surrounds both people, ensconcing them in a world of their own. It is an electric, bright, colorful, palpable, beautiful energy, very alive. Even when alone, the aura of a person newly in love is light and bright, though it is not particularly grounded. Also key for understanding the dynamics of new love, the personal auras of the two partners have not yet connected in the nuanced ways of a couple that has gone the distance.

A Stale Relationship

A collapsed energy is around each of them when they are together. These energies do not reach out for the partner. The energy around the two of them may still be there, but it is no longer animated. It has little movement.

A Renewed Relationship

The energies surrounding each partner are grounded and have become linked in ways not found in a new relationship. A great deal of connection has been established between their chakras, forming invisible lines of communication that are felt at a deeply emotional level. Their auras overlap—bridged with figure-eight patterns—but the energies surrounding them retain more of their individuality than in a new couple.

---

that the lack of spark between marriage partners who are great friends is far from unusual. Even as you may be aware or even fantasize that someone could sweep you off your feet, and perhaps someone could, the chemistry of that new love would inevitably be short-lived. The contrast between that fantasy and what you have is a common but misleading way of measuring what you have. That is not to say that the status quo you describe is acceptable. There are important ways it will not sustain you. But it is to say that the status quo need not define your future together." For taking the full and fulfilling ride of a committed relationship, we offered two mechanical suggestions: that they learn how long-term partners can still stimulate in one another the hormones of romance (pp. 111–113) and that they rediscover one another as sexual beings, as presented in this chapter.

"Just Do It" Doesn't Do It

If your time together has resulted in waning passion (if you are still hot for one another, just jump to the next chapter), the instruction offered here—that you say yes and then *create* the wanting—is vastly different from the simpler advice of a generation of sex therapists who counseled, "Just do it." "Creating the want" makes all the difference. The old theory was that having sex stimulates hormones and brain chemistry that make you want to have more sex. While biologically accurate, it does not take into account that such prescriptions (1) promote impersonal sex, (2) breed further alienation if a lack of intimacy was the source of the low desire, (3) are asking at least one partner to ignore his or her feelings, and (4) are robbing the person who is more desirous of sex of the chance to feel wanted.[12] Meanwhile, there is much to look forward to. Interviewing 150 women ages 20 through 90 about their sex lives, Iris Krasnow found that many in the after-70s group claimed that they are having the best sex of their lives.[13]

A challenge in writing about good sex is that one of the most important principles is to counter expectations, judgments, and notions *about* "good sex." Recipes don't support your spontaneity or internal authority. Nicole Daedone, author of *Slow Sex*, tells a story of bringing home to her grandmother a dish she had prepared in her home economics class that had gotten her an A. Her grandma took a taste and spit it out, saying, "You killed the food with the recipe!" Daedone goes on to explain that recipes don't work for sex either, because women:

want smooth, silly sex; we want climactic sex and we want slow undulating sex. We want range. We want gradients. We want sex to move from slow to fast, from hard to exquisitely soft. We want to be surprised by nuance and subtlety. . . . We want to communicate our sensations and hear about yours.[14]

This chapter would be much easier to write if we could just tell you how to "do it," but no matter what recipe you follow for good sex, you will be removing the spontaneity, variety, and surprise. To retain these over time requires communication, an easy flow of information between one another. "Give us the time, space and permission to taste a bit of every possible sensation," advises Daedone, "and to communicate which ones we like."[15] Many women have been systematically trained to deny what they desire, even to not eat when they are hungry, and cultivating an atmosphere that invites her to put into words what she may not even have been acknowledging to herself opens new worlds for both of you.

When you meet at this deep level, each encounter is new and fresh. We originally thought this chapter was going to describe energy techniques that are easy turn-ons to intensify everything from sexual desire to wild orgasms. Push this, feel that. As we delved into the topic, however, we realized that physical techniques that enhance sexual energy are just the icing on the cake. The foundation that lets us soar together over a distance needs to be built on a sense of safety, trust, communication, and deep encounter, all fueled by our ability to enjoy the sensations that travel through our own bodies. As Schnarch puts it, "Techniques make you a technician . . . not a lover."[16] We read and experimented with so many books and taped programs that had good techniques that we know that information is readily available. What we want to encourage you to do is learn to recognize and communicate about how the energies flow in your body and communicate about them (verbally and non-verbally) so you are able to surf the waves of your sexual energies in harmony and as shared erotic adventure.

Entering the Sexual Zone

Marianne Williamson cautions that "when sex is merely a substitute for communication," the emotional gap between two souls who long to connect is not bridged. But when sex "deepens conversation," the body "becomes a door to a realm that the body can't even enter . . . joining is of the spirit."[17] The sexual act opens energetic pathways that can bring us into states of consciousness that transform the collective field between us. Through sex, your shared biological, psychological, and spiritual energies have an opportunity to align themselves and build on one another. This allows the energies that form the matrix of your relationship to come into greater harmony and depth and for disruptions to be healed. Sex is indeed nature's "energy medicine for couples." Yet so often in long-term relationships, its power for pleasure, healing, and transformation is neglected.

Creating the Wanting

Saying yes and then "creating the wanting," Armstrong's advice, can turn this around. For us, the practical demands coming our way were unceasing, calling more loudly than the whisper of spiritual possibility or even the opportunities for momentary pleasure. Reflecting on this as we settled into writing this chapter, it became quite clear that if we waited until our to-do list was empty, a future of marital celibacy awaited us. So we started experimenting—with the guiding principle being "be creative, not rote." Using what we know about energy and passion, we innovated many intimacy dances that will never be repeated or even recalled. One we did jot down as possibly being useful for this chapter was designed for people who, like us, are so busy that some tricks may be needed to break the inertia and get with the program. It is brief and playful, signaling to our libidos that they are on deck. There are a thousand kinds of foreplay. This is just one of them. We found that it quickly shifted our mental states from busy and distracted to connected and ready for more.

PART I: RELEASING THE DISTRACTIONS

Our first step was to clear our psyches of competing thoughts or nagging responsibilities in order to get on with the business at hand. Energy medicine offers an excellent tool for quickly shifting from a cluttered mental state to a clear one. When you've said yes but haven't yet created the desire, turn to one another and state, honestly and courageously:

> "The most compelling thing that is, right now, keeping me from wanting to be in rapture with you is . . ."

This is what you will release with the energy technique. For instance, for Donna last night: "I am finally beginning to unpack from this last trip." For David: "I feel a lot of pressure to prepare for my talk tomorrow."

Once you have recognized what is pulling you away from wanting rapture (and how trivial it probably is in relation to feeding yours and your partner's soul's longing), you can make an informed choice for intimacy. The distraction may, however, still have an energetic hold on you. To release it, do the Blow-Out/Zip-Up/Hook-Up technique (pp. 86–88), blowing out obligations or other distractions that are preventing you from being able to bring yourself toward intimacy. Situate yourselves so you aren't expelling these energies onto your partner.

Do this a second time, or more if you wish. Then turn toward one another, let your eyes meet, and bring your hands, with one hand on top of the other, up the center of your body until they come to rest on the middle of your chest. From here, you can go in any number of directions, and with less energetic pull from your day-to-day responsibilities. We suggest you move right on to "Playing in Rhythm."

PART 2: PLAYING IN RHYTHM

In this shared movement game, one of you will lead and the other will follow, while you both maintain eye contact. Your energies will begin to dance as you stay in sync with one another. It is ridiculously simple but gives a structure from which you can be playful.

1. Put on music that makes you want to move. We still come alive to our old *Flashdance* and *Dirty Dancing* albums.
2. Make eye contact and again place your hands over the centers of your chests. When one of you is inspired to move to the music, the other follows, maintaining the eye contact.
3. Continue for as long as you wish, and then return to center, hands still over your chests, keeping eye contact. The other partner can then lead. Continue leading and following as many rounds as you wish.

Without touching one another, you can play with the motion, the speed, and the form. In summary, these two brief exercises—Releasing the Distractions and Playing in Rhythm—can create an energetic space that *beckons the wanting*. The next step is up to you.

Skin on Skin

Use your body to bring into manifestation the fullness of your love for your partner. Let every stroke whisper with your longing, every expansion of your iris bring through more light, let every brush of your lips administer the healing nectar of the reunion. Imagine . . . that you have been separated for eons, through all time and space, and that this moment has been given to you so that you may discover one another again in the flesh.

—ANAIYA SOPHIA, *Sacred Sexual Union*[18]

Sex invokes such powerful energies that many couples turn the whole encounter over to their bodies. Your body knows what to do with little discussion. But you can also open your consciousness to your partner's experience, create inroads into one another's vast interiors, and pave the way for your spirits to connect at ever deeper levels. You can begin at a very basic and concrete plane, which is to learn about one another's sensations. Your sensations are the language of the energies that move through your body, connecting your outer world and your inner world.

In the simplest terms, touching and being touched generates sensation. Touch, the first sense you acquire, can tell you much about your partner's inner experience. A great deal of intimate communication is nonverbal. In an experiment where people were blindfolded and touched by someone, they were able to identify the feeling the person had been instructed to express—anger, fear, disgust, love, gratitude, sympathy, happiness, or sadness—78 percent of the time through touch alone.[19] We are wired to correctly interpret the touch of our partner.

A Kiss Is Not Just a Kiss!

While we are wired to correctly interpret touch, sexual touch can still lead to misunderstandings. Not only can we misread or totally miss our partner's signals, the honesty inherent in touch may convey information that is awkward or ambiguous. For instance, Schnarch asserts that even foreplay is much more than it appears: "We like to think that . . . foreplay is where couples establish emotional connection and instill feelings of love, arousal, and desire in each other. Too often, however, foreplay establishes *disconnections*."[20] Take kissing, for example. Pointing out the many meanings that may be conveyed in a kiss, Schnarch describes a range of kissing varieties that can be turn-offs:

- The mushy, limp kiss of passivity and withheld eroticism.
- The impatient kiss of a partner preoccupied with more important things.
- The sloppy, soupy, wet kiss that triggers repulsion rather than desire.
- The rigid-tongued kiss of the mechanical lover.
- The smothering kiss that rekindles childhood fears of an intrusive, engulfing parent.
- The begrudgingly given kiss of the "you can't take me for granted" lover.[21]

Kissing is, of course, more often a turn-on, but turn-on kisses also have their own vocabulary, which Schnarch describes as follows:

- The soft but electric kiss of a familiar lover.
- The hard kiss of passion.
- The breathy, languid kiss of tasting and smelling each other's body.
- The gentle bite on the lip from someone begging to be "rode hard and put away wet."[22]

Think of the ways you and your partner kiss. Do you know how your partner experiences your kisses? Does your partner know your experience? If not, this can be fun to remedy.

Conscious Kissing

Of course you are aware of your own experience during a kiss. When you are also relatively aware of your partner's, an alchemy occurs that brings another dimension to your kiss. Ellen Eatough is a sex educator who understands the energetic dimension of sexuality. We found her audio CD program "Four Keys to Sexual Ecstasy: Experience Soulful Connection with Spine-Tingling Sex"[23] to be one of the best home-study programs available. She explains how kissing is the most intimate activity two people can do. Many prostitutes, for instance, who will have intercourse and engage in all kinds of other sexual acts refuse to kiss their clients on the lips. It is too intimate. The lips and tongue are among the most nerve-rich and sensitive areas of the body. Since we have an enormous amount of control over them, this allows for splendid "variety, and variety makes our brains light up with arousal."

Because people in long-term relationships often take kissing for granted, Eatough suggests that couples bring renewed attention to this staple of intimate contact. It can be as simple as the following, for starters:

1. Show your partner how you like to be kissed.
2. Ask your partner to kiss you as you've just explained or demonstrated.
3. Tell and show your partner what felt right and what needs adjustment.
4. Have your partner give it another try.
5. Continue until your partner is able to kiss you *just like* you wanted.
6. Switch roles so you learn how your partner likes to be kissed.

You can also experiment with new ways of kissing one another. For instance, you could explore the inside of your partner's lips with your tongue and then receive your partner's tongue on the insides of your lips. Or gently nibble and suck your partner's upper lip. Envision the energy that is moving within you and between the two of you. Let your partner know what feels good. Ancient teachings say there is a subtle nerve connection between the woman's upper lip and her clitoris. Find out if this is true for anyone in your relationship who has an upper lip and a clitoris.

Ask for What You Want

Use kissing as your training wheels for discovering what pleasures your partner sensually and sexually. Even healthy, relatively enlightened couples often have difficulty communicating what they want sexually or in allowing themselves to be creative in moving beyond established patterns. Among the most important skills for maintaining sexual satisfaction in a long-term relationship is to be able to ask for what you want, to ask for it without a lot of justification, and to ask for it without inadvertently conveying criticism. Your partner wants to give you what you desire. Since your partner usually can't read your mind, you need to ask for it with words, sounds, gestures, or touch. Crossing the barriers of shyness, modesty, shame, habit, self-judgment, or sense of not being deserving is the path toward ever greater sexual satisfaction.

Talk About Your Energies

Words may not come easily when you step into the realm of describing sensations and energy, but it can be enticing while opening new vistas of intimacy. Be curious. Notice the sensations in your body and describe them. You can focus your attention in ways that make this easier. For instance, put your hands over your chest, your Heart Chakra. This is the home of many emotions. Are the sensations heavy, fluid, agitated, calm? Do you feel flooded? Do you feel empty? Do you feel happiness? Sadness? Grief? Joy?

Still with your hands on your chest, let your eyes meet. Drop your hands. The energies of your Heart Chakras will naturally touch and engage one another, with or without your awareness. Notice what you feel in the center of your chest, what you feel coming out toward your partner, what you feel coming in from your partner, and what you feel between you. Use words that describe the sensations stirred by the energies that are continually moving through your body: *warm, cold, liquid, flowing, tingling, pulsating, intensifying, calming, spinning, stretching* . . . If words do not come, just gently notice what enters your awareness, moment by moment, as you keep your attention on your Heart Chakra and the space between you.

Knowing Your Partner Intimately

Many couples never really explore one another's sexual anatomy. In a new relationship, such exploration might push boundaries of intimacy and propriety. However, long-term partners who have never crossed this bridge and developed a comfortable familiarity with one another at the most intimate physical levels have left standing an unnecessary barrier to easy communication about their physical relationship. To be sure, such sharing can feel highly vulnerable and requires that your sense of safety with one another is well established, but it is an exploration well worth taking on.

Start with the conscious kiss and the communication it requires. Then other kinds of touch. (A note from our Etiquette Department: If you are going to enter anything delicate and sacred, be sure your hands are clean and fingernails short.) Knowing that you will be sharing and exploring your most intimate landscape with your partner may also motivate you to learn more about your own sexual anatomy and physiology. You can't count on what you learned growing up. Nor, until recently, was the wider culture particularly forthcoming on these topics. For instance, the clitoris, the only human body part that exists solely for pleasure, was not even correctly described by scientists until 1998.[24] Cultural inhibitions aside, nature was in high gear when designing your sexual physiology, and detailed information about her handiwork is finally readily available.[25]

Three Kinds of Sexual Energy

As we attempted to pull together our own understanding of sexuality from an energetic perspective, we discovered that teachings about *sacred* sexuality can be found in at least the Taoist, Tantric, Sufi, Buddhist, Jewish, Pagan, Wiccan, occult, Native American, and Afro-Caribbean traditions. We were particularly drawn to the Taoist and Tantric teachings because of their profound understanding of the relationship between sexuality and the body's energies in terms that we already use, such as the meridians and the chakras.

The Taoist physicians understood that an active sex life is a vital part of health and longevity, and they studied it with the same determination they applied to every other area of health. In Taoist sexual practices, the focus is on the way energy moves through the meridians, particularly the Governing and Central Meridians that flow along the spine and up through the center of the torso. The Taoist "Arts of the Bedchamber" have been beautifully systematized in a book for Westerners called *The Multi-Orgasmic Couple: Sexual Secrets Every Couple Should Know.*[26]

In the Tantric sexuality practices of India, the focus is on an energy known as *kundalini energy* that is channeled upward from the chakra at the base of the spine, up the spine, through each chakra, and finally reaching the chakra at the crown of the head. The most accessible yet authoritative book we have found on Tantric sexuality as it has evolved in the West is, dare we name it, *The Complete Idiot's Guide to Tantric Sex.*[27]

While it is not possible to present these bodies of wisdom and technique for working with sexual energy within the confines of a chapter, we will provide a few insights and exercises that give you a taste of each system. Also, along with the meridians and the kundalini energy that can move up the chakras, another vital energy is involved in sexual activity. It is called the *radiant circuits*. We will offer a brief introduction to this energy system as well.

The Meridians

The meridians—the pathways that bring energy into every organ of the body—are as basic to sexual activity as blood flow and breath. The primary meridians involved in sexual arousal are different for a woman than for a man. A woman's energy begins to climb along her inner thighs up into her genitals as well as reaching downward through her abdomen. This energy is carried upward on the Spleen, Liver, and Kidney Meridians and downward on the Stomach Meridian. The lightest upward touch on her inner thigh or downward touch on her abdomen moves the energy along these meridians, building a sexual response. Write that down, fellas. And remember, it's a feather touch!

For a man in his prime, the Kidney Meridian, which is considered the "Wellspring of Life," is always at the ready to stream large quantities of vital energy directly to the prostate and genitals, bypassing all logic, reason, or other distractions. It can be triggered by a lover's seduction, an erotic touch, or a cereal box. Not only are men and women aroused differently in these core energies, they also reach orgasm in different ways. For women, the energies that build toward orgasm are usually slow and not as easily separated from the energies of the relationship. For men, the buildup toward orgasm can be very rapid and less dependent on the energies of the relationship. As Billy Crystal famously quipped, "Women need a reason to have sex; men just need a place." However, as a relationship develops, these differences recede as the energies of the relationship bring both partners into a more natural harmony.

Two energy channels, the Governing and Central Meridians, connect in both men and women and form a circuit of energy that runs from the sexual organs, up the spine to the head to the back of the tongue to the lower lip, down the front of the body, and back to the sexual organs. Various practices can enhance the flow of this circuit—called the *Microcosmic Orbit* in Taoist sexual tradition[28]—which connects the reservoirs of energy in the brain, heart, abdomen, and genitals. Gaining control of the flow in the Microcosmic Orbit is a key in Taoist sexual tradition for progressing from genital orgasms to full-body orgasms to "soul orgasms."[29] In a full-body orgasm, the sexual energy is moving freely and fully through the Microcosmic Orbit. In a soul orgasm, the energy is not only moving freely through your entire body, but the energetic boundaries between the two of you dissolve. The exchange can profoundly expand and transform your consciousness and bring your love to deeper levels.

The energy that flows through the Microcosmic Orbit when it has been activated includes not only the electromagnetic energies that can be detected by scientific instruments but also the more subtle life force called *chi*. Chi is the vital energy inherent in all of life, though with no instruments that can detect it, Western science denies its existence. But there *is* an instrument. When you are alive, chi is flowing. When you are dead, it isn't. Is that so complicated?

The unimpeded circulation of chi, along with balance in its energetic polarities (yin and yang), is considered essential for good health. We can influence the flow of chi in many ways. An old Taoist saying instructs, "The mind moves and chi follows."[30] The converse is also true: Chi moves and the mind follows.

The electromagnetic energy that comes out of your hands can move chi. To explore the Microcosmic Orbit, you can trace it with your hands. Sitting comfortably, bring either hand to the bottom of your sacrum. Very slowly and with a light touch, move your hand up your spine. The electromagnetic energy coming off your hand, not the pressure, is moving the chi. Remember, feather touch. When you have gotten as high on your spine as you can reach, bring your other hand over your shoulder and back to your spine while imagining the energy moving up the gap between your hands. Continue to slowly move your hand up to your head, over your head, down your forehead, and to your upper lip. Now bring both hands to your lower lip and continue down the front of your neck, down the center of your body, to your genitals, underneath the trunk of your body, and back toward the base of your spine. You have just traced the Microcosmic Orbit.

How much you felt or didn't feel depends on a number of factors, including how kinesthetic you are in your sensory style (chapter 1) and how practiced you are at attending to your inner sensations. The sensations you may feel as the Microcosmic Orbit is activated may be warmth, tingling, or pulsating. If you go over the Orbit a number of times, the energies are likely to become more vivid in your mind, but simply doing the exercise activates these energies whether or not you consciously experience it. The energy generally moves very slowly, particularly at first, so your hands should keep pace. Once you are able to consciously move the energy through the entire circuit by tracing it with your hands, you can experiment with moving it with only your mind.

A series of Taoist practices begins with exercises (such as the one just described) that are designed to bolster the Microcosmic Orbit in your own body. They then progress to sharing the experience with your partner. Unimpeded by clothes, one partner sits on the bed and the other (usually the lighter) partner sits on the other's lap, maximizing the amount of contact from the pelvis up, supporting each other to the extent you can with your arms around one another's backsides (see Figure 8-1). Alternatively, you may sit facing one another in chairs or cross-legged on the bed or floor. Each partner activates the Microcosmic Orbit in his or her own body. While this may lead to intercourse that is primed for full-body orgasms, first take the time to get your own energies flowing and share the experience. In the more advanced forms, you bring the energy up your own spine and send it down the front of your partner's body, meet it at your partner's genitals, and bring it up your partner's spine so your energies are merging, facilitating an even more profound exchange.

There is of course much more to the Taoist sexual practices of cultivating spiritual connection. For instance, the man learns how to have orgasms without ejaculating (yes, the two can be pleasurably separated) so that the couple can become "multi-orgasmic." *The Multi-Orgasmic Couple* promises that learning how to have "multiple whole-body orgasms" can open the way for you "to harmonize your sexual needs and to reach ever more fulfilling levels of intimacy and ecstasy together."[31]

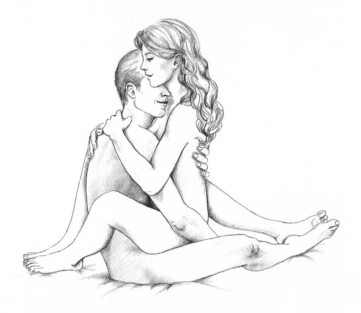

FIGURE 8-1 *Joining Microcosmic Orbits. An alternative position is to find balance so you can meet your hands palm to palm instead of around one another's backs.*

The Chakras

Whereas Taoism concentrates on the meridian pathways, Tantric sexual practices focus on the chakras. The seven major chakras are situated at the pelvis (First or *Root* Chakra), lower abdomen below the navel (Second Chakra), solar plexus (Third Chakra), center of chest (Fourth or *Heart* Chakra), throat (Fifth Chakra), forehead (Sixth Chakra or *third eye*), and the top of the head (Seventh or *Crown* Chakra). According to most texts, sexuality originates and is expressed through the Second Chakra. But Donna sees it differently. She sees the Root Chakra as the seat of sexuality. Wide agreement does exist that the Root Chakra is related to safety and survival. Donna indeed sees primal fear, traumatic memories, and survival strategies as being stored in the Root Chakra. When a person is feeling relatively safe, the Root Chakra is a source of stability, drive, and vital energies that move up the body, feeding the other chakras and empowering them. The genitals and other sexual organs are bathed by the energy of the Root Chakra, so it is not surprising that the survival chakra would be involved with sex, nature's sweet enticement for actions that ensure collective survival.

Here's a possible source of the confusion. In many situations, a woman's Root Chakra will not shift into a sexual response without a sense of emotional safety. A report that the safety check has been passed must be sent downward from the Second Chakra. The Second Chakra is the guardian at the gate that must usually be passed through before a woman becomes sexually aroused in the presence of a potential partner. It is receptive, creative, and full of feelings. The Second Charka has even been referred to as the "second heart." Babies develop while bathed in its energies. Romance, love, affection, admiration—or at a minimum, a sense of emotional safety—are required before the Second Chakra sends energy back down to the Root Chakra that clears the way for a full sexual response to be generated. Men do not require this two-stage clearance process to become aroused. This basic difference can be traced to the divergent sexual anatomy of males and females.

For men, sexual activity occurs outside their bodies and, once the act is biologically over, it is biologically over. Seed planted. What's next? Women, however, are not only taking another person's anatomy *into* themselves; once the act is completed, a baby that will grow in her body for nine months and eventually be asking to borrow the car may have been conceived. In the wisdom of the body's energies, which evolved into complex systems with decision-making capabilities, it would seem natural that the chakra that holds the womb (Second Chakra) has some say in who is going to help choose the car the baby will be borrowing. The Second Chakra assesses the potential partner in the moment and decides to send sexual energy into the Root Chakra . . . or not. Of course she can override the wisdom of her body, but indiscriminate sex can be much more costly to her than to him. Just as the meridians function differently in men than women in regard to sexual responsiveness (with the Kidney Meridian capable of bringing men into instant arousal but women needing the energy to also build in their Heart, Spleen, Liver, and Stomach Meridians in particular), the chakras conspire with the meridians in dictating a slower and more studied response in women than men.

The word *Tantra*, from ancient Sanskrit, means "expansion through awareness." A core attitude in Tantra is mindfulness: "You pay attention to what you're doing in the exchange between you and your partner. Being mindful induces a sense of respect and reverence for the experience, which lends itself to honoring each other as god and goddess."[32] Tantra itself is a profound spiritual philosophy and discipline. In its original form, many years of meditation, chanting, and postures that channel subtle energies are combined with initiation and purification ceremonies for worship and expanding spiritual awareness. The Tantra sexual practices that have been adopted in the West "use breath, sounds, movements, and symbols to quiet the mind and activate sexual energy, directing it throughout the body to achieve states of consciousness and bliss."[33]

Many Tantric practices are reminiscent of the Taoist joining of the Central and Governing Meridians to activate the Microcosmic Orbit (after all, they are both working with the same physical and energetic anatomy). These Tantric practices use the breath and the mind to move the powerful kundalini energies that are coiled at the base of the spine, raising them up along the chakras. As the kundalini energy moves up the chakras, it can lead to different levels of awakening and mystical insight until it reaches the Crown Chakra at the top of the head, where it can produce profound mystical experiences. Kundalini is an intrinsic, libidinal force that resides in the Root Chakra. For this reason, Donna sometimes refers to the Root Chakra as the "pilot light" of the chakra system. As the kundalini energy slowly rises through the chakras, it is often accompanied by a wave of euphoria and happiness as well as spiritual opening. We must also note, however, that in rare cases it is possible for it to rise so quickly and powerfully as to overwhelm a person who is unprepared, resulting in a psychological or physical crisis that has been termed a *spiritual emergency*. Untold numbers of people have been stigmatized and medicated or hospitalized when this has spontaneously occurred in an unusually powerful manner. Counseling that is attuned to this complex dynamic has, on the other hand, been shown to turn spiritual emergencies into opportunities for *spiritual emergence*.[34]

Thinking of the Root Chakra as the pilot light that can ignite each of the other chakras and open them to spiritual energies is a vivid metaphor for understanding the Tantric practices designed to raise the kundalini energies. Here is a basic Tantric practice that uses both breath and imagery. Sitting comfortably:

1. Tune into the Root Chakra at the base of your spine. It spins in a circle, creating a powerful, vital force. Think of it as a pilot light igniting the chakras above it. With a deep, slow in-breath through your nose, draw the energy from your Root Chakra up the center of your body, vividly imagining it activating, in turn, the chakras in your lower abdomen, solar plexus, heart, throat, and third eye, and the top of your head. As you breathe out through your mouth, send the energy down your spine to your Root Chakra. On the in-breath, again draw the energy up your chakras. Continuing this loop creates a clear channel in your body through which you can imagine or sense a stream of energy traveling past your chakras, "cleansing, feeding, and fueling"[35] them. A variation you may want to try is to take the energy up your spine with the in-breath and *down* the center of your body with the out-breath.

2. Once you have learned to consciously loop the energies through your chakras as described above, you can use this skill with your partner in some exciting ways. Sit comfortably facing your partner with your spine straight and using the position shown in Figure 8-1, in chairs or sitting cross-legged on the bed or floor. Do the chakra breath while maintaining eye contact and, if your position allows it, with your palms touching your partner's palms. This practice has three variations—called the "synchronizing breath," the "reciprocal breath," and the "circulating breath"—which can be learned in the order presented to get you "connected in a powerful, loving exchange."[36]

    a. The Synchronizing Breath: Do the breathing simultaneous with your partner. If it isn't obvious, signal in some way when you are starting the in-breath and the out-breath. Once you are in rhythm with one another, close your eyes and sense into one another's energy patterns.

    b. The Reciprocal Breath: Again breathe in rhythm with your partner, but this time one of you inhales as the other exhales.

c. The Circulating Breath: As you do the reciprocal breath, imagine that you are inhaling your partner's breath and energy. With your in-breath, consciously bring the energy up from your Root Chakra through the other six chakras as you have been doing. With your out-breath, however, imagine you are sending your energy down your partner's spine. With your next in-breath, imagine you are picking up your partner's energy at your Root Chakra and bringing it up through each of your other chakras, and then again sending the energy down your partner's spine with the out-breath. You are making a loop inside yourself and into your partner.

Such practices, basic to Tantric sex, are applied in creating many forms of loving connection that may or may not involve intercourse or orgasm. Like Taoist sexual practices, Tantric sex is a spiritual path that is oriented toward using sexual energy "as a means to *sacred love*."[37] Both the Tantric and Taoist sexual systems are disciplines that teach couples to open their hearts and manage the masculine and feminine energies within each partner so orgasms are prolonged and become sources of healing, ecstasy, and sacred love. This is not to say that you should or need to pursue the highly disciplined sexual practices found in Tantra or Taoism to have a satisfactory sex life. These are not paths we ourselves have followed. Rather, we have sought to inform our natural instincts with our understanding of the body's energies, and we love our sexual relationship. Nonetheless, as Marianne Brandon put it after reviewing a variety of sexual practices and arrangements, "If you wish to engage your partner in a spiritual ride of a lifetime, Tantra may be for you."[38]

The Radiant Circuits

The radiant circuits are the energy system of ecstasy. Called the "strange flows" or "extraordinary vessels" by ancient Chinese physicians, they were not given nearly as much emphasis as the meridians. Donna, however, sees them as an exceedingly important system that is directly tied to a person's health and happiness.[39] In addition to activating ecstasy—sexual or otherwise—they also promote healing, generate joy, and orchestrate all the other energy systems into a coordinated dance for maintaining your health. Each of the eight radiant circuits has a pathway that, like a meridian, can be traced on the surface of the skin. Unlike the meridians, however, the radiant circuits are able to jump their paths and go to wherever they are needed or attracted.

All eight radiant circuits are activated during any ecstatic experience, but one of them, the Penetrating Flow, plays a special role in sexual activity. As its name suggests, the Penetrating Flow *penetrates*. It directs energy into every cell, muscle, bone, organ, meridian, and chakra in your body. It may be active or dormant at any given moment. When it is weak or blocked, people feel depressed or empty inside and sex may feel hollow. When the Penetrating Flow is strong, sex will be ecstatic as the energies deep inside you are catapulted throughout your body, activating your emotions and your love, and awakening you to your spiritual depths.

You are stimulating your Penetrating Flow whenever you feel joy, gratitude, or curiosity. Savor a sunset; delight at a seashore; contemplate the stars; appreciate your partner. The stronger your Penetrating Flow, the more that sexual activity can catapult you to extraordinary realms. In addition to seeking mental or emotional states that cultivate the Penetrating Flow, you can strengthen it like a muscle using some simple physical exercises. You and your partner can get a feel for the Penetrating Flow if one of you lies facedown and the other places one hand on the sacrum and the other at the top of the back. Gently rock the sacrum for three to five minutes. When you have finished, lift both hands simultaneously and let your partner bask in the tingling feeling. You are experiencing the physical activation of your Penetrating Flow.

Here is an exercise you can do for yourself that also strengthens your Penetrating Flow (breathing slowly and deliberately):

1. Lying down, place your palms on your back at your waist with your fingertips touching.
2. Lightly move your fingertips down to the bottom of your sacrum.
3. Slowly draw your hands up over your hip bones from back to front and down to either side of your groin. Rest in this position for two deep breaths.
4. On the next in-breath, slowly draw your hands straight up your body, over your stomach, to your breasts, up your neck, to the bottom of your jaw.
5. With a slow out-breath, let your hands slide back down to your Heart Chakra, with one hand on top of the other. Rest them there as you take several deep breaths and experience the sensations of your Penetrating Flow after having been activated by physical touch.

These three energies—the meridians, chakras, and radiant circuits—are always working behind the scenes, but they become charged and operate in a powerful natural harmony during sex. This brief introduction to the role of each in your sex life gives you a peek into these invisible forces and a few simple techniques for exploring and enhancing each.

Before Your Bodies Touch, Your Energies Meet

With a dozen women's magazines at checkout counters giving sexual advice on any given day, we feel a bit squeamish about offering the following little bits of guidance, but some basics are not obvious to everyone and they do make a difference. These are a few brief tips from hundreds that could be mentioned, selected because they are so important to understand and because they can have an immediate impact on your personal and shared sexual energies.

Don't Make Her Orgasm Another Job for Her

As the culture turned a valuing eye on a woman's sexual pleasure, an extra premium was placed on her orgasm. This may, paradoxically, have become a formidable obstacle to her pleasure. The energies of sex are, at their best, a full-bodied unscripted experience, and feeling pressured to have an orgasm works against everything that orgasms are about. As Alison Armstrong put it, "Men could have more sex if they would let women have fewer orgasms."[40] Because his partner's orgasms have become a source of validation for a man, "he will keep you up all night until you get this 'treasured result.' It leads to women faking it just so they can get some sleep." The pressure for a woman to have an orgasm makes sex a job. The underlying lesson for a man is to understand that women want far more to feel treasured than to get that orgasm. Ask your partner which she would choose: having an orgasm every time or feeling loved, adored, and precious every time.

Don't Let the Tabloids Define Your Satisfaction with Your Sex Life

Just as the culture's valuing of a woman's sexual pleasure inadvertently turned having an orgasm into an expectation and a job, widespread media discussion of "good sex," "great sex," "making her scream," and "driving him wild" can cause us to negatively compare our sex lives with what everyone else seems to be doing or at least is expected to be doing. Holding expectations that are not based in the reality of who you are and who your partner is, of what you need, and of what you really want is a powerful way of draining the energy and joy from your love life. Intimacy counselor and media columnist Mary Jo Rapini closes an article titled "5 Ways to Keep the Sparks Flying in Your Marriage" with fair warning about this issue:

> Just as beauty is in the eye of the beholder, sex, whether it is hot or not, is the opinion of the couple. Many couples have sex once a month in the same position and *love* it! Others feel unloved if it isn't every day. . . . You don't need to swing from a chandelier to be happy.[41]

If you and your partner are both satisfied with your sex life and have persuasively conveyed that to one another, that is enough. When either of you feels it is time to amp it up or spice it up or give it more time and attention or change patterns that have developed, the need for new talk or new action has entered your interpersonal field.

There's a Place for "Quickies"

John Gray points out that a woman is generally open to occasional "quickie sex" when she feels emotionally supported in the relationship and knows that at other times she will experience regular healthy "home-cooked sex" and occasional "gourmet sex."[42] Your own energies and your partner's energies not only fluctuate within each of you, but they meet in a thousand different ways. Sex also has its seasons. You are likely to go through dry spells as well as periods of increased passion. Sex has many paces. Let the energies of the moment influence your sexual experiences rather than relying too heavily on familiar patterns. Although there is comfort and value in familiar or habitual ways of having sex, they do not necessarily propel you to encounter one another at the deepest levels.

Soft Touch; Hard Touch

While sexual energies move through the body spontaneously, partners can direct and intensify their flow through touch. Most people, however, assume their partner likes to be touched the way they themselves like to be touched. While this may sometimes be true, physiological differences between men and women make it less likely. Men have tougher skin; a woman's skin has more sensitivity. Many men like deep, firm strokes while many women like a lighter touch. Find out what your partner likes. Know that this may also change depending on the area of the skin, the level of arousal, and simply his or her mood at the moment. So develop some verbal and nonverbal cues that help you to *know* if you are delivering what your partner desires and to help you let your partner know what you desire about this many-splendored thing called touch.

Awaken Your Energetic Awareness

By attuning yourself to the energies that move through your body, you can awaken your awareness about them. Build a habit of mindfully noticing your inner world. Sit still and note the subtle sensations that move through your body. If they are too subtle for you to register, physical movement activates the flow of energy. Here are three simple ways to make it easier to focus on your energies: (1) Follow your breathing with your awareness and notice how your breath enlivens your body; (2) flex your back to stretch your spine (think of a cat stretching) and notice how your energies respond; (3) contract your abdomen with each in-breath and notice how heat begins to build. What does this have to do with sex? The more you are in touch with the energies that stir in your body, the more that energy guides you as you build, control, and release waves of passion in harmony with your partner.

Correcting Your Partner About Sex May Not Be the Correct Way to Correct

No one likes to be criticized. Judgment about your partner's sexual skills or performance is particularly sensitive. It tends to bring out the person's worst rather than best performance. How do you convey, without the jab of criticism, that you want something that is *different* from what is happening? If you can energetically attune yourself with your partner, the whole interaction changes. You are not breaking into someone else's space but participating in high-level teamwork. Suppose you want your male partner to caress you in a certain way. If you have established a harmonic energy between you, it is not jarring to gently move his hand to the spot where you want to be touched or to whisper what you would like him to do. You can convey what you like with words, gratified sighs, or movement so that there is reliable communication about what you are liking. For sex to stay hot, much is about maintaining the quality of your relationship, but it is also about how you communicate about the mechanics.

The Pleasures of Slow Sex

One of Donna's nominees for Most Instructive Song of All Time Is "I Want a Man with a Slow Hand." The key is attunement. His impulse may be to generate more sensation. Her need is to be met at the shores of the slow undulating waves flowing from her Root Chakra. Met. Not hastened. Not forcing the waves to be anything but exactly what they are. When she is saying, "Don't move, don't move," she actually means, "Don't move!" Don't go faster. Don't increase the pressure. Just believe her. Don't move.

Holding Hands Is Foreplay

In more than one language, the term for sexual relations translates into English as "going on a journey together."[43] It's an apt image, and foreplay prepares the emotional path for that journey. Intimacy counselor Esther Perel observes, "Foreplay starts at the end of the previous orgasm."[44] Speaking about the "myth of spontaneity," she notes that "we like to believe that sex arises from an impulse or inclination that is natural, unprompted, artless."[45] In our busy lives we become impatient when time, effort, and consciousness are required to cultivate what we think should be spontaneous. But in a long-term relationship, preparation ignites sex more often than spontaneity, and that preparation doesn't usually start in the bedroom. Caring touch generates oxytocin in men and women. Holding hands is foreplay. Hugs are foreplay. Loving words are foreplay. Smiles are foreplay. Unexpectedly doing a job your partner usually does, like washing the dishes or taking out the trash, is foreplay. Keeping your energies in sync with one another is foreplay. Agreeing to protect the time and space for intimacy is foreplay.

Trust and Safety Are Foreplay

Trust and a sense of safety develop with the accumulation of experiences demonstrating that you each hold positive intentions for one another and that you convert those intentions into effective actions. Enhanced cooperation, freely shared information, mutual problem solving, and intimacy are emotional prerequisites for a rich sexual relationship. Being made to feel safe and loved throughout the day is foreplay. Ellen Eatough points out that trusting yourself and feeling safe with your partner as you open to pleasure are necessary if you are to surrender control, which is "ultimately required for orgasm."[46] Safety allows you to let go without fear of being judged or being taken advantage of as orgasm brings you beyond the familiar boundaries of your ego to the vulnerable space of uncontrolled excitement.

Keeping Your Energies in Sync Is Foreplay

When you and your partner are in harmony, in sync with the nuances of one another's behavior, your brain waves begin to oscillate in rhythm with each other. You literally get onto the same wavelength. When your biological rhythms resonate, you feel intimate, even without saying a word. An intimate conversation, deep eye contact, and breathing in rhythm, in or out of the bedroom, are three ways that people can attune to one another. Why is this foreplay? As Eatough cautions, if you don't get in sync early on during lovemaking, "you may feel a sense of being oddly disconnected and unsatisfied even if you had a great orgasm."[47]

Foreplay in the Bedroom

As you enter the arena for naked intimacy, foreplay becomes the art of arousal. We have seen how a woman's physiology—as well as her chakras and meridians—do not usually bring about sexual arousal as quickly as a man's. Discussing how skills in building and circulating sexual energy apply to every stage of the sexual act, from arousal to the many kinds of orgasm that are possible, Eatough notes that foreplay can "close the typical gap in arousal rates and meet in the erotic middle." She tells men that "verbal expressions of love and tender caresses, gradually becoming more sexual, are more likely to arouse than a direct hit to our genitals. In fact, touching our breasts or genitals too soon can make us unconsciously contract, and then we have to work harder to get over that, before we can really get 'into it!'"[48] So start even bedroom foreplay by expressing appreciation to her. See her well and let her know what you admire. Take the time to let her feel your love. Move slowly into touching and kissing, starting with her extremities, perhaps stroking her hand or kissing her cheeks. Only move toward her center as her excitement has started to build. It is in opening a woman's heart that her sexual energies begin to flow.

What to Do with Your Mind during Sex

The mind can go to a million places, from checking off things on the to-do list to being totally absorbed in the passion of the moment. Sex at its best is an exquisite dance between skilled control and no control. If you are swept away by the passion of the moment, surrender to it. If not, you can direct your mind to numerous juicy choices. Erotic fantasies are a popular choice, but as Nicole Daedone cautions, "fantasy is a way we step *out* of our experience of sex, rather than stepping further *into* it."[49] You can, instead, focus on the energies in your body and let them tell you what is next. If that is too subtle, you can enhance your breathing. Your breath is a powerful tool for circulating sexual energy. Take a slow, deep in-breath through your nose. Fill your belly and lungs. Release it even more slowly through your mouth. Continue breathing in this rhythm until you become lost in whatever occurs next. Deep breathing not only circulates pleasure, it also keeps you attuned to your body and makes it easier to stay in sync with your partner.

Sexual Wounds and Their Healing

Sexual intimacy is inextricably linked with emotional vulnerability. The Root Chakra—the root of sexual energy—also governs safety, danger, and threat. It will close down to sexual pleasure if sex becomes associated with threat, criticism, or abuse. When a woman takes a partner inside her body, it is her Root Chakra that is entered. She is immediately opening herself to the possibility of being impregnated and dependent on a partner. As a result, if the male's pattern is seduction-sex-abandonment, for many women, this amounts to a form of abuse. She is wired for seduction-sex-partnership, and when partnership is not the outcome, a deep sense of betrayal may be the lasting impression even if her conscious mind can fully understand and accept the rules by which the man is playing.

In Donna's practice, innumerable female clients confided to her that while they enthusiastically participated in the free love movement of the 1960s and 1970s, they came away damaged. Swept up in the excitement and freedom of the times, they overrode their deeper instincts. They wound up with hurt, self-judgment, and a diminished capacity for sexual pleasure. A more subtle form of this scenario can occur even within a marriage. If there is little emotional connection, having sex can feel like a violation. In one woman's words, "Our foreplay leaves me feeling 'played' and manipulated. He thinks that if he touches me in a certain way, that will turn me on. If he kisses me in a certain way, that will turn me on. But when we are so distant from one another in every other way, I don't want to be turned on by him. Sometimes if the foreplay does get me aroused and we go on to have sex, I feel that my body has betrayed me." She is not alone. Many women report that they don't want to have sex with someone who has been an emotional stranger all day.

Sexual encounters with men who are disrespectful, mean-spirited, or more overtly abusive can leave lasting harm on a woman's ability to be free and enjoy sex, even if she subsequently establishes a relationship that is loving and deeply respectful. Many of Donna's female clients complained that their sexual energies were turned off. Their work with Donna didn't erase the lessons of the past but rather was focused on reversing the damage. Sexual energies can be reawakened. Donna's book *Energy Medicine for Women* presents several simple energy techniques that can reopen a woman's sexual channels.[50] A case history described in that book shows how a therapist used energy psychology to help a woman overcome the wounds of severe childhood abuse. It follows to demonstrate the power of an energy approach.

Sandy and her partner came to one of our colleagues for premarital counseling.[51] Among the issues they were concerned about was their sexual relationship. Although Sandy had been married before, she found herself reacting with uncontrollable negative feelings when her fiancé initiated sexual play. He was willing to be patient, kind, and understanding, and he seemed genuinely interested that sex be a shared experience. While she freely acknowledged that she had no problems with his attitude, she still would usually become upset and turned off by his overtures. They asked for help with this problem, and a private session with Sandy was arranged.

When she came in, the therapist gently asked, "Is there something in your earlier years that you could talk about?" She immediately burst into tears. Red blotches appeared on her skin, and her words were punctuated with heavy sobbing and gasping as she began to relate her story: "When I was seven years old, we lived in [a small rural town]. One day my stepfather took me for a walk down a country road. It was in the summer. We hiked up the side of a hill. Then we stopped. Then he took off all my clothes. Then he took off all his clothes."

At this point she was scarcely able to breathe. The therapist stopped her and said that it was not necessary to go any further. He had her state her distress rating about the memory, which obviously was a 10. He then led her through the Tapping Sequence. Her intensity dropped from 10 to 6. At this point, an Acceptance Statement that began "Even though I still feel overwhelmed . . ." was used, followed by another round of tapping. This time the intensity fell to 2. Then another Acceptance Statement was introduced, beginning with, "Even if I never get completely over this . . . ," and a last round of tapping.

By this time, Sandy was breathing quietly. Her skin was free of blotches, her eyes were clear, and she was looking at her hands, lying folded in her lap. The therapist said, "Sandy, as you sit there now, think back to that hot summer day when your stepfather took you for that walk down that country road. Think about how you hiked up the side of that hill until you stopped. Think about how he took off all your clothes. Think of how he took off all his clothes. Now, what do you get?"

She sat there without moving for maybe five seconds, then looked up calmly and said, without excessive emotion, "Well, I still hate him." The therapist, after agreeing that hating him might be a reasonable response and possibly a useful one to keep, then asked, "But what about the distress you were feeling?"

Again she paused before answering. This time she laughed as she said, "I don't know. I just can't get there. Well, that was twenty years ago. I was just a little girl. I couldn't protect myself then the way I can now. What's the point in getting upset about something like that . . . I never let that man touch me again, and my kids have never been allowed to be near him. I don't know, it just doesn't seem to bother me like it did."

After this single session, she no longer experienced negative feelings in response to her partner's sexual advances. On a two-year follow-up, she reported that the problem was "good and gone," and her partner, now her husband, confirmed that there was no sign of the former difficulties. Notice, also, that by the end of the session she was speaking of the trauma almost casually, and she was placing it into a self-affirming framework: "Well, that was twenty years ago. I was just a little girl. I couldn't protect myself then the way I can now." Such shifts in relationship to a traumatic memory that has been emotionally cleared with a therapist who uses an energy approach are not unusual, and they can give you a new lease on your sexual life.

Men's Ancestral Programming; Women's Ancestral Programming

The old quip that "God gave men two brains but only enough blood to run one at a time" has been excruciatingly played out in innumerable broken relationships and the downfall of many a politician. It is also a source of tension in the psyches of men and women and even many happy relationships. Marianne Williamson describes the dilemma in evolutionary terms: For our distant ancestors, "nature needed men to go from one woman to another, impregnating us as they went along to propagate the species. And women needed to settle down with the children, to nurture them so that they would grow into adulthood. Those impulses running through our systems for at least a few hundred thousand years turned man's instinctive response after sex into, 'I gotta go,' while a woman's still tends to be, 'Let's settle down.' "[52]

Whatever the evolutionary contributions to tension in male-female relationships, nearly half of marriages in the United States end in divorce,[53] and infidelity is one of the most frequently stated reasons for divorce.[54] In one survey, 74 percent of men and 68 percent of women said they would consider an affair if they knew they would never get caught.[55] Attraction to others is a powerful and often unacknowledged energy in many relationships. It plays out differently in men than in women, and it can be a challenging issue for couples who are committed to going the distance with one another. This closing section of the chapter grapples with the biological underpinnings of this energetic conundrum.

Why Men Stray

A study that interviewed 120 young men about their relationships found conflict about fidelity to be a common theme. Emotionally they wanted to be monogamous, but their brains still craved sex outside their relationship. After a romantic phase of six months to two years, despite the love and intimacy they had come to share with their partner, their discontent grew until it felt like the relationship had placed them in a "form of socially compelled sexual incarceration."[56] They did not want to break up with their partners, but even as the emotional bonds deepened, a cognitive dissonance occurred (in this case, wanting two things that are mutually exclusive) as they tried to reconcile their sexual desires with their desire not to hurt their partner and honor the social mandates of a committed relationship. Simply stated by the investigator, they "want something they do not want."[57] Making matters worse was that they feared telling their partners about their desire for sex with others. Because of cultural beliefs that equate such desires with depravity or at least no longer being in love, regardless of the strength of the emotional bond, they feared that their partners would break up with them if they were honest. Cheating seemed less risky to the stability of their relationships than honesty, giving them a chance to have sex outside the relationship while maintaining emotional intimacy with their partner.

According to neuropsychiatrist Louann Brizendine, "both men and women have a deep misunderstanding of the biological and social instincts that drive the other sex."[58] For starters, a human male produces enough sperm in two weeks to impregnate every fertile female on the planet,[59] and men have two and a half times as much space devoted to sexual drive in the brain area where lust originates as women.[60] With forefathers who pursued fertile females having been selected to pass along their genes, modern men are physiologically primed to respond to appealing sexual opportunities independent of their values or druthers. Across all cultures, men evolved to focus on features that indicate health and fertility. Firm ample breasts, a small waist, flat stomach, full hips, clear skin, and facial symmetry add up to a look that "tells his brain that she's young, healthy, and probably not pregnant with another man's child."[61] His primary "mate-detection circuit comes prewired" to notice women with these physical characteristics, and when it does, "his brain's 'must have' sequence" is, at least for a moment, triggered.[62] A high-octane mix of testosterone and dopamine bathes brain regions that fuel his cravings for the blissful euphoric experience promised by the raw data his eyes are sending to his visual cortex. The attraction is magnetic. Like it or not, these rude physiological facts are ingredients in the male's side of the physical-psychological-interpersonal-social-spiritual-energetic stew called marriage. In energetic terms, it takes, as we showed earlier, little provocation for a man's Root Chakra energies to rush up to his Heart Chakra and surge "out of his body like a heat-seeking missile speeding toward a near stranger" (p. 108).

Why Women Stray

Our culture's assumptions about monogamy are captured in the popular ditty (often incorrectly attributed to William James), "Higamous, hogamous, woman is monogamous; hogamous, higamous, man is polygamous." For more than three decades, David has invoked this to explain peculiarities of his gender as well as to give himself license to keep some measure of self-respect amid feelings and urges he would prefer to no longer be experiencing. For Donna, it gave license for her to assume that males were an inferior, lascivious, unconscious lot, not wired to really love. David wanted to counter this viewpoint, sensing that it somehow did not reflect favorably on him, but he would be muted when the discussion would progress to rapists, plunderers, and philanderers as cases in point.

For the umpteenth time in our long relationship, we were having the higamous/hogamous discussion when David, who had been reading about the biological underpinnings of sexual behavior in animals and humans for this very chapter, decided to take a new tack in trying to defend himself from Donna's "holier than thou" attitude. Donna was not aware of any urge to not be monogamous within her primary relationship (unless she had been abandoned—physically or emotionally), and she viewed men who didn't hold to the same standard with contempt. That is not to say that she wasn't aware of her attractions to other men. She was, and she had no compunction about freely sharing such feelings. She had, in fact, recently mentioned how drawn she was to the mathematician and cosmologist Brian Swimme while we were watching a DVD of his, *The Universe Story*.

David said, "Okay, let me give you a hypothetical. Imagine us living as we do, happy with each other. Brian Swimme is living next door. He lives alone. He has respectfully signaled to you that he finds you attractive. I am getting old and able to make love only occasionally. I also travel a lot. Are you still monogamous? Or say we're younger. . . . We've had two children with severe congenital health problems. You desire a third child and everything in you wants this child to be healthy. You are walking by Mr. Swimme's home one day while I am at work. He looks *so* healthy and *so* strong. He invites you in. You are in the fertile time of your cycle. Are you still monogamous?" Donna: "Okay, okay, I get it! A woman's hogamous can go higamous. But men who fool around are still jerks!"

After working intensively with hundreds of women, we believe that women stray outside their primary relationship most often because they feel unloved or seek affirmation their partner is not providing. Variety, excitement, waning passion, and revenge are other reasons women give for cheating. Personal histories that include parental or other abuse can also make commitment to one partner difficult. Beyond these more obvious explanations are biological predispositions that may influence a woman's motivations in ways that are outside her awareness. Females in the wild generally choose their mate based on whether he has "what it takes to be a good

---

→ THE ENERGY DIMENSION ←

While everyone is unique, here are some features that stood out when, at a party, Donna compared the energies of men and women who were obviously "on the make."

Men on the Prowl

If men only knew how unattractive their energies are when they are trying to be suave and debonair for the purpose of seduction, they would take a different tack. The strongest energy emanating from a man who is making an uninvited pass comes from both his Root Chakra and his Third Chakra, which is at the solar plexus. The energy feels aggressive yet strangely impersonal. It has an air of manipulation and dishonesty and a desire to overpower and win at all costs. Part of what makes it so unattractive is that it is not deeply connected to him—it starts on the surface of his body and moves out from there. Its color is usually in the range from sharp yellow to brown. The energies of a man who is genuinely and deeply attracted to a woman have a very different quality. While they also come out of his Root Chakra, they come out of his Heart Chakra as well.

Women on the Prowl

I usually see a receptive rather than aggressive energy. The energy coming out of her heart is large and open, ready to take in and embrace the energy of a suitor. This energy has an air of hope and excitement. Once she is interested in someone, however, this energy becomes more focused. It moves out from *her* Third Chakra, which carries strategic energy, often geared toward playing to the man's ego. I can't exactly describe it except to say that I have seen women follow this energy in their behavior. And, embarrassing as it should be to men, it often works.

protector and provider."[63] That is still our basic programming. Interestingly a woman is not necessarily primed to select the genetically superior man.

In fact, dominant males who are genetically superior often "have a tendency for lower parental investment."[64] Single women can smell this, literally. Subtle body odors provide women with a surprising amount of information as their brains respond to cues about whether a man is nurturing and will stick around to help raise his offspring. Preferences also change with the time of the month and with marital status. Yes, scientists actually study these things! Dominant, genetically superior males (who are less likely to help with parenting) literally smell better to women who already have stable partners than they do to women who are unpaired, particularly during the time of the month that they are fertile.[65] Why might that be?

One of nature's first priorities in designing women was to favor the survival and success of their young. Once having secured a reliable partner, a woman who is open to a dalliance with a genetically superior man can improve the chances of genetically superior offspring. With nature having set it up so that men don't know if their partner's child is theirs, combined with a bit of deception, she can pass on better genes while being supported by the unsuspecting and characteristically more faithful partner. Given all of this, it is not surprising that a good deal of human history has been shaped by fuss about paternity. Another practical reason for a woman to indulge in secret liaisons, beyond psychological benefits such as adventure and affirmation of attractiveness, is to ensure that she will indeed be impregnated. Another is that a clandestine lover may bring gifts that will benefit her and her children, which in our ancestors' time usually meant food. Her genetic programming not only drives her to find a mate who will help her raise her young, it then drives her to see that those young have the best genes and resources she can attract.

These Forces Play Out within You in a Way That Is Unique to You

To become conscious of these forces in a manner that will be useful, the starting point is not only to read about their place in human evolution, as presented above, but also to recognize how they may or may not influence you at this point in your life and in your relationship. They do not operate in equal measure in all people or consistently across time. For instance, you may be a man whose sexual interest focuses only on your partner, or you may be a woman who can enjoy multiple sexual relationships with no emotional commitment.

Instructive here is a story Brizendine likes to tell of the side-blotched lizard. The males use three different mating strategies, and the tactics they use match the color of their throat. Males with orange throats guard a group of females, and they mate with all of them. Males with yellow throats sneak into the "harems" of the orange-throated males and mate with their females whenever they can get away with it. Males with throats that are a brilliant blue are wired for an entirely different strategy: They mate with only one female and guard her ardently. From a biological perspective, Brizendine concludes, these are three "successful mating strategies for lizards and for human males, too. I affectionately call my husband a blue-throat."[66] With humans, however, whose throats are not conveniently color-coded, the truth is that imprints for more than one mating strategy are probably fighting it out, or have fought it out at least at some point in your life. Bringing your consciousness to the battle makes a beneficial resolution more likely.

Does Monogamy Best Serve the Man, the Woman, Both, or Neither?

The above discussion shows that higamous/hogamous may not be the final words about male and female sexual drives after all. In *The Myth of Monogamy*, evolutionary biologist David Barash and his wife, Judith Lipton, a psychiatrist who specializes in women's issues, note that the traditional belief is that in nature as well as in civilized society, the female's "yearning for cozy monogamous domesticity was supposed to be as strong as the male tendency to mate with as many different partners as possible."[67] DNA analysis and related technologies have, however, found that even in the relatively few animal species that were believed to be monogamous, "females are not nearly as reliably monogamous as had been thought . . . they are active sexual adventurers in their own right."[68] Bird species that had been seen as being among nature's prototypes for monogamy often have eggs spawned by more than one male in the same nest, "tell me it ain't so" sentiments notwithstanding.

If aspiring toward monogamy, as Barash and Lipton and many other social scientists have concluded, goes "against some of the deepest-seated evolutionary inclinations with which biology has endowed most creatures, Homo sapiens included,"[69] why is it the bedrock of our culture? Not only does the Sixth Commandment demand "Thou shalt not commit adultery," the Tenth Commandment prohibits you from even enjoying the fantasy. This has, however, proven to be difficult to legislate. Anthropologists and historians of family and sexual arrangements have had to recognize that "the triumph of monogamy" has also been the "triumph of" unfaithfulness, marital deceit, and dishonesty.[70] The title of the section of our workshops that addresses these issues is called "What Was God Thinking?!"

Given the power of the male's proclivity for conspicuous and relatively indiscriminate fooling around, monogamy is often thought of as an arrangement that benefits women more than men. Historically, however, monogamy actually protected the interests of men more than of women. According to Barash and Lipton, having no restrictions on male sexual activity "is a disaster for most men."[71] The reason is that, unchecked, a small number of dominant males tend to reign over most of the females. While modern laws and mores counter this tendency, it was dramatic in many preindustrial societies. One of the most beautiful love poems ever written, *The Song of Songs*, is attributed to King Solomon. He was apparently writing from experience. The Old Testament reports that he had seven hundred wives and three hundred concubines, an innovative strategy for not being tempted to break the Sixth Commandment. Among the Incans, the four top political officials in a region (from petty chief to chief) were allotted seven, eight, fifteen, and thirty wives, respectively, while the emperor kept thousands of women.[72] Those of you who are good at math can see the problems this might cause for men in the middle or lower ranks. Monogamy also helps ensure a man's paternity and the inheritance rights that go with it. In addition, monogamy keeps the father around to protect his offspring against the little quirk in the brains of male mammals to kill the infants of other males,[73] a credible threat when living in nature "red of tooth and claw."

Meanwhile, Barash and Lipton go on, if a woman plays her hand well, the arrangement allows her to be impregnated by men with superior genes and higher status than her own while ensuring that she and her offspring will be provided for by a man inclined to make a strong investment in progeny he believes to be his. Oxytocin is a powerful propellant for women to bond with one partner, but the historical record as well as evolutionary biology suggest that both men and women are wired, though in very different ways, for sexual liaisons outside their primary relationship. As we look at these scholarly conclusions, we ask ourselves, "What's wrong with this picture?" A lot, actually, if you are wanting your relationship to take you to the most profound depths that two people can reach together.

Will Self-Defeating Impulses Always Run the Show?

Here's some good news. In a carefully documented scholarly paper called "Is Biology Destiny?," philosopher Phil Gasper concluded that "the key to our ancestors' success was their enormous flexibility and ability to learn, not patterns of behavior hardwired into their brains."[74] The male inclination to spread his seed far and wide may be powerful, but it is not a biological imperative. The female inclination toward suitors other than her partner may be powerful, but it is not a biological imperative. As our brains evolved and increased in size, no longer were rigid biological programs the basis of social behavior. We are endowed with the neural connections, logic, and memory to steer beyond the hazards inherent in our biological instincts. We are capable of navigating in ways that are not bound to outmoded strategies in our hardwired biological programming. Even as legions of conflicting biological and social forces are scurrying around in our psyches when we commit ourselves to "till death do us part," the evolutionary advantage of the human brain is in its enormous flexibility. Polygamy is a choice. Monogamy is a choice. Most of the women we know are less driven by the pursuit of better genes than by the pursuit of attention, love, and affection.

Monogamy vs. Monotony

Monogamy, if from the heart, is an agreement to enter into deep communion with another human being. . . . While the mortal mind sees monogamy as a feast for guilt, the divine mind sees it as a feast for love. At the level of our souls, we do not want monogamy in order to imprison each other, but to free each other—to create a context where the deepest level of safety might occur . . . that the deepest level of growth might occur.

—MARIANNE WILLIAMSON, *Enchanted Love*[75]

Our teen years were shaped by the sixties. As our outlooks were developing, we were exposed to free love, women's lib, open marriage, and the impact of contraception on sexual attitudes and behavior. We will admit to having considered numerous arrangements during our long and tumultuous relationship. But we are fully convinced at this point, and have been for many years, that every attempt to support freedom and variety through sexual liaisons outside our relationship had high potential for creating pain and distance. The damage would far outweigh the fleeting pleasures and even the deep soulful connections. In whatever way they operate within you, sexual drives are powerful forces that can be (1) squandered, (2) used in ways that are divisive to your primary relationship, or (3) channeled in ways that deepen it and make it more wondrous. This is why we have learned to enjoy sharing any attractions with one another—recall Brian Swimme—rather than trying to suppress them or allow them to take us in directions that divert us from intimacy.

We realized long ago that if we want our partnership to grow closer and more profound, our priority, even when things become strained or stale between us, needs to be on renewing the vitality of our own relationship. While it requires some chutzpah to broadcast that we have discovered what was right there in the Sixth Commandment all along about sexual relationships outside a marriage, we are also broadcasting the deep but elusive truth that monogamy need not equal monotony. Keeping our relationship fresh and vital keeps each of us fresh and vital.

Marriages that have gone the distance in a manner that supports each partner's growth tend to remain interesting and exciting. Sue Johnson, who developed the most effective approach to couple counseling that has been investigated by scientific research, observes that "hot sex doesn't lead to secure love," but rather "secure attachment leads to hot sex" as well as to "love that lasts."[76] Couples whose love does last have developed a sense of deep understanding, safety, and soul connection—all of which play into the fact that many women report that they enjoy sex more after years of marriage than they did when they were first married.[77] As Mary Jo Rapini observed: "My husband says things and touches me now in a way that is much deeper than when we first married. . . . Our way of communicating is different than it was. I get him, and he gets me. Couples who have been happily married for a long time understand the concept of feeling 'freer' with marriage than they were being single."[78] Asked about his many opportunities to stray while discussing his fifty-year marriage with Joanne Woodward, Paul Newman replied, "Why go out for a hamburger when you have steak at home?"[79] Channeling your passion into your relationship brings out the beauty in your partner and your partnership.

We are not saying or even feeling that our path should be your path. If you have found a better arrangement, go for it! We know of polyamorous arrangements that were done in a manner that felt sacred to the participants. But if you want to use your sexuality as a sacrament for the deepest spiritual connection available to you and your partner, monogamy paves a path that can lead there. Writing about sacred sexuality, Anaiya Sophia states it strongly. To enter "the space of deep communion" allowed by "the penetrating process of sexual intercourse . . . there must be no other man or woman on the sidelines . . . The back door of your sexual exchanges needs to be firmly closed for this sacrament to work alchemically. . . . Energetically this sacred act can only take place when we close the back door and cast instead a sacred circle."[80]

On to Chapter 9

Your sexual relationship is the first of the mutually created aspects of love we are addressing in this final section of the book. Building a conscious partnership is next.

9

Conscious Partnership

Staying Awake through the Highs and the Lows

The highest purpose of intimacy
is to call forth the beloved's soul.

—MARIANNE WILLIAMSON[1]

THE TERM *CONSCIOUS PARTNERING* IS BANDIED ABOUT A GOOD DEAL IN COUPLE self-help books, teleseminars, and workshop descriptions, yet we were unable to find a good definition of what it means. *Conscious* partnering as contrasted with what? *Normal* partnering? *Unconscious* partnering? To put "consciousness" into context, only a fraction of your brain is dedicated to conscious thought. In a typical waking moment, in fact, the parts of your brain involved with conscious thought process about forty nerve impulses per second while the brain areas involved with activity outside your consciousness process forty *million* nerve impulses per second.[2] However complicated your life may seem, it would be even worse if you were consciously tracking each instruction your brain generates.

This suggests, with no insult intended, that "unconscious partnering" plays a much larger role in your relationship with your beloved than conscious partnering. Fortunately, much of this works to your advantage. You may have, for instance, eventually learned to automatically leave the TV clicker in the agreed-upon spot. Your subconscious mind is a storehouse of the lessons life has taught you as well as your natural abilities and intuitive wisdom. Along with countless automated actions as mundane as putting on your shoes, your subconscious mind holds innumerable instructions for more complex actions and has access to transcendent sources of inspiration for solving the bewildering problems life presents and for pursuing your most creative aspirations. While your subconscious mind is an enormous source of sound guidance that is available 24/7, it also stores past hurts, self-limiting beliefs, unresolved conflicts, and dysfunctional behavioral strategies. So it doesn't *always* work to your advantage. Because a large percentage of our cognitive activity is controlled by outmoded genetic or acquired programs downloaded into the subconscious mind, explains Bruce Lipton, we are compelled, despite our most sincere conscious intentions and desires, "to lunge for the Krispy Kreme donuts in the refrigerator or fall for the biggest jerk at the party—again."[3]

In this chapter, we will explore the nature of conscious partnering and describe seven qualities of consciousness that you can cultivate, using energy techniques, to make your journey together a richer one. We will also identify outmoded biological programming and habitual patterns that undermine conscious partnering as well as happiness and suggest ways of overcoming them.

A Glimpse into a Conscious Partnership

In trying to make the concept of conscious partnering more concrete, we could think of no better way than to interview a couple who illustrate its principles in their living experience. We asked ourselves, of all the couples we know, who do we think really "walk their talk" in terms of what they strive for in a relationship? A couple came immediately to mind. Both are noted musicians. We sent an e-mail asking if we could interview them for our book on love. They were actually leaving the next day for a recording in New York City where the husband, Paul Horn, was going to accompany his old buddy Tony Bennett, who was performing with Lady Gaga! It promised to be an interesting mix. We got to conduct and record our interview with them over Skype just before that trip.

Paul is a jazz hall of fame flautist who, in addition to Tony Bennett and now Lady Gaga, has played with Duke Ellington, Nat King Cole, and Paul McCartney, among many other world-class musicians. He was first known to us through his haunting meditative solo flute recordings, done inside the Taj Mahal, the Great Pyramid, and other sacred sites beginning in the 1960s. Donna first met Paul in 1963 during the successful healing of a grieving, dying killer whale while Paul played to it. Paul is married to Ann Mortifee, a dear friend to both of us since we met her in 1990. Ann is a singer, composer, and playwright. During the first Earth Day festivities in Vancouver, in 1970, she sang her songs to eighty thousand people. David and Ann have worked together. Their first project was an album for people facing death, *Serenade at the Doorway,* which is still used by many hospices throughout the world. Ann closed the 1994 Commonwealth Games with "Healing Journey" from that album, heard by hundreds of millions of people worldwide.

Different Temperaments

Ann and Paul first met when Ann had written a musical score for the Royal Winnipeg Ballet in 1971 and Paul was one of the musicians, but they did not become a couple until after they had raised their own families. We asked, "We know that you, like us, have very different temperaments—how do you make that work?" With her wonderful dramatic flair, Ann described an image she once saw in a temple in India:

> In the middle of the temple, there stood a sculpture of Shiva [one of the major Hindu deities] and dancing around him were statues of the sixty-four dakinis [forms] of Shakti [the goddess of female creative energy]. On one of the statues she has blood dripping from her mouth. She holds a sword in one hand and the head of Shiva in the other. In another, she's a beautiful Madonna. In another, she's the sexy lady. And Shiva, in the middle, remains always the same. It's like he's saying: "Whoa, look at her go!" And I remember thinking, "If I am ever with a man who can let me be all the selves that I am, that would be marvelous!" And Paul lets me! He doesn't hold me to some expectation. Perhaps I have come to a brink where I physiologically need a good cry or I will explode. I burst into tears, weep deeply, and he is right there saying, "Let it go, let it go!" Maybe at some point he'll say, "I love you," or "I'm here," but it doesn't wrangle him in the slightest. He doesn't worry about me. He is simply there. [Paul interrupts, "I might say, 'What a woman! There she goes! Hold on! Let me get my camera.'" We all laugh. Ann continues:] We both simply recognize that one of my dakinis has just gone by! And so I feel a tremendous permission to be as extreme as I am. Being loved like we love each other has changed my physiology. Something has relaxed in me so that now I

almost never go to those extreme emotional places anymore. I have become more balanced than I ever thought would be possible for me. The little voice in me that always believed someone was judging me, which they usually were, is completely gone with Paul. So whatever I go through passes very quickly and a new pathway is being created from my subconscious mind and into my consciousness. Old patterns simply fall away.

Sharing Separate Paths

PAUL: "Both people have to do their own work, walk their own path. The path is about the big questions. 'What am I here for?' 'What's important?' Of course common interests are also necessary, but when people have done their own work on these big questions, or at least have made a good start on them, then the relationship is going to be based on their deeper journeys, not on externals."

ANN: "Both of us have done an immense amount of work. I was not looking for someone to complete me. I wasn't hungry for someone to give me something that would make me feel good or fill a void. I was content to live alone for the rest of my life if that was what was meant to be. So was Paul. But I was open for a true partner to continue evolving with me. I already came with a basketful of my own Self, as did Paul. Both of us have gone through the joys and agonies of love with other people, and we've both come to a place of having made a clear decision to either live alone or to create something truly splendid."

PAUL: "Having had other relationships in our lives, we would often say, half kidding, 'If it's going to be fun and rich, I'm in. Otherwise, I'm not interested.'"

The Real Purpose of Marriage

Paul spent time in India with Maharishi Mahesh Yogi at the Maharishi's ashram in 1967 and then again in 1968, the year of the Beatles' famed stay. He returned as one of the first teachers of Transcendental Meditation. The Maharishi had said something to Paul that has become a cornerstone of Paul and Ann's relationship: "The purpose of marriage is to help each other grow to cosmic consciousness as quickly as possible." They took that on as their motto—that their real purpose together is to help one another evolve to their fullest potentials.

Allies, Not Enemies

ANN: "That's been right at the center of our relationship from the beginning. When we are at the edge of old patterns, of misunderstandings, we pull out. We say, 'This does not serve us. We are allies. I am never going to look at you as my enemy. You are my ally.' Anytime that an argument comes up, we immediately stop and say, 'Okay, *I* need to learn something here.' We don't point fingers at one another. We're very disciplined in that. Paul never calls me on things in a negative way. He sees when I'm overwhelmed, and he's very tender with me, very sweet with me, and it dissipates like that [snaps fingers]. Sometimes, when you've got so much to do, it's easy to forget that there are things that are more important than changing the hydrofilter [laughter]. It's very sweet to be so kind to each other. Speaking the truth with kindness brings out the best."

PAUL: "Or as Maharishi used to say, 'Speak the *sweet* truth.'"

Another Damned Opportunity to Evolve

ANN: "We have opposite difficulties and learning edges. Usually for me it's got to do with discernment. Not being clear enough, not being focused, not using my best judgment. And for Paul, it's usually about not being as accepting or compassionate as he could be with others. So we know this about each other. I know the little quirks that Paul has. He knows mine. When something comes up that causes me to react in a negative way, I always ask myself: 'What is it in *me* that triggers this reaction? Why do *I* lose *my* equilibrium when this comes up?' If you have a higher purpose, it's not about the other person anymore. It's about your own evolution."

PAUL: "Yes, another damned opportunity to evolve!"

ANN: "And your partner usually can see something in you that you cannot. This is a great gift not to be squandered. This is the relationship that can make all the difference in your journey toward self-realization, the most important journey of all. I've often thought: If you can stay conscious in a love relationship, you can stay conscious anywhere!"

It's Not Easy Living with Your Guru

ANN: "Regarding my challenge with discernment, oh my God, this is the most difficult learning for me. I meet someone who is hurting or in need. I know I shouldn't get involved. I warn myself not to get involved. But they share their sorrow with me and, suddenly, I am involved. I lose all perspective. My heart goes out to them and I'm off to the races. It's been tough to learn boundaries and edges. It's been tough on both of us. But the fact that Paul understands how difficult this is for me, and doesn't judge me for it, is helping me to move through it and evolve. And I do want to evolve. I want to leave this planet very awake, and that's what we bring each other. Paul has been my teacher, my mentor, my guru in discernment. He understands my challenges with it. When I'm not being discerning, I can feel that old feeling, the impulse to jump into an unwise decision, but I can't hide anymore. I can't get any mileage out of the old excuses."

PAUL: "And Ann has been my teacher in love and forgiveness. I lived alone for many years and got into the habit of ruminating about what or who might be bothering me at the time. Ann has helped me to see that these conversations with myself were not serving me or anyone else. As Ann said, 'You can't hide anymore.' It's not always easy living with your guru."

Taking Full Responsibility

PAUL: "It's your partner who can help you the most in growing and knowing about yourself. Rather than being annoyed or defensive when something comes up, we discover together how to use the situation as an opportunity to evolve."

ANN: "I take a hundred percent responsibility for how we're doing. Not fifty percent. If we're not doing well, then I am one hundred percent personally responsible for it, instead of the unproductive need to deflect the blame from myself onto him, that tit-for-tat thing that couples do."

PAUL [PLAYFULLY]: "It's an opportunity to grow twenty-four hours a day!"

ANN: "It's not about him 'learning' from me. If there is something for him to learn, that's his department. If he doesn't see something I offer as being useful, I have to accept that. Consequently, because I'm always working with myself, if I feel agitated and annoyed, it's got nothing to do with him. I'm agitated. I'm annoyed. It's my nervous system going haywire. How do I work with that? Sometimes I might say, 'I'm losing it here. I'm having an irritation that is really getting to me. I need time to work this out.' Or I might say, 'Would you scratch my back?' And he's just right there, willing to help."

PAUL: "We have a basic respect for one another's intelligence and for what each of us has learned throughout our lives. Because there's no judgment in the field, we simply work together to help each other. We are not in competition with each other. I can look at Ann as my teacher, which she is in so many ways, and it doesn't diminish my sense of self at all."

Cultivating the Great Virtues

ANN: "We have an overlaying awareness that through our relationship we are cultivating the Great Virtues. This aspiration helps you to understand why the Great Virtues always take so long to cultivate and bring to flower. Patience is very difficult. It takes a lot of patience to cultivate patience! It's not easy to allow yourself, or the other person, to grow at the rate you or they need to grow. Acceptance is another great virtue. To accept your partner's little flaws and the things they wrestle with. To not expect them to do things the way you would like them to be done. Surrender is another. To surrender to whom the person really is. To not be wishing they were a little bit more like this or more like that, but to truly surrender to the person your partner actually is. To love and appreciate them as they are, not as you wish them to be. Forgiveness is another great virtue. Just forgive. Forgive everything. Get to a state where you don't even need to forgive anything because there was no judgment there in the first place. This is sometimes called 'witness consciousness.' Cultivating these Great Virtues is a central motivation for us in our relationship."

Losing It

ANN: "I have a lot going on, and I sometimes become overwhelmed. What's made a difference is Paul's steadiness. He doesn't get taken down by my overwhelm. In fact, what I've been discovering in our time together, and really, I've been stunned by it, is that I don't lose my temper anymore. At all. Do I? [asking Paul, who confirms, "No."] No. I didn't think so. I still get antsy. I get overwhelmed. But I never take it out on Paul. Never, never, never. Every time I feel an emotional upset, I immediately become alert. I know my body is communicating to me that my energetic field has become disturbed, and I look for the truth I'm not getting. Where am I in denial? I just dive into it because there is something I need to understand. This helps me to accept life as it is. To be equanimous no matter what is going on. To be in the moment rather than in the past or the future. What helps us is that we are also mirrors to one another. When we look at each other, what is shining back at us is a full acceptance and love and awareness. We are being seen in our highest while at the same time we are being witnessed in our weakness. This is very liberating. Thank God I have a partner who wants me to succeed, who wants me to evolve, and who helps me."

When Your Partner Can't Be Consoled

ANN: "I have given Paul the power to console me. I welcome his help because we are very mindful of each other. If there is a disturbance in the field, we acknowledge it right away, but we are very considerate in how we do that. We don't have harsh words with one another. I truly say this with great surprise knowing how I've been in other circumstances [laughing]."

PAUL: "Me too."

ANN: "One of us might get irritable, the other just notices it and says, 'How about a cup of tea.' Or 'Why don't we sit down for five minutes and meditate.' If it's Paul saying that to me, I will probably say, 'MEDITATE!?!?! At this moment! You gotta be kidding!' And he'll say, 'Come on, I know you'll feel a lot better.' And I go . . . [makes protesting sounds]. Then I say, 'Okay.' Then I finally sit down, and sure enough, 'Ahhhhh.' The anxious, trying-to-get-everything-done fades away."

Meeting the Dark Side

PAUL: "We have a lot of respect for one another."

ANN: "But respect can be tricky. With people out in the world, it's easy to be respectful, usually. But with a partner, the dark side can come up so quickly. That's fine, that's what partners do for each other. This lets you have a good look at what is sometimes invisibly under the surface, running the show. But to respect it! To accept it! To welcome it! That's not so easy. But you can do it. If you remind yourself, 'This is an opportunity to see into the darkness, and I have a witness who loves me, who is with me, who is my ally,' everything shifts."

The Gift of Limitation

PAUL: "Getting older helps. People fear getting older, but you have to see the value in every stage of your life. There are great benefits to getting older. You have more wisdom. You're not so driven by hormones."

ANN: "Paul is eighty-three. Our time together now is very limited, and we know that. There is a real blessing in limitation because we don't take our time together for granted. We realize it is going to be over so soon. It's made me very cognizant of the preciousness of time and how fleeting it is. I ask myself every day if I am loving Paul to the extent I would if I knew this was our last day on earth together. Am I really here, really present, really taking advantage of this relationship while I have it, of this lifetime while I have it? Everything is finite in this realm, and I'm learning the gift of limitation. We are building the eternal aspects of our relationship. It's not focused so much on the day-to-day external world but on building a powerful inner spiritual foundation between us as we live moment by moment on this amazing planet."

Practices

PAUL: "It's important to have a quiet time of day where you are quiet and share appreciation for the gift of life. It's as simple as that. And your appreciation gets extended to your partner: 'I've found someone I really love who is my best friend and I get to hang out with my best friend every day.' So we do that. We start the day with focused time with one another. We might read together. We talk together. We meditate together. Meditation is our practice. Meditation soothes the nervous system tremendously. It stills and connects us to a realm of Silence, which is the source of creative potential. Maharishi didn't give me an answer. He gave me a technique by which I could get answers for myself."

ANN: "We also every so often will take an evening, dress in our best, light all the candles, and sit together and tell each other in so many ways how much we love and appreciate each other. We give thanks for one another. It's like a prayer of gratitude. Things like that keep love alive and pure and real. Lord knows, that's the space I want to be in during our last moments together. So we tell each other we love each other fifty times a day."

PAUL [LAUGHING]: "Maybe sixty. We were reflecting on that the other day, how many times we just spontaneously say 'I love you.' It keeps us connected. We have lived together, under the same roof—morning, noon, and night—for many years now. It could be easy to take one another for granted. We simply don't."

Every couple must find their own ways of supporting one another's evolution, turning their differences into strengths, and keeping their relationship fresh and vital. Still, Paul and Ann's reflection on their own development as a couple is worth reviewing from time to time. It contains inspiration and wise instruction about the day-to-day interactions that build intimacy and more conscious ways of relating.

Seven Qualities of Conscious Partnering

Just as Paul's and Ann's open sharing invites you to reflect on the possibilities of conscious partnership, we have done our own reflection—both as a couple and as professionals who work with couples. We have identified seven qualities that characterize our own relationship when we are at our conscious best. In articulating them, we have also reaffirmed our intention to further cultivate these qualities. Energy follows intention. These seven intentions are stated here in a manner that allows you to consider them for your relationship as well. Qualities of consciousness that support a richer relationship can be cultivated through:

. . . an intention to bring the vast resources of our subconscious minds into our relationship. Even in our darkest times, if we have stayed open to the possibility that a new and deeper understanding is going to emerge—rather than becoming locked in stagnation or hopelessness—something fresh and sustaining usually takes bloom. Rather than a mental state you have to work hard to attain, this gradual opening to ever-deeper parts of your being is a natural, though uneven part of personal evolution. Expect it; welcome it; cultivate it; relax into it.

. . . an intention to bring into consciousness unacknowledged impulses, motivations, and beliefs. When we find ourselves caught in self-defeating patterns, our commitment is to look deeper and courageously stare them down at their source. Beneath your personality and defenses dwells a universe of unnamed forces and vulnerabilities that are revealed in your unconscious proclivities and automatic

behaviors. Creating with your partner a context where it is safe to share your deeper workings brings them into your awareness. Recognizing and accepting them may sometimes seem overwhelming, but it ultimately makes you and your relationship stronger, not weaker.

. . . *an intention to address these internal conflicts and outdated learnings that had been operating beneath our consciousness.* Not only are we committed to recognize deep sources of conflict or dysfunction tracing to our personal histories or simply our lack of wisdom, we are determined to utilize that information for our evolution. When internal conflicts and outdated learnings are brought into the light, they become less onerous and can be creatively and actively resolved or transformed. Energy medicine and energy psychology give you particularly powerful tools. Accepting and working with your foibles also builds trust and intimacy with your partner.

. . . *an intention to keep focusing on what is beneficial and empowering.* We are committed to recognizing the strengths within us and the resources around us even when feeling lost, judgmental, or uncertain. You and your relationship flourish when your personal strengths and the strengths of your partnership are registered and acknowledged—far more than when your shortcomings get the focus. A tendency to scan for what is right rather than what is wrong can, as is discussed later in this chapter, be cultivated.

. . . *an intention to process the past and envision the future in ways that bring out the best in each of us and in our relationship.* We are committed to viewing our own and our partner's needs for change and growth as opportunities rather than liabilities. Relationship is a challenge to completely accept and appreciate what is. Relationship is *also* a challenge to actively transform what is into what can be. The visions you hold about what is possible and desirable become the maps that will lead you into your future.

. . . *an intention to bring up tough topics in a loving and constructive way.* We are committed to processing our own negative feelings in a manner that allows us to treat one another with kindness. Studies on the characteristics of marital success have shown again and again that it is not the amount of conflict couples have between them—all couples have areas of friction—but rather the way they resolve their differences. Specifically, the quality of the partners' *emotional responsiveness* to one another predicts longevity in a marriage. Register the way your actions impact your partner's feelings and use that understanding to treat your partner like a king or a queen.

. . . an intention to stay receptive to one another's evolving beauty. We are committed to using the power of our minds and imaginations to see one another anew and with profound appreciation and respect for the other's journey and challenges. When you deeply witness another's struggles and the person's striving to bring forth into the world that which is beautiful and worthy within them, love is ever renewed.

While good intentions have gotten a bad rap—you know which road is paved with them—you can use your understanding of the body's energies to make these seven affirmations more than just platitudes. Doing a round of energy psychology tapping (chapter 6) while mindfully stating one of the intentions as you tap on each point embeds the words and their meaning into your energy system. An even simpler way for incorporating the meaning of a statement into your nervous system is to say the words out loud, as an affirmation, while you slowly and consciously do a Zip-Up (p. 87). Choose a quality from the above list that you would particularly like to develop, adapt the first or second sentence in the description to your liking, and "tap it in" or "zip it in" every day for a week. You will notice its expanding role in your mental outlook. If an internal objection to incorporating the quality arises (e.g., "I am too angry to want to bring up these tough issues in a loving way"), give the intensity of the internal objection a zero to ten rating and use the energy psychology protocol to bring that intensity down to zero. This may not fully resolve your anger or other emotion, but it will allow the affirmation to begin to take hold. Conscious partnering is within your grasp.

A Tidy Relationship vs. Your Wild Self

Conscious partnering is not a *product* but rather a day-to-day *process*. It requires a willingness to set aside adolescent images of love as a magic elixir and to embrace a much more complex, challenging, and ultimately fulfilling vision. In a wonderful book, *Undefended Love*, Jett Psaris and Marlena Lyons describe a familiar dilemma:

"Many people have absorbed something of the cultural belief that if we find the right partner and love each other enough, the outcome will be the passionate yet secure relationship we have always hoped for. When we don't achieve this, as is so often the case, we believe something is wrong with the relationship, with us, or with our partner."[4]

Psaris and Lyons develop a powerful concept: Our yearning for deep love and our yearning to express the most profound and untamed aspects of ourselves are often at odds. The ways you and your partner successfully adjust to the demands of a relationship can, paradoxically, keep you from deeply knowing one another and supporting the raw beauty that lies within each of you. In conscious partnership, on the other hand, the form and rules are never orderly and are forever changing.

This is necessitated by one of nature's more irritating interpersonal paradoxes: The adjustments and agreements we make so our relationship will run more smoothly often require that we suppress our deeper, wild nature. How do you resolve the tension between the requirements of your relationship and the elemental core of your being? This lifelong project involves building a partnership in which your messy, juicy, deepest self is continually informing the relationship. The solutions we come to in order to keep our relationships peaceful and tidy prevent the deep encounters with one another that keep relationships fresh and vital, so "instead of helping us find ways to dismantle the walls between us, making agreements leaves them unchallenged and intact."[5]

Compromises and agreements are, of course, necessary for a relationship to operate. They build a context of safety and support within which the relationship can flourish. The challenge is to not hold on too tightly to these arrangements so the journey of the self is not shut down by the practicalities of the relationship. In the process, each is enhanced. One way of supporting both your partnership and the most authentic parts of each of you is to be alert for when an agreement breaks down. Use that as an opportunity to further your personal evolution and take the relationship to a deeper level of engagement. Rather than rush to plug the hole in the relationship with new promises or a revised agreement, or to compulsively try to meet each other's every emotional need, take the time to discover and honor the impulses in each of you that have led to the breakdown of the existing agreement. Digging below the surface in this way may cause some short-term discomfort and may even temporarily bring you onto shaky ground with one another, but it is a route to more profound engagement that opens you to the vast resources within each of you.

Habits of Thought That Undermine Conscious Partnering

Habits of thought that keep our attention running along fixed pathways even if they limit or harm us are the antithesis of conscious partnering. Ron Siegel, a psychologist at Harvard Medical School, describes five "neurobiological mechanisms that make us miserable."[6] These trace to the harsh lives our ancestors survived millions of years ago. Simply becoming aware of evolutionary tendencies that have become self-defeating is a step toward freeing yourself from their grip, so we list them here.

Focusing on What Is Bad

Our ancestors were attuned to danger. Anticipating what could go wrong was an effective survival strategy. Being alert for whether a hungry lion was in the vicinity had more survival value than finding the tastiest berries. We, as the distant offspring of the survivors, are still wired to give more weight and attention to problems than to pleasures. As Siegel quips, "We evolved minds that are like Velcro for bad thoughts and Teflon for good ones."[7] In short, we are programmed to obsessively and painfully focus on what is wrong.

Stress Arousal System Stuck in the "On" Position

To compound the tendency to focus on what is wrong, our highly developed cerebral cortex makes the fight/flight/freeze response to threat—which is so remarkably effective in the wild for mammals with less complex lives and brains than ours—problematic for us. Other creatures get past the danger when the danger has passed, but we get caught up thinking about it. Our arousal systems get stuck in the "on" position as we obsess about "what went wrong in the past and what might go wrong in the future, experiencing painful emotions each time."[8] We transform even problems we have handled effectively into worry about what will go wrong next.

Self-Comparisons

Another vestige of our evolution that makes the psychological equipment we have inherited challenging is our predisposition to compare ourselves with others. Higher-ranking ancestors got to mate with healthier partners with better genes, and this history fuels our compulsion to "constantly fill our minds with comparisons to others."[9] We can always find someone to whom we can compare ourselves negatively and are compelled to do so, though it undermines our personal sense of well-being.

Avoiding What Is Unpleasant

Much of our psychological suffering, according to some mental health experts, paradoxically involves our efforts to avoid unpleasant experiences at the expense of taking needed actions. From not confronting difficult tasks or relationship problems to the abuse of drugs and mind-numbing media, the problem, Siegel observes, "is that many things that make us feel better in the short run make us feel much worse in the long run."[10] One of our most instinctive strategies for avoiding suffering tends to backfire. Even physical pain, when met with mindful awareness and acceptance, changes in texture and becomes easier to bear.

A Future Framed by Awareness of What Can Go Wrong

We are wired to anticipate famines, wars, and other threats to our well-being and very existence. Making our propensity for worry and self-generated misery even worse, we, unlike other creatures, know we are going to die. We know that no matter how well we live we are headed toward either sickness and decline or a gruesome premature ending.

These psychological predispositions, whose roots often trace more to the twists and turns of our jagged evolutionary heritage than to our upbringing, not only undermine our capacities for joy and fulfillment, they sabotage our ability to form secure, healthy relationships. An effective approach to interpersonal bliss does not include (1) emphasizing what is wrong rather than what is right about your partner and your relationship, (2) maintaining perceptions and expectations about your partner or your relationship that keep you in a threat alert mode, (3) comparing your partner or your relationship negatively with others, (4) not dealing with difficult issues within your relationship, and (5) expending your energies and good spirit worrying about that which neither of you can control.

Our Capacity to Change What Isn't Working

The reason for the above cheery discussion about our inborn tendencies for making ourselves and our relationships miserable is that recognizing a predicament is the first step in finding ways to move beyond it, and we can also suggest steps beyond mere recognition. Recall from our discussion in the previous chapter about whether we are destined to act out the sexual proclivities of our ancestors. The answer was, "No, we are not." And so it is for each of these inborn habits of thought. The keys to our success as a species are our flexibility and ability to learn—based on our logic, memory, and enormous neural network—rather than rigid biological programs that are hardwired into our brains. Brain researchers use the term "self-directed neuro-plasticity" to describe your brain's built-in ability to change itself based on what you do with your mind.[11] It is an empowering concept. Even as the parts of our brain that cause us to act like reptiles battle it out with the parts that are "in apprehension how like a god" (*Hamlet*), evolution gave us the capacity to enter the fray and counteract dysfunctional remnants of our prehistoric past.

Mindfulness

Siegel advocates mindfulness as a way of overcoming self-defeating psychological predispositions, and we will add an energy psychology approach as an additional way of replacing self-defeating habits with more adaptive patterns of thought, feeling, and behavior. Research has demonstrated that mindfulness influences gene expression, providing direct health benefits as specific as the reduction of activity in pro-inflammatory genes.[12] Psychologically, it brings about beneficial neurological changes leading to improved regulation of emotions, enhanced perspective, better memory, greater well-being, and a more fluid sense of self.[13]

While mindfulness is many things, it is also an energy technique, a highly sophisticated approach that establishes new energetic habits in the brain. Focusing your attention leads to shifts in your energies that lead to changes in your neurochemistry. The patterns by which your energies flow are the first process influenced by mindfulness. The practice aligns your energies in ways that correspond with the experience of inner peace, and it establishes energy habits that will be beneficial to you as well as to your relationship. From that energetic shift, stress is less likely to trigger a threat response, your partner's behaviors are less likely to send you into fight/flight/freeze mode, and the rational part of your brain will have greater influence over your primitive brain centers.

At the core of mindfulness is awareness and acceptance of your inner experiences, moment by moment. Mindfulness is the art of recognizing and accepting what is. With this awareness, our responses to what life presents soften, naturally and organically. By noticing your thoughts and emotions with curiosity and acceptance, rather than clinging to or acting on them, you come to understand how they regularly appear and then fade. In mindfulness practice, Siegel explains, "we begin to see our thoughts as secretions of the mind, arising and passing like clouds moving across a vast sky. We stop believing in them as we once did. That, in turn, lessens their grip and reduces our emotional reactivity to them."[14] The T-shirt slogan "Don't believe everything you think" nails it. Siegel discusses how mindfulness counters the self-defeating habits of thought that trace back to our ancestors by helping us "see more clearly the habits of our minds that create unnecessary suffering—and offers a way to change them."[15] An introduction to mindfulness, along with free audio instructions for several practices, is generously provided on Siegel's website, http://www.mindfulness-solution.com.[16]

Energy Psychology

Energy psychology also begins by recognizing *what is* (the SUD rating, p. 193) and accepting it (the Acceptance Statement, p. 196), but then goes on to use acupoint tapping to send signals to the brain that rapidly change our emotional response to difficult thoughts and memories. While changing your consciousness shifts your energies, shifting your energies changes your consciousness. Each of the five self-defeating psychological dispositions discussed above is stated next in terms relevant to both the individual and the relationship. Each is then followed by (1) a sentence summarizing the way that mindfulness might shift the pattern and (2) an energy psychology Acceptance Statement and Reminder Phrase that can be used, along with acupoint stimulation, for shifting deep habits of thought and emotion.

1. EMPHASIZING WHAT IS WRONG RATHER THAN WHAT IS RIGHT ABOUT YOURSELF, YOUR PARTNER, OR YOUR RELATIONSHIP

Mindfulness: Deeply recognizing how your psyche automatically produces thoughts that focus on what is wrong powerfully challenges the authority of those thoughts.

Acupoint Stimulation: Massage the points on the Central Meridian (p. 198) while stating, "*Even though I keep focusing on* [name the thought] . . ." Then place your hands over your Heart Chakra as you say, "*I deeply love and accept myself.*" Then do a round of tapping (see Figure 6-3), stating the thought as you come to each acupoint. [For this and the four subsequent acupoint stimulation instructions, you can simply do them as written or, to address the issues involved more deeply, do them within the complete energy psychology protocol presented in Chapter 6, starting with a zero-to-ten SUD rating about the distress you feel when you bring the self-defeating thought or habit to mind.]

2. MAINTAINING PERCEPTIONS AND EXPECTATIONS ABOUT YOURSELF, YOUR PARTNER, OR YOUR RELATIONSHIP THAT KEEP YOUR STRESS AROUSAL SYSTEM STUCK IN THE "ON" POSITION

Mindfulness: Accepting whatever thoughts or emotions your psyche produces without clinging to them defuses their power to endlessly evoke the stress response.

Acupoint Stimulation: Use the physical procedures described in #1 while stating, "*Even though I become anxious when I think of* [describe the situation], *I deeply love and accept myself.*" Then do a round of tapping, describing the situation in a few words as you come to each acupoint.

3. COMPARING YOURSELF, YOUR PARTNER, OR YOUR RELATIONSHIP NEGATIVELY WITH OTHERS

Mindfulness: Noticing our self-judgments without overidentifying with them is a way of offsetting our culturally reinforced preoccupation with our selves, our status, and the market value of our personal qualities.

Acupoint Stimulation: Use the physical procedures described in #1 while stating, *"Even though I judge myself* [or *my partner* or *my relationship*] *for* [describe], *I deeply love and accept myself."* Then do a round of tapping, briefly naming the judgment as you come to each acupoint.

4. AVOIDING WHAT IS UNPLEASANT

Mindfulness: Being present with and experientially embracing every thought and emotion, whether pleasant or unpleasant, prepares your nervous system to meet whatever life presents with equanimity and to deal with it effectively.

Acupoint Stimulation: Use the physical procedures described in #1 while stating, *"Even though I avoid* [describe], *I deeply love and accept myself."* Then do a round of tapping, briefly naming what you avoid as you come to each acupoint.

5. EXPENDING YOUR ENERGIES AND GOOD SPIRIT WORRYING ABOUT THAT WHICH NEITHER OF YOU CAN CONTROL

Mindfulness: Experiencing your thoughts and feelings as passing events while holding an open, curious attitude about how they, like your breath, rise and fall, is a potent way to prepare for transitions, large and small.[17]

Acupoint Stimulation: Use the physical procedures described in #1 while stating, *"Even though I worry about* [describe], *I deeply love and accept myself."* Then do a round of tapping, briefly naming the worry as you come to each acupoint.

Both mindfulness and energy psychology techniques can help us break the trance that our reflexive thoughts and emotions are the only valid reality in town. This allows us to engage our lives, moment by moment, at more profound and genuine levels. While the energies in your body are to a large degree governed by habits, you can willfully affect their flow. When you do—in fact, when you do almost anything that is outside your habitual repertoire even once—it will be easier to do it again. That is how quickly your energies and your brain can begin to establish new habits and new neural pathways.

Conscious Partnering Means Telling
the Microscopic Truth

Conscious partnering is both an inside job and a shared creation. Cultivating a relationship that can serve as a creative container for the conflicting and shifting feelings and perspectives that characterize everyone's inner life is an ongoing adventure. Psychological development is all about one set of worldviews and related preferences and strategies making way for another. How has your vision of marriage changed since you were younger? Your senses of calling, destiny, and purpose and your methods for fulfilling them are in a process of continual evolution as you move from one phase of your life to the next (and as the culture changes around you). This process does not, however, unfold in a neat and orderly fashion, and you and your partner are one another's closest witnesses in this messy piece of personal evolution. To fully embrace this dimension of conscious partnering requires profound acceptance as well as radical honesty.

Radical Honesty

A long-term relationship that can contain two people's passions, beliefs, and desires freely expressed and fully respected is an evolutionary landmark. In their classic book, *Conscious Loving*, Gay and Kathlyn Hendricks describe an essential skill for a conscious relationship as the ability and commitment to tell one another the "microscopic truth."[18] They explain that most people learn to conceal or distort the truth of their inner experience during childhood. The job of a parent and a culture is to mold a child's motivations and behavior toward certain preconceived ideals, and the job of a child is to pretend that it is working. Some feelings (and the behaviors that grow out of those feelings) are acceptable in the family, the school, and the society and can be freely expressed; other feelings lead to ridicule, shame, or punishment and are concealed. Was that the case for you? It is for most people, and it carries into our adult relationships. Donna got the message that she was not to cause trouble, and she learned to quickly dismiss or not even recognize feelings within herself that might cause problems for others. David learned to define himself by his achievements and to convert every impulse for play into this drive to achieve before it might divert him into actually having fun. These messages become so firmly embedded that many people, the Hendrickses explain, "simply do not know themselves deeply enough to tell the truth at a meaningful level."[19]

While telling the truth would seem an obvious part of conscious partnering, telling the "microscopic truth" is a skill that requires practice not only in stating what your partner might not want to hear, but also in recognizing just what is your deeper truth. Rather than a broad philosophical position, this is a moment-by-moment endeavor. The Hendrickses define truth, in the sense of the *microscopic truth*, as "that which absolutely cannot be argued about."[20] And the only thing that absolutely cannot be argued about is your experience. David might notice that his beloved has become the center of extreme chaos when packing for a trip and helpfully observe, "Donna, after all these years, you are still totally disorganized." This, however, is *not* the microscopic truth.

If he could see inside her head how many considerations she is balancing in trying to figure out what she needs for another month-long teaching tour with two dozen stage appearances, he might realize that even one as obsessively organized as himself might be challenged by the task. So his statement not only isn't a truth that is informed by compassion, it isn't even the truth at the surface level. The microscopic truth, on the other hand, reports only your experience, not your judgments or interpretations. So David might have said, "I get uncomfortable when I see your clothes and accessories and papers covering the bed and the kitchen table and every chair in the house." Or, looking deeper, he might say, "When I see you struggling to get packed, the part of me that likes to keep everything neat and organized gets nervous." Telling her that she is totally disorganized does not provide information Donna can use other than to feel bad about herself. On the other hand, the microscopic truth that David's organized part is threatened amid the disorganization opens the way for Donna to say, "Well, don't just sit there wallowing in your digital sense of superiority, you bastard! Help me pack!"

The microscopic truth, the description of your inner experience, might be a straightforward report of something that occurred. For example, as a husband, you might say to your wife, regarding your son: "I heard Billy swearing at you." It might describe your sensations: "My neck tightened when I heard Billy swearing at you, and my heart started to race." It might name your feelings: "I'm angry with Billy and feeling protective of you." It might describe an image or thought or desire: "I want to ground Billy for the rest of the week." It might portray an anticipation or internal conflict: "I'm afraid that you are going to disagree about grounding Billy." As you develop your ability to tell the microscopic truth with your partner, you may find it amazing how much can be communicated by limiting yourself to the truth of your immediate experience and how that discipline can make your communications so much more pristine and effective.

In developing this discipline, keep in mind also what microscopic communication is not. It does not include slipping in a disguised judgment, justification, explanation of cause-and-effect relationships, or a bit of self-righteousness, as in: "I want to ground Billy for the rest of the week because you haven't managed to teach him an ounce of respect." It is not even about the outside world. It is, rather, about "the deepest and most subtle truth you can see and feel inside yourself."[21] You are telling the truth for one purpose and one purpose only: *to communicate your internal experience.* Telling the truth for its own sake rather than to justify or manipulate is what conscious partners do. At the energetic level, the Hendrickses explain, "hiding the truth blocks energy at a very fundamental, cellular level." Telling the microscopic truth "liberates energy that has been trapped [leading to] the clear, high feeling that is the payoff" for telling the truth at the deepest levels of which you are capable.[22]

One of the great things about telling the microscopic truth is that conveying your inner experience instead of indulging in judgment produces empathy rather

---

→ THE ENERGY DIMENSION ←

Telling the Microscopic Truth

When tension emerges, energies become blocked within each partner and in the flow between the partners. Triple Warmer (p. 162) is activated. When you begin to tell the microscopic truth, the blocks are still there and Triple Warmer may even become more active. But as the process brings you into deeper touch with your own truth and your partner receives you, those blocks begin to melt away, the energy becomes transparent, and Triple Warmer backs off. Safety is in the air, and a deep connection becomes possible, which allows the original source of difficulty to be addressed effectively.

---

than defensiveness in your partner. However, there are some topics where extra sensitivity is required.

"DO I LOOK FAT?"

These four words can infuse terror into the heart of the strongest of men, and replies like "Do I look stupid?" do not tend to set the conversation onto a positive course. If the microscopic truth for these men be told, however, it might begin with something as transparent as, "I feel nervous hearing that question." So far, you've told your inner truth and she's interested but wary and perhaps expecting the worst. While you are certainly not off the hook, you are paving the way for an interchange that brings you closer to one another rather than to where it might have been headed. The next step involves where you direct your consciousness. Your first statement came, honestly and openly, out of your negative anticipation and sense that there is no right answer here. If you continue down that path, however, your knee-jerk negative anticipations are likely to become self-fulfilling.

The act of consciousness that is required at this moment is to call up your empathy and your love and speak from that "sweet truth" (p. 302). This is not your enemy poised to create havoc in your life after you give the wrong answer. This is your life partner in a vulnerable moment. This is where David might use the brief, practical, heart-centering meditation, "notice breath; soften belly; open heart" (p. 65). The microscopic truth emerging from this awareness might be, "I care that you are concerned about how you look right now." You are not passing a judgment, you are affirming your collaborative alliance. Suppose the situation is that she is getting ready for an important meeting, has just put on an outfit she is thinking of wearing, and you feel it really isn't very flattering. Your next statement might continue to confirm your collaborative alliance ("You know I wouldn't hurt you for anything") and could at the same time respond to the original question ("but I don't think this is the outfit for you"). This is also an opportunity to stay constructively engaged in the tenderness of having just moved through a possible rupture: "I'd like you to feel you are looking your best for this meeting. How about if we go back to your closet and pick out something that makes you look great?"

Weight is a particularly delicate topic.[23] Research on couples where one partner is obese and the other is not ("mixed-weight" couples) has found that these marriages have greater conflict than "matched-weight" couples.[24] This conflict was mediated, however, when the "healthy-weight" partner provided support rather than judgment, nagging, or teasing. With your collaborative alliance as the bedrock, your partner can feel and deeply know that you are on the same team, rooting for your partner's well-being in all ways. Beyond weight, another touchy area involves permanent flaws. Learning to love your partner's physical imperfections or character foibles is part of learning to love your partner, and it may be as challenging as learning to accept your own flaws. You can accomplish both. While energy psychology tapping can push you through some of the challenges in accepting your partner's flaws as well as your own, telling the microscopic truth can build your collaborative alliance to give you a stronger foundation for addressing even the most delicate areas of your partnership.

A few caveats beyond weight and permanent flaws are also in order. As powerful and constructive as you may find it to tell the microscopic truth, it does not mean that you should volunteer every thought that occurs to you, particularly if it might be hurtful to your partner. The seven qualities of conscious partnering (pp. 307-309) offer guidelines for processing your inner experiences in a manner that is supportive of your relationship. Each individual and each couple must find their own way of addressing issues that are particularly tender.

Cultivate Your Curiosity About One Another

When David was in high school, he began to drive and to date at about the same time. One of his nightmares was taking the hourlong drive into Los Angeles to see a play and discovering that the radio wouldn't work after he had run out of conversation. He has since learned that it is not that hard to cross the silence barrier by cultivating his curiosity about what is going on in Donna. "What were your favorite parts of the conference?" "What did you feel when Joan told you she was resigning?" "It's your dad's birthday—what are you remembering about him?" "Are you missing Tiernan?" These openers can lead to discussions that reach deeper and deeper levels. If your partner is appreciating the invitations, keep asking questions: "I'm surprised you feel that way. Tell me more about it." "I'm wondering how that feels."

It is easy to begin to take for granted that you know your partner well enough. Successful couples, however, take an active, ongoing interest in learning more about one another's history, preferences, friends, stresses, aspirations, activities, injuries, triumphs, and dreams. This may seem like an obvious feature of conscious partnering, but having someone express genuine curiosity about you is a gift from the soul. In an ongoing partnership, it keeps the relationship fresh when you are continually adding greater detail to the knowledge you have about one another. With each new discovery, your bond deepens. Conscious partnership is a moment-to-moment adventure, but it is far more than that. You each become a wellspring of information about the other, deepening your connection. Be curious about your partner and pursue that curiosity.

And, Finally, "Make Not a Bond of Love"

"Let there be spaces in your togetherness and let the winds of the heavens dance between you," advises Kahlil Gibran's *The Prophet*: "make not a bond of love."[25] We, Donna and David, are both strongly conditioned for independence. Since independence is the easier part for each of us in the dependence/independence/interdependence dance of relationships, we have placed less emphasis on it than perhaps we should have. Retaining your autonomy and freedom no matter how close you grow to another is critical if both partners and the relationship are to stay vital over the years.

Energetically, this means that in addition to the words and hugs and intimate contact that allow the energies to build over time and become a palpable, lasting force between you, there is also space for your own sense of connection with others, with the universe, and with the path of your soul. Gibran's passage on marriage ends, "the oak tree and the cypress grow not in each other's shadow."

Psychologically, retaining your freedom and individuality within the most intimate relationship of which you are capable means many things, from pursuing the callings of your heart to taking time for personal reflection and renewal. It can begin with fairly mundane considerations. In cross-cultural interviews with couples from more than twenty different countries, Esther Perel asked people what was occurring when they felt the most drawn to their partner. The answers were uniform in that it was not when they were eyeball-to-eyeball close to one another but when there was some degree of distance. For instance, people felt strong desire when the partner was away or when they were observing their partner with other people or in a setting where the partner was radiant and confident, such as when giving a performance. People were also more drawn to their partner when there was novelty, such as when a dormant part of the partner would emerge or when both would go to an edge, which was often reflected in laughter.[26] Again, integrating the parts of yourself you have developed independently back into your relationship makes your relationship richer.

At its core, healthy autonomy within an intimate relationship emerges from developing a well-grounded sense of self that gradually replaces one that is based on reflections from others. The *reflected* sense of self is defined by others beginning in infancy, and it continues to be defined by your partner. David Schnarch explains that a *solid* sense of self "develops from confronting yourself, challenging yourself to do what's right, and earning your own self-respect. It develops from inside you, rather than from internalizing what's around you."[27] Living from a wholesome identity requires self-reflection and a level of maturity that is hard-won. It is not just granted with age, and without a healthy sense of self in both partners, marriages tend to become stagnant and rigid. For a marriage to stay passionate—sexually and otherwise—an essential ingredient is that each partner takes a journey from a reflected sense of self into one that retains its own psychological "shape" no matter how physically and emotionally close to one another the two of you become.

On to Chapter 10

Conscious partnering involves using your mental and emotional capacities to keep your relationship fresh and vital, day by day. Spiritual partnering brings your awareness into the eternal realms of soul and spirit. Chapter 10 explores what that might be about.

10

The Beckoning
of the Possible

Your Evolving Relationship
Is a Spiritual Journey

*We have entered a new kind of spiritual partnership
where we are being asked by the universe to create a
whole new form of relationship and possibility.*

—JEAN HOUSTON

AS WE BEGIN THIS CHAPTER, MORE THAN THREE-AND-A-HALF DECADES INTO OUR partnership, we are sitting in our home, which was built in 1896, looking out a window at the rafters. Donna mentions that whenever she sits in this spot, she is for a moment drawn into a reverie about the people who built those rafters, sensing where their souls must have traveled by this time, and then thinking of the destinies of all the other people who might have sat in this spot and rested their eyes on these same rafters. This brings her into the realm where imagination meets spirit, and her soul is uplifted. David looks at the rafters and wonders how long it will be before they need to be painted again. All couples have areas in which one partner's proclivities and aptitudes are different from the other's. It is good that David is in charge of maintenance and Donna is in charge of woo-woo.

Despite these clearly defined roles, long-term relationships create an alchemy that changes each partner. Donna can now WD-40 a squeaky hinge with the best of them, and David can gaze at a quartz crystal and get lost in the ways it reflects the patterns of the universe. As you become deeply involved with another person, the energy field that was established when you first connected emotionally takes on greater texture, nuance, and complexity. This energy matrix not only expands each of you, it can also be a bridge into the invisible world of spirit that surrounds your relationship. Topics that are even further from the reports of your senses than the energies that have so far been the domain of this book are difficult to convey with words, yet the elusive realms of soul and spirit are always involved when creating the deepest, most loving, long-term partnership possible.

While we were reflecting on how to open the chapter, David had a dream. It seemed quite mundane. We were both in the dream and had a list of tasks we needed to complete. We had ample time to complete them. But we kept getting caught up in other activities until we suddenly realized that we had only half an hour to finish what would require far more than that. The meaning of the dream seemed obvious. We do have a deadline to finish this closing chapter and send in the completed manuscript—that deadline is approaching quickly. Other projects have indeed been getting in the way, and David woke with his motivation redoubled to keep our focus on completing the chapter. But in the brief journey from bedroom to computer, he realized that the dream had a deeper message than just being about pedestrian dead-lines and distractions.

David had just turned sixty-seven, and he was continually being pulled away from the richness of his inner life by the demands of his outer life. This was not new. For years, if not decades, he had been promising himself and Donna that he would soon shift his priorities toward a much more soulful existence. Now that he was about to embark on writing a chapter telling others how to do this, the dream was urging him to reckon with his own lapses as the clock ticked on. He was not follow-ing the urging of his deepest wisdom.

The dream, in its own metaphoric way, had also perfectly laid out the theme and challenges of this chapter. So many of us live our lives always intending to come into greater spiritual fullness within ourselves and our relationship—but always a bit later—when we are better prepared, or when we have the time, or when conditions are right. If you don't start now, however . . . well, tomorrow is always a day *away*. After reflecting on these deeper meanings of the dream, David realized that it was also letting him know that a way to enter the topic of the eternal realms of soul and spirit is to speak of dreams. While some of you reading this will be highly skeptical about concepts such as an immortal spirit, dreams are a familiar (if mysterious) ex-perience for most people.

Somehow, in dreams, "the *average sleeping brain* becomes massively creative [so] the dreamer with no prior experience or education becomes a script writer, actor, director, costume and set designer, prop maker, lighting expert, and many other things to produce a complex dream."[1] Even "neuroscientists who insist the mind is identical with the brain will generally acknowledge that the waking brain has many limits on its creative capacity," and dreams far exceed those limits.[2] People who systematically work with their dreams know that often enough dreams will provide a solution or a more useful perspective for life's dilemmas than the mind had been able to reach. Dreams let you peek around a corner that shows there is much more to your psyche than what you identify with during your typical waking hours. There is also much more to your relationship than it might seem. That is the topic of this chapter.

A Shared Spiritual Journey

About the time we were beginning to envision the chapter, we were off to the Omega Institute in upstate New York to teach workshops on energy medicine and energy psychology. We had been very pleased with the way that our interview with Ann and Paul set the tone for chapter 9 and were wondering about taking a similar approach in opening this chapter. As synchronicity would have it, also teaching at Omega at the same time were Alberto Villoldo and Marcela Lobos, an inspiring couple we'd long known about as two of the most grounded and effective voices bringing ancient shamanic wisdom to the contemporary Western world. We had only gotten to know them personally the previous year when we had them as featured speakers at our first annual convention on Donna's approach to energy medicine. They made a profound impression on our community, and we were delighted to see them again. As we spoke with them, it dawned on us that they were exactly the couple we were looking for. While we will be suggesting that all couples, whether or not they realize it, are on a shared spiritual journey, Alberto and Marcela are extraordinarily conscious about it. They draw on ancient illumination techniques such as shamanic ceremonies and vision quests in regularly creating "sacred space" for themselves and their relationship. They graciously agreed to allow us to interview them about their personal relationship as a spiritual journey.

From the start of the interview, it became clear that conventional concepts are too limiting to permit an accurate understanding of the way Alberto and Marcela experience their partnership. For instance, they described their wedding as having not only the familiar features of family and such, but as establishing a contract for being together not just during this lifetime but a "marrying of our souls." They were making a commitment to a journey that is beyond the physical body, "which takes us into conversations of where we want to live when we leave this body." Not just "till death do us part" for Alberto and Marcela! "While the physical body changes and dies, we are connecting to one another's essence, so we do practices that will help us find one another on the other side." One of the practices we found to be the most remarkable is that they have cultivated the art of "lucid dreaming" and are sometimes able to find the other and enter his or her dreams. During lucid dreams, people are aware they are dreaming and are able to exert a degree of control over the experience, exploring or directing the way the dream unfolds. This is well documented and is an ability that many people have naturally or have developed. Entering one another's dreams takes lucid dreaming into yet another dimension. In the morning, when they describe their adventures together in the night, they find that their stories match!

We were curious about their contract, "the marrying of our souls." Does this mean that they are now and forever after soulmates, traveling to the other side together, and reincarnating back into this world together, having made a perpetual contract into eternity? This was the first place it became clear that conventional concepts are not adequate for understanding Alberto and Marcela's spiritual partnership. The mind-bending answer was that "in the invisible realm, which is spiritually even more real than the visible realm, there *is no time*. So it is a contract written in *timelessness*. It's not till tomorrow, till you die, till I get bored. It's not forever. It simply means that it's *established in timelessness*. And we share spiritual practices so that we spend a lot of our lives together in that timelessness, in the invisible realm, in the dream realm. Because we do this consciously, we are able to see that this physical world is actually the dream we are dreaming together. It is very real in clock time. But then we close our eyes and enter infinity, clockless time. That's where the essence we see in one another resides, and we find each other there." Having trouble with these concepts? Both shamanism and quantum physics—take your pick—come to the same counterintuitive conclusion that time is an illusion.

As the conversation went on, two of their core commitments were discussed: (1) dedication to one another's spiritual development and (2) dedication to being of service. "We live in both the world of clock time and the world of clockless time. So we see each other in the morning and our mood might be, 'Namaste, I salute your divine essence. *And* I'm pissed at you!' Our lives have this dual manifestation. What is not negotiable is that our relationship never gets put on the table. It never becomes a bargaining chip. That's because it is not only about fulfilling one another's emotional needs; it's also about furthering one another's spiritual growth." As they spoke of the way they hold their relationship as a commitment "to be in service to life, to the world," they made an interesting observation. They said that it is as if there is "something that understands that Alberto and Marcela together are so much more than Alberto and Marcela alone, and it is as if the universe colludes to support our service to the world. The opportunities that come our way are remarkably harmonious. Synchronicities happen in amazing ways when you're in tune at a deep level and committed to service."

The largest part of our discussion focused on Alberto and Marcela's shared spiritual practices. One that is readily available to any couple is that they routinely take the time to share and reflect on their dreams. This has them regularly returning to sacred space in one another's presence. Because of the depth of their backgrounds in shamanism and other spiritual traditions, it would be overly simplistic and misleading to try to convey here in just a couple of pages the quality of their shared practices. For instance, saying that they meditate and pray together is easy enough to grasp, but their prayers are more than that. They are spontaneous ceremonies of gratitude and blessing informed by traditional practices using elements like fire and earth and honoring the earth's four directions. These practices keep their consciousness at the edge of the larger spiritual story that for them is the real story of their relationship.

Are All Long-Term Relationships Spiritual Partnerships?

Alberto and Marcela are attuned to a truth that eludes many people who were bred in Western technological cultures. Daily life is part of a larger story than our senses can detect. At the interpersonal level, when you build a life with another person, your energies merge to form a new field that is unique to your relationship. This field carries the deeper patterns inherent in each of your personal stories and blends them into a shared adventure that is influenced by forces that usually transcend your conscious awareness. Glimpses into this larger interpersonal story and beyond shed a light on the earthly story of your day-to-day experiences. Touching into this perspective has several times kept us on track when our entire relationship might have derailed.

When Donna first saw David, before he had even looked her way, she distinctly heard words that told of a deep and profound love, including—and she remembers this verbatim—"This man will spend the rest of his life with you." That it took David some seven years of tumultuous on-again, off-again romance and tension to fully grasp that there "may have been something to that" reflects a great deal about the interplay of the earthly realm and the forces beyond it (not to mention what it reveals about the dynamics between us). The realm of the senses is the reality that stares us in the face every day. Recognizing the invisible forces influencing that reality requires a different kind of perception and consciousness, and these can be cultivated, as you will see later in the chapter. When you cultivate them in collaboration with your partner, your relationship can enter spaces that your rational minds could not have conceived.

Body and Soul

The familiar world of your physical body is connected to the ethereal and mysterious realm of your soul through layers of invisible energy. Some of these energies have been scientifically mapped (for instance, neural pathways that are electrochemically activated during a moment of inspiration have been identified) while others remain as unfathomable as the forces that designed Creation itself. A remarkable historical fact is that a coherent explanation of the relationship between *body* and *soul*, or even *body* and *mind*, has eluded science, philosophy, and religion. By what mechanism can an ethereal soul or mind move a physical body (the "mind-body" problem[3])? How does a physical brain produce subjective experience (the "*hard* problem of consciousness"[4])? Answers to these questions may rest with increasing understanding of multi-layered energies connecting body and soul, but deeper mysteries about soul and spirit will remain.

Soul and Spirit

What can we know of the invisible orders of soul and spirit? Our ancient ancestors needed a word to describe the animating force or vital principle they observed in all of life. The English word *spirit* traces to the Latin *spiritus*, which referred to the movement of air—the mysteries of the wind over the earth and the breath through the body. The ethereal realm was not conveyed through concrete metaphors like the wind or breath, but in a way that invites the mind to ponder the *sources* of the earth's wind and the body's breath. *Spirit* has now come to mean the animating force in all living creatures and, when capitalized, refers to the all-pervasive, intelligent energy of Creation. Whether you think in terms of God, the natural forces that put the bang into the Big Bang, an invisible unimaginable power, or the ordering principle behind the design of all we can see, something is going on beyond that which meets the eye. We will refer to *that something*, the force that is responsible for the consistent laws and order of the universe, as Spirit.

Soul, meanwhile, is the manifestation of Spirit at the *personal* level. In this rendition, widely shared by the world's mystical traditions, your conscious identity is but a sliver of all who you are. Your soul is not only the knowing, observing, experiencing, living essence that sees through your eyes and registers your thoughts. With its direct connection to Spirit, the underlying creative force in the universe, it is much more than what your mind can comprehend. Spiritual sages would have an initiate study the vastness of the night sky as a metaphor for the vastness within.[5] It is an illuminating exercise. While your personality does reflect your soul, it was also formed by your genetics, upbringing, and circumstances. It is the limited outer shell of your essence, and it may actually have little resemblance to your soul, which is at the core of your being. As we mature and gain wisdom, however, the ways of the soul often become more prominent and discernible in our daily lives. Nonetheless, Spirit and soul are the unfathomable, vital mysteries of our existence. Any attempt, such as this, to capture them in words is merely to point rather than describe.

Soulmates?

Reflecting on Spirit and soul raises two questions that have puzzled humanity throughout history: afterlife and fate. Are there soulmates who have traveled together in previous lifetimes and are somehow fated to continue their shared journey in this lifetime? Did Donna's hearing "This man will spend the rest of his life with you" establish us as *soulmates*? Was it the fulfillment of the promise that "some enchanted evening, you may see a stranger . . . across a crowded room"? Popular literature about soulmates suggests that "your soulmate makes you feel entirely whole, healed and intact, like no piece is missing from the puzzle," punctuated with

→ THE ENERGY DIMENSION ←

Spirit (Big S)

We have been using the term *Spirit* to describe the *primal energy* of the universe—the incomprehensible, eternal Source of all that is. While it cannot be understood, it can be and often has been experienced in direct mystical apprehension as a transcendent force that is orchestrating the universe and all within it.

Soul

We have called "soul" a manifestation of this primal energy. Soul *registers* experience and *evolves with* experience. This evolution is marked by expanding consciousness. Soul sits on a continuum of energies between the incomprehensible realm of Spirit and the more tangible energy that you know as your *personal* spirit.

spirit (little s)

In the way that "big S" Spirit spawns your soul, your soul spawns your spirit, and your spirit animates your body (economists might call this the "trickle-down effect" of universal energy). I (Donna) experience *soul* as a deep velvety energy that is highly stable—it evolves very slowly. I know *spirit* as the dynamic energy coming from deep within a person that interacts with the world. It is profoundly intelligent and courageous, doing your soul's bidding as you navigate your way through this world of matter, the densest known energy. Your spirit is in continual interaction with your body's physical energies—those on the electromagnetic spectrum as well as the more subtle dimensions of your aura, meridians, chakras, and radiant circuits—and it needs their support to thrive. A way to understand the distinction between the spirit and the body's other energies is that spirit leaves the body upon death while the aura, chakras, meridians, and electromagnetic energies slowly fade. The spirit of a young child is relatively pure, but the challenges of life transfigures it. One way to measure your success is in the degree to which you have maintained or recovered your natural strength of spirit.

flashbacks to past lives together, a profound wordless understanding of one another, easy acceptance of one another's flaws, and a reliable sense of security in one another's presence.[6] That's not, we must confess, quite how it happened for us (or anyone else we know, for that matter). We in fact marvel at our early years together and how it seemed we had to fight for every last shred of compatibility.

Nonetheless, there does seem to be a fated quality to our partnership. Once, after we had completely ended our relationship, we were living hundreds of miles apart from one another, and Donna had just gotten to the other side of a painful grieving process about our relationship. She was finally feeling free in her heart to welcome whatever was to be next in her life. She spent some time on a mountain in Oregon savoring the feeling. As she was driving down the mountain, feeling joyful and triumphant, she heard the same voice that she heard on the night we met, as clear as if it were coming out of the radio in her car, say, "Despite appearances, you will marry the man." Having just gone through the agonies of getting "the man" out of her system, she was furious and started to argue. She was living in Ashland, Oregon, and David was still in San Diego, where we had met. There was no likely way we were going to be running into one another. It was over, and she mentally but emphatically stated this fact! "You will be spending the summer in San Diego," said the voice. "That's ridiculous!" Donna's mind replied. "Besides, how would I support myself and the girls?" Undaunted, the voice replied, "Jobs will be coming!" That week Donna received in the mail offers to teach seven separate classes in San Diego during the following summer. Meanwhile, one of her closest friends in San Diego called her and said, "I'd love to spend the summer in Ashland. Would you like to come back to San Diego for a while? We could swap houses."

So Donna called David to inform him that she was going to be spending the summer in San Diego. She courteously told him that she wanted him to learn about this directly from her rather than through the grapevine, and she wanted to assure him that she was not coming back to reconnect with him in any way. Weeks went by after Donna returned to San Diego without us seeing one another. David had already become involved in another relationship. Then on June 21, 1981, in San Diego, four years to the day of our having met, David pulled into a gas station. As he stepped out of his car, who was there pumping gas into her car but Donna Eden! When our eyes met, there was an electricity that we both still remember. David almost screamed at her, "No! We can't do this. I'm practically married." His protests were, however, no match for the energies that were magnetically drawing us toward one another. After half an hour of talking, our relationship was firmly, irrevocably reestablished. When David got home, the woman who had just started to live with him was packing her stuff. She prophetically said, "I don't know what is going on, but I think you need some space." Incidentally, when David had pulled into the gas station, he was returning from a visit with his parents. As he was leaving, his father said, "I have a book for you. It's one that shaped a lot of my thinking about health back in the forties, and I just found an extra copy that I must have picked up somewhere along the way." The name of the book was *Back to Eden*.

Before all of that, while trying to reconcile the deep connection we felt with how damn hard it was to be together, David brought our birth information to an astrologer. The astrologer told him, in essence, to find somebody else; there was no way this relationship could flourish. Feeling quite silly about resorting to something with as unscientific a reputation as astrology,[7] he at least wanted to see if there was agreement among different astrologers. He took the same birth information to two other astrologers, who came to virtually the same conclusions. Donna was already living in Ashland at the time, and David decided to make one last visit to be sure that it was really unworkable. Meanwhile, Donna had befriended a woman, Kate Maloney, who had a local reputation as being a remarkably gifted astrologer with profound spiritual depth, and Donna arranged for us to have a reading with her. On the appointed day, however, Kate called Donna and told her that she had been sick and had not been able to do the joint chart. David was on his way back to San Diego the next day, so we never had that reading. While our time together in Ashland was actually quite profound, David decided that our history had been filled with so much strife, combined with the negative portents of the three astrologers, that it just wasn't the right path for him to pick up and move to Ashland. He ended our relationship with a phone call that was agonizing for both of us.

A few days later, Kate called Donna and told her she had completed the chart. Donna told her it was too late. She didn't want to see all that she sensed was right about the relationship now that it was over. The next morning, Kate called again and said she had just had a dream that she believed was telling her that Donna should come in for the reading. Donna still wasn't interested. A couple of days later, Kate called yet again and said that her "guides" were on her case to get the information to Donna. Donna still wasn't interested. About that time, we had a phone conversation to tie up some loose ends and Donna mentioned the astrologer's persistent attempts to share her interpretation of our joint chart. David, believing that the reading would corroborate the strikingly similar conclusions of the other three astrologers and thus make it easier for Donna to let go of our relationship, encouraged her to make the appointment.

When Donna went in, Kate described a profound harmony that was more important than the surface incompatibilities that were the themes reported by the other three astrologers. While Kate also saw what the others were focusing on, she felt there was a deeper story. She said, "You will not be having children together (we were both still in our thirties at the time), but your family will be the 'family of man.'" While we had no sense back then that we would ever work together, the shared journey that has emerged for us has involved offering healing services not just for the individuals whom we might have seen had we continued our work independently. Nearly a thousand energy healing practitioners who have completed our two-year certification program are giving sessions to many thousands of people at any point in time and teaching hundreds of classes all over the world. We had no ambition back then to expand beyond our own individual practices, yet providing healing for "the family of man" has since become the defining purpose of our lives.

Does this mean that we were destined to be together to carry out this work? It has seemed a number of times that the universe went to quite a bit of trouble to keep us together or to reunite us, such as getting Donna to San Diego in the summer of 1981 to head David off from most likely marrying another. We've always considered the appearance of the *Back to Eden* book a particularly nice touch on the universe's part. But most of the time, our lives are like everyone else's. There are no flashing lights in the sky spelling out our joint destiny. We still get irritated with one another and miss one another's signals in ways that can be inconvenient if not hurtful. So are we soulmates with a clear destiny together or just another couple inching our way forward day by day?

Our sense is that some of each is involved. After long careers in helping people live in greater alignment with their highest possibilities—what Abraham Lincoln referred to as "the better angels of our nature"—we believe that human destiny is determined by three essential factors: choice, fate, and chance. The choices you make every day are the most decisive ways you shape your future. The role of fate in your destiny is most obvious in your genetic inheritance. Your height, natural aptitudes, and vulnerability to certain illnesses—while they may each be mediated by your choices and your circumstances—are, to a considerable degree, determined by fate. Fate also selects your family and the conditions that shape your identity and personality. Beyond simple genetic inheritance and family and culture of origin, the concept of fate also implies that certain other circumstances in your life are also predestined. How might that work? Just as the structure of a maturing body is inherent in the energies that surround the embryo, as persuasively demonstrated by Harold Burr (p. 4), each of us carries an energy that may influence key events in predetermined ways. Even occurrences that appear to happen by chance may be orchestrated by the invisible hand of fate. Some things, however, appear to be the products of pure chance, such as when people are injured in an earthquake or other mass disaster. On the positive and creative side, the universe uses chance, down to random genetic mutations, as the engine of evolution and expansion.

We believe all three—choice, fate, and chance—play a hand in all people's lives. Whatever combination of choice, fate, and chance brought you together, your relationship is a journey of your souls, a meeting of the deepest sources of your being. As the saying goes, "We are not human beings having a spiritual experience but rather spiritual beings having a human experience."[8] In this sense, the term *soulmates* is useful as a constant reminder that more is going on between you than what is obvious and at the surface. The term is not useful, however, if you take *soulmate* to mean that in order for your relationship to be spiritually valid it somehow has to embody the qualities of ease and sense of destiny mentioned earlier. That concept does not provide a realistic set of standards against which your relationship can be measured. When you come together, your souls are mutually creating a new story on earth that is influenced by the older stories that propel each of you forward. The choice is not whether your relationship is a journey of your souls but how much you let that dimension of your partnership into your consciousness and mindfully foster it.

The Ways of the Soul

Why is it important for your relationship that you know about the invisible realms of Spirit and soul? Thomas Moore, author of the *New York Times* best-selling books *Care of the Soul* and *Soul Mates*, does not oversimplify, or glorify, his topic. Marriage, which he refers to as the "weaving together of many different strands of soul," is "filled with paradoxical feelings, far-flung fantasies, profound despair, blissful epiphanies, and bitter struggles, all signs of the active presence of soul."[9] Nor does he limit his sights to the psychological and romantic aspects of love:

> Marriage has less to do with conscious intention and will than with deeper levels of soul. In order to gain insight into marriage and its problems, we have to dig deeper than the familiar therapeutic investigation into parental influences,

childhood trauma, and the illusions of romantic love. The soul always reaches deeper than we expect, especially in marriage, which lies far beneath matters of communication and even interpersonal relationship, touching areas of absolute importance to a meaningful and soulful life.[10]

The soul loves to be in relationship with other souls via intimate partnerships, family, friendships, and community. Relationships call us into the realm of the sacred as we encounter "infinite and mysterious depths" in ourselves and one another.[11]

The overriding theme running through Moore's writing is that the ways of the soul are distinctly different from and often at odds with the ways of the mind. As captured in Blaise Pascal's penetrating observation, "The heart has reasons of which reason does not know." The soul is not captivated by ideals and aspirations. It is not interested in making life predictable and orderly. It is not on a quest to find the structures that will most efficiently advance your career or keep your marriage neat and tidy. It is not dedicated to perfection. Instead, the soul is wild and unpredictable, transcending rational understanding. It is a "mystery" rather than "a puzzle that can be solved."[12] The instrument of the soul is neither mind nor body but imagination, and love is its deepest expression.

⇢ THE ENERGY DIMENSION ⇠

The Energies of Love

Love has gotten good press: "God is love." "Love is the highest expression of the human spirit." "Love is the pinnacle of evolution." But just what, beyond the poetry, is the *energy* of love? Asked to describe love energetically, Donna said: "There are many kinds of love, and each has its own energy. Let me try to find some common denominators. What is shared, for instance, by romantic love and the love of a grandparent for a grandchild? A radiant energy swells out from the Heart Chakra and, with a rolling motion, actively seeks the aura of the lover or grandchild. The energy coming out the eyes looks to me like what beautiful music would look like if you could see the sounds. When I look deeper at mature love, it is as real a force as gravity. It pulls two souls together with stunning power or even a whole family or community."

Soul brings your awareness to the heart of a matter, seeing right through your intellect's take on the situation. Rather than being remote or ascetic, soul is oriented toward life and engagement with the world—it loves getting involved with "places, ideas, times, historical figures and periods, things, words, sounds, and settings."[13] At the same time, the soul requires "regular excursions into enchantment [just as] the body needs food and the mind needs thought."[14] Enchantment is "an ascendancy of the soul"[15] that allows us to connect intimately with the world and other people with direct appreciation of the sacred in every aspect of life. The soul "needs to live in a world of both facts and holy imagination."[16] To live a more soulful life is to discern the ways of the soul and to set about resolving their conflicts with the ways of the mind, beginning by recognizing and respecting the value in each.

Opening to the Ways of the Soul

In cultures all around the world and throughout history, enchantment is cultivated for the individual and the community through festivals, rituals, ceremonies, and celebrations. Practices that speak to the soul and its mysterious depths open us to "transcendent visions, experiences that swell the heart and stretch the limits of belief and understanding."[17] Of course no one is always in a state of rapture, "but we do have frequent, even daily opportunities to enter" levels of experience that elevate us.[18] These "daily opportunities" often have two shared properties: a sense of joy or delight and seeing the familiar with new eyes. Nature reinforces you for taking the time to let the realm of soul touch your consciousness. Even amid great suffering, observed the ancient Greek philosopher Epicurus, a modicum of pleasure lets a deeper order reveal itself and sustain us.[19] A gentle sense of joy can accompany something as simple as taking in anew the lavender bush you see through your window every day. Discovering for the first time what has always been there or in other ways encountering your partner and your world at a new level is usually pleasing and can be exhilarating. In our healing work, we may readily be transported into an elevated space. Known in clinical circles as "psychotherapeutic resonance"[20] or the "meld experience,"[21] many healers report a momentary merging of the boundary between themselves and a client that, in its intensity, exceeds empathy and rapport, including immediate nonverbal understanding of the feelings and even the physical sensations of the other. Couples can also enter this space with one another.

Entering Sacred Space

While this resonance occurs spontaneously, you can invoke the experience by dedicating protected time and directing your attention in specific ways, such as those described shortly. The more you call forth the sacred into everyday life, the more that being in sacred space becomes familiar and habitual. Because being in that zone is deeply nourishing, you will begin to look for additional opportunities, and you will find them in nature, people, behaviors, and events, as well as in an increased awareness of synchronicities, the meaningful coincidences that reveal the workings of a larger plan.

Recall the advice in chapter 8 for keeping sexual passion in your relationship: "*First* say 'yes,' *then* create the wanting!" You can also first say "yes" to entering sacred space together, and then create the pathway. Following are some structured ways that you can use your will and intention for creating pathways that move you both into the spiritual realm.

Shared Excursions of Your Souls—Easier Than You Might Think

Great music, poetry, drama, literature, sacred texts, paintings, choreography, and appreciation of nature speak to the soul. They can also be shared entries with your partner into the soul's realm. This can be as simple as watching a DVD of an uplifting or deeply poignant movie together. While there are many ways to watch a movie, even "passive" entertainment can be active and soulful. We sit next to each other, bodies touching in one manner or another, being transparent with our emotions and responsive to the other's experience. We'll also take time to share and reflect on our feelings afterward or even during, using the pause button. Art and nature offer doorways that you can enter together for nurturing the soul, and they are readily accessible. Uniting in creative expression, as we have been privileged to do in our joint writing and teaching, can add extra dimension to the shared journey of your souls, but anything that gets your energies flowing together in new ways may strengthen your soul connection. Taking our five-year-old grandson for an outing to the zoo or beach or a park is among our favorite ways of being carried into the world of imagination and soul.

Energies Mingle in the Shadows as Well as the Light

In addition to using art and nature as gateways for together touching into the domains of soul and Spirit, you are in each other's lives as catalysts for one another's growth and evolution. Your disharmonies are as vital to your relationship as your harmonies. As you push against the outer shells of one another's personalities, it may be painful, it may cause cracks, but it is sometimes through these cracks that your soul can find your partner's heart. The pain you cause one another and how you deal with that pain are ways your souls touch and intertwine. Recognize that those difficult times are as much part of your soul's alchemy and journey together as the high times. The poet John O'Donohue offers beautiful counsel for the hard times, while they're not as easy to welcome or embrace:

FOR LOVE IN A TIME OF CONFLICT[22]

When the gentleness between you hardens
And you fall out of your belonging with each other,
May the depths you have reached hold you still.
When no true word can be said, or heard,
And you mirror each other in the script of hurt,
When even the silence has become raw and torn,
May you hear again an echo of your first music.
When the weave of affection starts to unravel
And anger begins to sear the ground between you,
Before this weather of grief invites
The black seed of bitterness to find root,
May your souls come to kiss.
Now is the time for one of you to be gracious,
To allow a kindness beyond thought and hurt,
Reach out with sure hands
To take the chalice of your love,
And carry it carefully through this echoless waste
Until this winter pilgrimage leads you
Toward the gateway to spring.

→ THE ENERGY DIMENSION ←

When Your Energies Mingle in a Creative Activity

When you are creatively involved with one another, the energies of your auras overlap. In the area of overlap, a new energy with vital qualities from both your auras is temporarily created. This energy may actually grow and become a separate field of energy that surrounds you both, keeping you in sync and on a creative edge. Within this field, specific chakras may also reach toward one another, spark one another, and enhance creativity in the area or theme governed by that chakra. In addition, sometimes you can both be catapulted onto another frequency that is quite distinct from either of your separate energies. This frequency may be part of the "morphic field" of the topic you are mutually delving into, whether the courage shown in a movie, the farther reaches of human potential seen in an athletic event, or the inspiring handiwork that permeates nature. All of these mingling energies dissolve boundaries until your souls may be recognizing one another in a raw encounter that alchemically changes each.

When Your Energies Mingle in a Tense Activity

When there is a rift with the one you love, an urgent and overwhelming energy shoots out like a bullet, often blindly trying to right what suddenly feels so wrong. It may follow entrenched patterns like blame or self-blame, judgment or self-pity, aggression or withdrawal, shame or depression. Its deeper impulse, however, is for you to be seen by your partner at the soul level and to reconnect at that level. Even amid the static of unskillful responses such as blame or self-deprecation, however, the encounter with one another makes the field that surrounds you larger and more powerful. But unlike the field supporting creativity, this field can feel like bondage. An outside force comes into this field and holds you in the conflict with incredible intensity, but for a holy purpose. That purpose is to break through and reach your partner's soul. When you do break through and reconnect (that's what the Pact presented in chapter 3 is all about), your soul bond deepens with joy, relief, safety, and a sense of having come home.

A Daily Ritual

When we decided in 1999 to give up our comfortable practices in Ashland, Oregon, to embark on a life of travel and teaching, David promised Donna that he would give her an energy balancing each morning. The energy balancing has evolved into a daily ritual we both look forward to. While the energy techniques we use vary somewhat from day to day, they generally include many of the basic methods presented in chapter 3.

Here is an example from this morning. We have a massage table permanently set up in our bedroom (making things a bit crowded, but definitely worth it—when we are traveling we use the bed in the hotel room, which is workable but less comfortable for the one giving the balancing). This morning Donna was the first to receive, lying facedown with her head hanging over the edge of the table as David directed the full weight of his body into his thumbs to give her a deep Spinal Flush (p. 94). Then he did the Crossover Shoulder Pull (p. 89) on her back, but rather than stopping at her hips, he extended the pull all the way down her leg and off her foot. Then her other leg and foot. This often brings energy into the feet that can get caught there, so each foot received a quick but firm massage, ending with the energies being whisked off her feet, and finally pulled off each toe. Donna was already in a state of semibliss, which was accelerated with a thorough scratching of her back. The sounds coming out of Donna's mouth by this point were very reinforcing, but David finally backed off, indicating that it was time for her to turn over.

Now with Donna lying on her back, David started with the Four Taps (p. 84), though he massaged rather than tapped the points this time. He then stood at her head, placed his middle fingers in the indent in the middle of her neck where it meets the base of the skull (known in energy medicine as the Power Point), pushed in, and leaned back so he was pulling the point toward himself, stretching her neck and opening the connection between head and body for about half a minute. He then moved his middle fingers to the sides about an inch each (these are known as the Electric Points), pushed in, and again leaned back so he was pulling the points toward himself for about half a minute. Next, he did a Crown Pull (p. 89) and ended it with the Stress Release Hold (p. 90). Then he did another Crossover Shoulder Pull, this time over the front of her body, again off her legs and feet, and followed with a brief foot massage.

Next he gave her a Belt Flow, one of Donna's favorites. Standing at her side, he placed his hands under her back on the side of her body that was away from him and began pulling toward himself with pressure, with his hands going around her waist and then up and over her stomach, one hand at a time. As each hand completed this movement, he brought it back to under her back and repeated the pull, so that in twenty or thirty seconds he had done the motion a dozen times, ending again by pulling the energies down her legs and off her feet. Then he moved to the other side. Since the Spleen Meridian is a vulnerability for Donna, he traced her Spleen Meridian (with one hand on the inside of each foot at the big toe, he moved slowly up the inside of each leg with the flats of his hands, flaring out at the hips, going up the sides of her rib cage, and then down to the bottom of her rib cage).

This routine has become fairly standard for Donna, though the order may vary and she may request, or David may be inspired to use, other techniques. At some point, however, David will ask, "What else does this body need?" This morning Donna asked David to "bounce" her. She was feeling some tension in her back, and a technique that got the energies moving through her whole back area involved David putting his hands under Donna's back, one hand around each side, placing his middle fingers under paired points right next to the spine, and pushing up and down so that Donna was literally being bounced on the table. He did this on three or four different points, looking to her for feedback about the points that felt best. Finally, less than ten minutes into this little energy treatment, we ended it, as we typically do, by David doing a Zip-Up (p. 87) on Donna followed by a Hook-Up (p. 88). During the Hook-Up, we bring a more verbal element into our little daily ritual. David directed Donna to address three topics we touch into each morning:

"Say some appreciations" [statements of gratitude about what is right and good about your life, your partner, or your lives together].

"Bless your day" [find words to wrap your highest intentions around the coming day and specific elements about it that might be challenging or might have rich potential].

"Tune into your guidance" [listen for your internal wisdom about the day that is about to unfold and put what is there into words].

While all three points are usually addressed within a minute or two, they set the day for each of us. Not only do we come out of our ritual with our energies flowing and balanced, we are connected and aligned as we separate to go off into whatever the day is to bring. This ritual has become habitual. We rarely skip it, because when we do, we miss it. Daily activities that foster meeting one another at a higher plane, when cultivated, will be longed for. As you saw in our intimate glimpses into the lives of Ann and Paul and of Marcela and Alberto, rituals for bringing one another into shared sacred space can take many forms, but couples who devote the time and discipline to create and perform them are rewarded. We encourage you to design a daily ritual that will uplift your relationship and to carve out the time to enrich yourselves with it.

Connecting with Your Partner is a Model for Connecting with Spirit

Ann Mortifee (p. 300) is known for writing songs and theatrical productions that take her audiences deep into the world of spiritual imagination. When we asked her for some techniques that might help those reading this chapter to more readily enter sacred space, she put the question into a larger context:

> The more we identify with the Spirit world, the more the Spirit world can speak to us. It's like any relationship. If you love somebody, the more you tell them you love them, the more time you spend with them, the more you think about them, the more you communicate with them, the more they notice that you are there. I think it's the same with your relationship with Spirit. The more you state expressions of love for Spirit, for the unseen world, for the spiritual essence that gives you life, the more you communicate with it, the more it seems to notice you. So my daily life is a back-and-forth conversation with myself and what I cannot see.

Just as maintaining rich and active conversation with your partner is vital for your relationship, maintaining a conversation with the natural forces that are behind the design of all you can see makes your relationship with those forces more conscious and palpable. This spiritual attunement can be more basic and less highfalutin than you might think. It is as much an attitude as an action. Ann finds the natural world to be a powerful portal into the Spirit world, and she stays alert for opportunities to step into that portal. She might, for instance, be passing a tree and literally stop and say, with full and sincere appreciation: "I see you there. Look at how beautiful you are! Look at what Spirit has created!" Does Ann really say things like that out loud?

Yes, we have heard her. And her utterances have invited our consciousness into the realm of Spirit as well.

Your relationship can be another portal into Spirit. For instance, some of the actions required to nourish your relationship with your partner can serve as metaphors for staying connected with Spirit as well. Three practices we have explored in previous chapters for keeping your relationship vital:

1. Attuning yourself so you *notice* what pleases you about your partner and your relationship and regularly *putting this into words* (gratitudes and appreciations, p. 70)
2. Searching out the higher bands of energy that justify the most noble and empowering interpretations possible for whatever life presents (high-banding it, p. 74)
3. Staying emotionally and meaningfully connected throughout the day (p. 76).

Strengthening your relationship by using these practices with a focus on your partner gives you training for using them to strengthen your relationship with the invisible forces that embrace all of life. Adding shared prayers and invocations to these practices elevates them.

Shared Prayers and Invocations

By building upon the above three principles for cultivating conscious love with your partner—instilling gratitude for the life you have been given, attuning yourselves to the "higher bands" of possibility, and keeping yourselves meaningfully connected with the universe's majestic forces—your relationship is elevated. For this third principle, keeping yourself partnered with majestic spiritual forces, language, and imagination offer powerful bridges. In the form of prayer and invocation, they can align your energies to connect with the spiritual realm. While often melded with religious practices and tenets, no special beliefs or traditions are necessary for prayer and invocation to be meaningful and potent in bringing spirit into daily life.

In her book *Illuminata: A Return to Prayer*, Marianne Williamson speaks of prayer as a way of "focusing our eyes," dramatically changing our orientation, releasing us "from the snares of lower energies," and aligning "our internal energies with truth."[23] Her book presents prayers for every aspect of life, from loneliness to love to healing to encountering loss and death. Saying a simple prayer before a meal or delivering an inspiring invocation as part of a wedding ceremony envelops the event that is about to occur in a higher energy. It alerts your sensibilities to dimensions that your senses do not perceive. Invocations we have used in recent months and later transcribed for the purposes of this chapter include the following. As you read them slowly and deliberately, notice how the energies in your body shift.

FOR A NEW DAY:

New morning, I greet you with my eyes open and my heart eager.

I ask this day for opportunities to love, to flourish, and to heal that which thirsts for healing.

I ask for support so that which is purest within me can shine through.

May this day be kind to me and to all other creatures on this magnificent planet.

FOR YOUR LIFE PARTNER:

You are the one I choose to walk with and share my life.

May my love for you glow in *my heart* so I am always resonating with your Spirit.

May my love for you glow in *your heart*, bringing you pleasure and strength.

May my love serve in healing your wounds and uncertainties.

As we behold one another's sacredness, may we walk our love with a joy that radiates to all others on this planet.

FOR A BIRTH:

This child who comes into the world this day

Is surrounded by love, by awe, by hope.

May you grow in the bosom of peace and with the radiance of health

And blossom into a being of love, strength, and good deeds in the world.

While we prefer to make up our own invocations in the moment,[24] numerous books such as *Illuminata* are also available. John O'Donohue's *To Bless the Space between Us* (the poem "For Love in a Time of Conflict" is taken from that volume) has beautiful invocations for virtually every aspect of a shared life, and Rumi and Gibran are time-honored favorites for many. For us, our daily ritual, described above, ends with appreciations and consciously wraps our blessings around one another's coming day. Beyond that, we are not particularly consistent in our use of invocations, but when we do create them, they are meaningful. Meals are a natural occasion for invocations that avow our gratitudes and our intentions for how we might use the nourishment we are about to receive. Times when we are about to embark on a creative activity are another. Dozens of mini-prayers have infused the writing of this book, sometimes asking for wisdom, clarity, focus, and humor; other times asking that you, dear reader, receive guidance that gives your relationship greater ease, depth, healing, and joy. Often before a presentation we will ask that we touch people deeply and in ways that enhance their spirits, well-being, and mastery of their energies. More recently, we have begun to include our teaching assistants so the invocation takes on the quality of a group ritual. Combining an invocation with tapping on the energy psychology points is sometimes fitting and can give greater power to the words.

Finally, we close this section on the use of words to evoke each other's spirit by intimately sharing, from Donna's vows during our wedding in 1984:

> I join with you, David, to do our highest in our own unique way to help lift the vibration of the planet, to help restore the broken connections, and be a part of the healing of the earth. I surrender with you into this magnificent love space, and I know that the incredible strength of our bond, David, is equal only to its incredible fragility. I therefore give my word to do my best to speak my truth lovingly. I will love you well, and I align with you in the intention of joy and love for evermore. I pledge to sing, feast, dance, grow, and love with you, in sickness or in health, for better or for worse . . . By all that is holy, David, by this holy earth on which we are standing, in the name of ecstasy of the spirit and the joy of the earth, I take thee to my hand, my heart, my soul, and my home.

Mindfulness Practices

As discussed in the previous chapter, regularly focusing your attention on the present moment has been shown to have numerous potent psychological and health benefits. It also shifts your perspective in ways that are distinctly spiritual. Jon Kabat-Zinn, who has been bringing mindfulness practices to the attention of Western science and medicine since the 1970s, reflects: "Perhaps ultimately, spiritual simply means experiencing wholeness and interconnectedness directly, a seeing that individuality and the totality are interwoven, that nothing is separate or extraneous. If you see in this way, then everything becomes spiritual in its deepest sense."[25] With its health, psychological, and spiritual benefits to recommend it, you might wonder why mindfulness practice has not become the "universal elixir" of our culture; but as advocates of the method admit, it has not.[26] Uncounted numbers of would-be meditators have been wrestling with this dilemma for centuries. It is simply difficult to interrupt the inertia of daily life to introduce practices that take time and effort and whose payoffs may be subtle and less than immediate. Faith in the value of meditation is, however, now supported by science to the extent that increasing numbers are finding ways to incorporate the discipline into their lives.

David has found two tricks that make a difference for him. He set up his computer so it chimes every hour. With that chime, he raises his eyes to the window at the left of his work space, rests them on a magnificent eucalyptus tree, takes two very deep breaths (with a pause between each full exhalation and the next inhalation), and becomes absorbed in the eucalyptus or its surroundings. He then returns to the drivel he was composing when the chime sounded. Simple as it seems, and is, it brings him for a brief but influential moment into a state of mindfulness that punctuates his work.

A second practice builds on the fact that David swims almost daily. We have access to a nearby pool where we live and, when feasible during our travels, we stay in hotels that have pools. Each day, a component of David's swim is attending mindfully to the physical experience of swimming (he uses a snorkel and mask so he can stay in a meditative space), followed by more structured invocations silently but mindfully stated. Mindfulness does not necessarily mean sitting still in a lotus posture. It can be that, but mindfulness practice can involve a range of activities, from walking meditations to tea ceremonies. Combining it with something you already do makes you more likely to regularly incorporate mindfulness into your life.

For Donna, mindfulness is a different issue. Her default position is to be fully immersed in the here and now. Leaving that space so she can get something done is her challenge. Spirituality, rather than being a frame of mind she seeks, is where she lives. Her most natural state is appreciation and a sense of oneness with all of life. Mindfulness practices feel redundant to her. She is instead summoned to get out of the here and now, wresting herself away from bliss and into her head so she can respond to the practical demands of daily life. Helping to found and run an organization has been a great support to her for staying out of bliss.

Guides, Muses, and Sacred Medicine

When Donna heard on first glimpsing David's profile that he was going to spend the rest of his life with her, it was not an unfamiliar voice. She has received guidance from forces that seem external to her since childhood. In addition to hearing them, she would also sometimes see figures she has come to think of as her guides. They appear very tall, somewhat human, and somewhat otherworldly. Beyond the guidance they offer, she feels deeply loved and supported by them. Usually their guidance came unbidden, but it has proven to be remarkably accurate. On occasion, when faced with a difficult dilemma, she would ask them for help and often receive it. From the time we first got together, stories of these "guides" have been of great interest to David. He had read about such things, had even consulted a psychic once, but he had never felt he had direct access to information from the other side. Being the more structured of the two of us, he began to have us set time aside for Donna to enter into the altered states from which she could more reliably hear her guides, and we have spent many hours blessed by their presence and wisdom. For decades, these sessions were David's closest encounters with what he thought of as the world of Spirit.

David longed for more direct access to these other dimensions. His father had introduced him to mystical traditions that gave him a basis for understanding the plausibility of spiritual realms, but his first direct encounter was, dare we say it, with drugs. Too conservative to experiment with uppers, downers, and psychedelics like normal kids in the 1960s, David saved his drug virginity for when he was teaching at Johns Hopkins University School of Medicine. A research team had been awarded an NIMH grant to administer LSD to mental health professionals, providing them with training in experiencing altered states of consciousness. David volunteered. He met God along with the forces of evil in such overwhelming doses that he spent the next several years trying to put the genie back into the bottle. Donna's more balanced approach had much greater appeal. However, David's proximity to Donna wasn't wearing off on him in ways that gave him greater access to the world of Spirit. A second opportunity for a surprising mind-altering experience came his way a few years after meeting Donna.

David's first book, *Personal Mythology*, was coauthored by Stanley Krippner, one of the country's most colorful psychologists. In addition to a prestigious academic career that has included dozens of impressive honors, such as the American Psychological Association's Distinguished Contribution Award for helping to advance psychology on an international scale, Stanley was friends with and sometimes the informal counselor to the band members of the Grateful Dead. He had a standing invitation to get backstage passes any time he could get himself to a concert. We were doing a presentation at a conference at the University of California in Los Angeles, and the Dead were performing in nearby Long Beach the night before.

David continues:

Stanley invited me to join him. As we were sitting backstage with one of the band members, I was given a little sliver of mushroom just before the concert was to begin. I was not very sophisticated about mushrooms, but the piece seemed so small. What could it really do? Nor had I particularly appreciated the music of the Grateful Dead. An hour later, the Grateful Dead were, in my estimation at that moment, the wisest sages in the culture, showing us where we had gotten off the path as individuals and as a society, and they were there on that very stage instructing all of us about how to get back on the path toward love, peace, and fulfillment. Oh my God! These were the shamans of the modern era!

Profoundly stimulated and perhaps a bit crazed by this experience, the next day, at UCLA, I asked Stanley if I could open the two-hour presentation. Instead of my usual staid and academic introduction to the topic, I stood up on a table in front of the crowded room and said with my voice aflame: "For these next two hours, let me be your shaman! Come with us on this journey and your life will be changed forever!" I then set out with newfound passion to help people delve into their mythic depths. Stanley did not miss a beat. He was with me all the way, setting our usual design aside and going full throttle to create a breakthrough experience for everyone in the room. It was just one of those moments. That night Stanley received a call in his hotel room from Jeremy Tarcher, at the time the most visionary publisher in the country of leading-edge science and personal development books. He and his wife had attended our presentation and felt transformed by it. He asked if we could meet with him while we were still in L.A. When we did, he said, "You guys don't know what you have! This is profound! I want to publish your book!" He did, and the book became an immediate best seller for its genre and eventually earned us the *USA Book News* Best Psychology/Mental Health Book of the Year Award, along with innumerable speaking and teaching invitations.

However, writing the book from the consciousness that got us the contract during our performance at UCLA proved problematic. Jeremy was extraordinarily disappointed with the first draft, which he found to be dry, academic, and convoluted. He wanted us to streamline it to the heart of the way we had demonstrated in our presentation that lives can be transformed by working at the mythic level. As the primary author, many of the revision assignments landed on my plate, and I struggled unsuccessfully to do what was being suggested. Having had his editorial staff wade through five failed drafts, Jeremy finally assigned the book to Connie Zweig, his best editor. She offered excellent guidance, but I still couldn't get the sixth draft to the level that satisfied her or Jeremy that the book touched the promise of our two-hour presentation at UCLA, two years earlier by this point. It finally dawned on me that the difference between my consciousness as I plugged away at the manuscript every day that my consciousness leading to the UCLA presentation could be summed up in a single word. Drugs. I had never before tried to write on pot, but it was an amazing experience. While it required tenacious discipline and a good deal of subsequent revision with my cognitive faculties unaffected, by the time Connie read the seventh and final draft, she said, "I am amazed! It is like this was written by a much more spiritually evolved person!" In the process, I also found that I could meet Donna's spirituality more fully and deeply when assisted by the smoke of the cannabis plant.

It would not be honest to write this chapter without admitting the above. I found that there was a place for the grounded use of psychoactive substances in my own spiritual opening. I came to fully understand why indigenous people across time and throughout the world have used sacred plants to access a deeper opening to spirit. The existence of guides or muses is not a particularly far-out concept among writers and artists, and the marijuana seemed to open me to them. Even more exciting to me is that over time I began to have access to these same muses, especially early in the morning, without the drug. In fact, it is much easier to write with my brain unaltered. While my experience is not like Donna's, where my muses or guides seem like separate entities from myself, the subjective experience is that when they are there, I know it because my thinking seems so much clearer and more creative than when I am left to my own devices. Whether this access would have occurred as part of my natural development had sacred plants not served as a bridge, I cannot say. I can say that entering the realm of Spirit, and entering it with Donna, is one of the most precious recurring experiences in my life.

Sharing Your Dreams

An unexamined dream, goes a Talmudic saying, is like a letter from God left unopened. While not every dream is an excursion into the realms of Spirit, some have a distinct numinous quality. Dwelling on such dreams uplevels your consciousness, and sharing them with your partner uplevels your relationship. Dream interpretation is, however, tricky business. The tendency is to interpret dreams from the vantage of your conscious mind or according to the narrow agenda of your ego and personality. These lenses can obscure the dream's deeper spiritual message. So rather than limiting your exploration to the dream's surface meanings or consulting "dream dictionaries" or other superficial guides for dream interpretation, we suggest a more open-ended approach. Carl Jung said it simply: "If we meditate on a dream sufficiently long and thoroughly, if we carry it around with us and turn it over and over, something almost always comes of it."[27]

A variety of techniques for turning a dream "over and over" are quite dynamic. Our favorite is to role-play various elements of the dream. Dreams include characters, activities, settings, objects, sensations, and emotions. Identify a few that stand out for you or that hold a charge for you or that puzzle you. Even dreams that seem totally meaningless may hold unexpected treasures when explored. Describe the dream for your partner from the vantage point of that dream element. "Okay, now I am the cougar and . . ." Then as another element. "Okay, now I am David's sadness . . ." In describing the dream, you can also elaborate on the dream element you are exploring. Let it have words to express itself during various parts of the dream. Perhaps allow a dialogue to emerge between it and another element of the dream. You can do a full role-play by taking on physical postures that reflect the dream elements in the dialogue. When you play with your dreams in this manner, their deeper meanings begin to unfold. Energy tapping can also help you understand your dreams.[28] For instance, if a dream was particularly disturbing and you replay it in your mind while tapping to neutralize the distress, hidden meanings are likely to appear.

"Sharing your dreams" has another meaning beyond exploring your nighttime dreams together. How do you support one another in your dreams of the heart? Help your partner articulate his or her highest sense of calling and purpose and seek ways you can involve yourself so these deep and precious dreams may come true. Beyond all this, "sharing your dreams" has still another meaning. In what ways do the two of you create a force in the world that carries a shared purpose? Raising children together is the natural, archetypal shared purpose for couples, but you can ride this archetype for other purposes as well. Alberto and Marcela recognized that their commitment "to be in service to life, to the world" helped them touch into the realization of how much more they are as a couple than they are as their individual selves. This seemed to beckon larger spiritual forces "as if the universe colludes to support our service to the world." Such has been our experience as well. Manifesting your dreams together is a blessing to be savored.

Sabbaths

The Fourth Commandment begins: "Remember the *Sabbath* day, to keep it holy. Six days shalt thou labor, and do all thy work, but the seventh day is the *Sabbath* of the Lord thy God" (Exodus 20). Whatever your religious orientation, the instruction to keep one day a week "holy" is worth contemplating. With the Sabbath, explains Rabbi Abraham Heschel, "we learn how to consecrate sanctuaries that emerge from the magnificent stream of a year."[29] These sanctuaries exist in time, not place. Rather than building physical monuments, Heschel notes, "the Sabbaths are our great cathedrals."[30] The regular sanctification of a period of time is a core spiritual challenge. Not a mere "interlude" in the week, the Sabbath is, rather, considered "the climax of living."[31] Heschel likens the Sabbath to "a palace in time, a dimension in which the human is at home with the divine . . . a window in eternity."[32] What more worthy challenge than to create a sanctified period each week where time as measured in the workaday world ceases and life is infused with the sacred?

The Sabbath also reminds us of the need to rest. "In six days the Lord made heaven and earth, and on the seventh day he rested, and was refreshed" (Exodus 31:17). Wayne Muller, a minister and graduate of Harvard Divinity School, emphasizes the "rest and refresh" dimension of the Sabbath in his book *Sabbath: Restoring the Sacred Rhythm of Rest*: "In our bodies, the heart perceptibly rests after each life-giving beat; the lungs rest between the exhale and the inhale. We have lost this essential rhythm. . . . Because we do not rest, we lose our way. . . . we bypass the nourishment that would give us succor. We miss the quiet that would give us wisdom. We miss the joy and love born of effortless delight."[33] The Sabbath's rest is not merely to refresh yourself for the next round of labor. "To observe the Sabbath," Heschel notes, "is to celebrate the coronation of a day in the spiritual wonderland of time."[34] With the Sabbath, emotions of joy and delight are evoked as gateways into the heavenly realm.

If your religious or spiritual tradition offers you practices that bring you into periodic, passionate communion with the sacred dimensions of life, it is serving you well. Many people who are not buoyed by such practices feel a spiritual hunger but do not know how to satisfy it. Any of the practices described in this chapter may be used during times that you set aside for nurturing your higher nature and opening your consciousness to the realm of Spirit. To forge regular spans of time that are dedicated to this purpose—to create a Sabbath for yourself, your partner, and your relationship—takes the individual practices to a higher level. The Sabbath provides a context for using those practices for greater communion with your own spiritual essence and for better perceiving the god/goddess in your partner.

Heschel reflects that the Sabbath "is not a date but an atmosphere."[35] This atmosphere is characterized by "*tranquility, serenity, peace, and repose.*"[36] Repose is the freedom from work, strain, or responsibility. Explaining why the orthodox Jewish Sabbath may seem as much a list of prohibitions from worldly deeds as a pronouncement of the splendor of the day, Heschel draws an analogy. Just as the mystery of God can never be captured in words, our rituals and other human practices can never fully replicate the spirit of the Sabbath. What better way, he asks, to open us to "glory in the presence of eternity" than with "the silence of abstaining" from the "noisy acts" of our daily affairs?[37] Our ordinary words and thoughts tend to obscure and distract us from the spiritual realm.

As the traditions for observing the Sabbath developed, the laws for abstaining from one's usual activities became prominent.[38] Not only does work cease, one does not talk "in the same manner in which one talks on weekdays. Even thinking of business or labor should be avoided."[39] Heschel admits that as the Sabbath rules of observance developed, "law and love, discipline and delight, were not always fused,"[40] and the strictest practices might seem oppressive. But as we (Donna and David) have learned (because we have so often failed), imposing a firm discipline for carving substantial portions of sacred time out of busy lives may be exactly what is required for regular self-initiated journeys into the higher realms that are always there if we but open the door.

In Closing

The Energies of Love has taken you on a journey through the biochemical, psychological, social, and spiritual dimensions of love, always with an eye on the vital role your body's energies play in each. Chapter 1 opened by showing you how core differences in organizing information and managing conflict are based on Energetic Stress Styles that are inborn and underlie many of our psychological differences. We went on to explore energy techniques that can change the course of arguments that could be devastating to the energies of your partnership. We have learned energy techniques for healing old emotional wounds, defusing triggers, addressing resentments, bridging differences, and cultivating skills for successful bonding. We have seen how sex is nature's energy medicine for couples and how, by staying attuned to your own and your partner's energies, you can keep your sexual relationship vital. We have sensed into the multilayered energies connecting body and soul that allow a deeper love to grow out of conscious partnering and fostering your relationship as a spiritual journey. For the two of us, garnering these lessons has been an amazing ride, and we thank you for allowing us the privilege of sharing them with you. May the energies of love smile on all your days.

References

Introduction

1 Sue Johnson, Hold Me Tight: Seven Conversations for a Lifetime of Love (New York: Little, Brown, 2008), 15.

2 Brian Thomas Swimme and Mary Evelyn Tucker, *Journey of the Universe* (New Haven, CT: Yale University Press, 2011).

3 Ibid., 13.

4 Barbara L. Fredrickson, *Love 2.0: Creating Happiness and Health in Moments of Connection* (New York: PLUME/Penguin, 2014), 4.

5 Ibid., 6.

6 Ronald E. Matthews, "Harold Burr's Biofields: Measuring the Electromagnetics of Life," *Subtle Energies and Energy Medicine* 18, no. 2 (2007): 55–61.

7 Rollin McCraty, "The Energetic Heart: Bioelectromagnetic Communication within and between People," in Paul J. Rosch and Marko S. Markov, eds., *Clinical Applications of Bioelectromagnetic Medicine* (New York: Dekker, 2004), 541–562.

8 Ibid.

9 Rollin McCraty, Raymond Trevor Bradley, and Dana Tomasino, "Our Heart Has a Consciousness of Its Own," n.d., http://newearthdaily.com/our-heart-has-a-consciousness-of-its-own/.

10 Claude Swanson, *Life Force: The Scientific Basis*, 2nd ed. (Tucson, AZ: Poseidia Press, 2009).

11 Laurel Thatcher Ulrich, *Well-Behaved Women Seldom Make History* (New York: Knopf, 2007).

12 Hanna Rosin, "The End of Men," *The Atlantic* 306, no. 1 (2010): 70.

13 Ibid., 64.

14 Ibid., 60.

15 Ibid., 58.

16 Ibid.

17 Ibid., 60.

18 Andrew J. Cherlin, *The Marriage-Go-Round: The State of Marriage and the Family in America Today* (New York: Vintage, 2010).

19 Ibid.

20 Ibid., 15.

21 Robert N. Bellah, *Habits of the Heart: Individualism and Commitment in American Life* (Berkeley: University of California Press, 1985), 108.

22 Eli J. Finkel, Chin M. Hui, Kathleen L. Carswell, and Grace M. Larson, "The Suffocation of Marriage: Climbing Mount Maslow without Enough Oxygen," *Psychological Inquiry* 25 (2014): 1–41.

23 Ibid.

24 Ibid.

25 Ibid.

26 W. Bradford Wilcox and Jeffrey Dew, *The Date Night Opportunity: What Does Couple Time Tell Us about the Potential Value of Date Nights?* (Charlottesville, VA: National Marriage Project, 2012).

27 Stephen Larsen and Robin Larsen, *The Fashioning of Angels: Partnership as Spiritual Practice* (West Chester, PA: Chrysalis Books, 2000).

Chapter 1

1 Ayala M. Pines, *Falling in Love: Why We Choose the Lovers We Choose*, 2nd ed. (New York: Routledge, 2005), 58.

2 The system being taught that evening builds on the cognitive functions identified by Carl Jung (and popularized in the Myers-Briggs Type Indicator, http://www.myersbriggs.org/my-mbti-personality-type/) as *thinking, feeling, sensing,* and *intuiting,* which in varying combinations form basic psychological types. The terms we have adopted—*visual, tonal, kinesthetic,* and *digital*—are also used in Richard Bandler and John Grinder's neuro-linguistic programming (NLP), although our use of these terms is somewhat different from Bandler and Grinder's. We have also gained instruction and inspiration from Virginia Satir's genius in working with stress-based communication styles (blaming, placating, distracting, and computing) as demonstrated in her workshops and recordings.

3 For more information on the prenatal development of hearing, visit http://birthpsychology.com/free-article/importance-prenatal-sound-and-music.

4 Daniel J. Siegel, *The Developing Mind: How Relationships and the Brain Interact to Shape Who We Are,* 2nd ed. (New York: Guilford Press, 2012), 6.

5 Ibid., 187.

6 Beverly Rubik, "The Biofield Hypothesis: Its Biophysical Basis and Role in Medicine," *Journal of Alternative and Complementary Medicine* 8, no. 6 (2002): 703–717.

7 The Energetic Stress Style Assessment is based on a questionnaire first developed by Dana How after she took one of our seminars. It has proven useful in its various evolutions over the years in our own work with couples. We are grateful to Dana for generously allowing us to use and build on her work. Insights from Peg Elliott Mayo are also reflected in the questions and gratefully acknowledged.

8 David Schnarch, *Passionate Marriage: Love, Sex, and Intimacy in Emotionally Committed Relationships* (New York: Holt, 1997).

9 John M. Gottman, *The Science of Trust: Emotional Attunement for Couples* (New York: Norton, 2011), 203.

10 Kim T. Buehlman, John M. Gottman, and Lynn F. Katz, "How a Couple Views Their Past Predicts

Their Future: Predicting Divorce from an Oral History Interview," *Journal of Family Psychology* 5, no. 3–4 (1992): 295–318.

11 John M. Gottman, *Why Marriages Succeed or Fail* (New York: Simon and Schuster, 1994).

12 Ibid., 40.

13 Ibid., 46–47.

Chapter 2

1 Daniel J. Siegel, *The Developing Mind: How Relationships and the Brain Interact to Shape Who We Are*, 2nd ed. (New York: Guilford Press, 2012), 75.

2 This final part of the technique is adapted from Harville Hendrix's Imago Dialogue, which is outlined in his book *Getting the Love You Want: A Guide for Couples*, rev. ed. (New York: Holt, 2008), 268–271.

3 Roger Walsh and Shauna I. Shapiro, "The Meeting of Meditative Disciplines and Western Psychology: A Mutually Enriching Dialogue," *American Psychologist* 61, no. 3 (2006): 227–239.

4 Rollin McCraty, Raymond Trevor Bradley, and Dana Tomasino, "Our Heart Has a Consciousness of Its Own," n.d., http://newearthdaily.com/our-heart-has-a-consciousness-of-its-own/.

5 Doc Childre and Howard Martin, *The HeartMath Solution* (New York: HarperOne, 2000), 10.

6 Taught to David by Stephen Levine in the early 1980s.

7 John M. Gottman and Joan DeClaire, *The Relationship Cure: A 5 Step Guide to Strengthening Your Marriage, Family, and Friendships* (New York: Crown, 2001), 70.

8 John M. Gottman, *The Science of Trust: Emotional Attunement for Couples* (New York: Norton, 2011), 24.

9 Gottman and DeClaire, *The Relationship Cure*, 71–73.

10 Ibid., 30.

11 Gay Hendricks and Kathlyn Hendricks, *Conscious Loving: The Journey to Co-Commitment* (New York: Bantam, 1990).

12 Patricia Love and Steven Stosny, *How to Improve Your Marriage without Talking about It* (New York: Random House, 2007).

13 Ibid.

Chapter 3

1 David Schnarch, *Intimacy and Desire: Awaken the Passion in Your Relationship* (New York: Beaufort, 2011), 268.

2 Ibid.

3 John M. Gottman, *Why Marriages Succeed or Fail* (New York: Simon and Schuster, 1994), 110.

4 William Doherty, *Bad Couples Therapy: How to Avoid Doing It*. 2006. Online course. https://www.psychotherapynetworker.org/store.

5 David Feinstein, Donna Eden, and Gary Craig, *The Promise of Energy Psychology: Revolutionary Tools for Dramatic Personal Change* (New York: Tarcher/Penguin, 2005), chap. 7.

6 Tiffany Field, *Touch Therapy* (London: Churchill Livingstone, 2000).

7 John M. Gottman, *The Science of Trust: Emotional Attunement for Couples* (New York: Norton, 2011).

8 Ibid.

9 Ibid.

10 John M. Gottman, *The Science of Trust: Emotional Attunement for Couples* (New York: Norton, 2011), 25.

11 Ibid., 26.

Chapter 4

1 Helen Fisher, *Why We Love: The Nature and Chemistry of Romantic Love* (New York: Holt, 2004), 98.

2 Edward O. Laumann, John H. Gagnon, Robert T. Michael, and Stuart Michaels, *The Social Organization of Sexuality: Sexual Practices in the United States* (Chicago: University of Chicago Press, 2000).

3 Marion Solomon and Stan Tatkin, *Love and War in Intimate Relationships* (New York: Norton, 2011), 5.

4 Donatella Marazziti, Hagop S. Akiskal, Alessandra Rossi, and Giovanni B. Cassano, "Alteration of the Platelet Serotonin Transporter in Romantic Love," *Psychological Medicine* 29, no. 3 (1999): 741–745.

5 Fisher, *Why We Love*, 87.

6 Larry J. Young, Zuoxin Wang, and Thomas R. Insel, "Neuroendocrine Bases of Monogamy," *Trends in Neurosciences* 21, no. 2 (1998): 71–75.

7 Louann Brizendine, *The Male Brain* (New York: Random House, 2010), xix.

8 Ibid., 60.

9 Fisher, *Why We Love*, 94.

10 Ibid., 92.

11 William Shakespeare, *Two Gentlemen of Verona*, act I, scene 3 (New York: Folger Shakespeare Library, 2006), 35.

12 Fisher, *Why We Love*, 96.

13 John M. Gottman, *The Science of Trust: Emotional Attunement for Couples* (New York: Norton, 2011), 19.

14 Circulated by e-mail. Author unknown.

15 The primary sources for the "Men's Brains/Women's Brains" section are Louann Brizendine's *The Female Brain* (New York: Random House, 2006) and *The Male Brain* (New York: Random House, 2010).

16 Specific brain differences have, however, been observed between gay and straight individuals. For instance, a part of the hypothalamus is twice as large in gay males as in straight males, and the nerve bundles connecting the right and left brain hemispheres are larger in gay men. At least "35 percent of sexual orientation" can be attributed to genetic influences that have already been identified (Brizendine, *The Male Brain*, 135).

17 Brizendine, *The Female Brain*, 13.

18 Ibid., 8.

19 Brizendine, *The Male Brain*, 81.

20 Ibid., 129.

21 Brizendine, *The Female Brain*, xix.

22 Ibid., 137.

23 Ibid., 4.

24 Brizendine, *The Male Brain*, 67–68.

25 Ibid., 64.

26 Brizendine, *The Female Brain*, 31.

27 Brizendine, *The Male Brain*, 10.

28 John Gray, *Venus on Fire, Mars on Ice: Hormonal Balance—The Key to Life, Love, and Energy* (Coquitlam, BC: Mind, 2010).

29 Ibid., 26.

30 Ibid., 51.

31 Ibid.

32 Ibid.

33 See chapter 3 of Donna's book *Energy Medicine*, rev. ed. (New York: Tarcher/Penguin, 2008) for more in-depth discussion of the benefits of a daily energy medicine routine.

34 Gray, *Venus on Fire, Mars on Ice*.

35 Ibid., 54.

36 Ibid., 56.

37 Martin Schulte-Rüther et al., "Gender Differences in Brain Networks Supporting Empathy," *Neuroimage*, 208, 42(1): 393-403.

38 Gray, *Venus on Fire, Mars on Ice*, 54–55.

39 Ibid.

40 Ibid., 53.

41 Ibid., 67.

42 The concept that undeveloped feminine aspects of a man are projected onto women and undeveloped male aspects of a woman are projected onto men is captured in Carl Jung's notion of the *anima* and *animus*. John A. Sanford describes this concept in *The Invisible Partners: How the Male and Female in Each of Us Affects Our Relationships* (New York: Paulist Press, 1980).

43 The descriptions of the Five Elements build on the descriptions presented in chapter 7 of *Energy Medicine* (New York: Tarcher/Penguin, 2008). Also see Leta Herman and Jaye McElroy, *The Energy of Love: Applying the Five Elements to Turn Attraction into True Connection* (Woodbury, MN: Llewellyn, 2014).

44 Carl R. Rogers, *On Becoming a Person: A Therapist's View of Psychotherapy* (Boston: Houghton Mifflin, 1961), 17.

Chapter 5

1 John Bowlby, "The Growth of Independence in the Young Child," *Royal Society of Health Journal* 76 (1956): 589.

2 Bowlby summarized his earlier work in the preface to his three-volume Attachment and Loss series. *Attachment (Attachment and Loss, Volume 1)* (New York: Basic Books, 1969), xiii.

3 Harry F. Harlow, "The Nature of Love," *American Psychologist* 13, no. 12 (1958): 673–685.

4 Daniel J. Siegel, *The Developing Mind: How Relationships and the Brain Interact to Shape Who We Are*, 2nd ed. (New York: Guilford Press, 2012).

5 John Bowlby, "Maternal Care and Mental Health," *Bulletin of the World Health Organization* 3 (1951): 355–534.

6 Alan Sroufe and Daniel Siegel, "The Verdict Is In: The Case for Attachment Theory," *Psychotherapy Networker* 35, no. 2 (2011): 34–39, 52–53.

7 Amir Levine and Rachel S. F. Heller, *Attached: The New Science of Adult Attachment and How It Can Help You Find—and Keep—Love* (New York: Tarcher/Penguin, 2010).

8 Mary Sykes Wylie and Lynn Turner, "The Attuned Therapist: Does Attachment Theory Really Matter?" *Psychotherapy Networker* 35, no. 2 (2011): 19–27.

9 Mario Mikulincer and Phillip R. Shaver, "Security-Based Self-Representations in Adulthood," in W. Stephen Rholes and Jeffry A. Simpson, eds., *Adult Attachment: Theory, Research, and Clinical Implications* (New York: Guilford Press, 2004), 162–163.

10 Ibid.

11 R. Chris Fraley and Phillip R. Shaver, "Adult Attachment and the Suppression of Unwanted Thoughts," *Journal of Personality and Social Psychology* 73 (1997): 1080–1091.

12 Various writers have estimated the percentage of adults who have a secure attachment style. All the estimates we have found show greater than 50 percent and up to 70 percent, with two-thirds being a frequent estimate. This happens to be the percentage of one-year-olds with a secure attachment style that Van IJzendoorn and Kroonenberg found in their review of cross-cultural studies of infant attachment. Marinus H. van IJzendoorn and Pieter M. Kroonenberg, "Cross-Cultural Patterns of Attachment: A Meta-Analysis of the Strange Situation," *Child Development* 59 (1988): 147–156.

13 Rollin McCraty, Raymond Trevor Bradley, and Dana Tomasino, "Our Heart Has a Consciousness of Its Own," n.d., http://newearthdaily.com/our-heart-has-a-consciousness-of-its-own/.

14 Levine and Heller, *Attached*.

15 Mikulincer and Shaver, "Security-Based Self-Representations in Adulthood," 166.

16 Mario Mikulincer and Phillip R. Shaver, *Attachment in Adulthood: Structure, Dynamics, and Change* (New York: Guilford Press, 2007).

17 U.S. Department of Health and Human Services, "The Effects of Marriage on Health: A Synthesis of Recent Research Evidence" (June 2007), available online at http://aspe.hhs.gov/hsp/07/marriageonhealth/rb.htm.

18 Daniel J. Siegel and Mary Hartzell, *Parenting from the Inside Out: How a Deeper Self-Understanding Can Help You Raise Children Who Thrive* (New York: Tarcher/Penguin, 2004), 84.

19 Joanne Davila and Rebecca J. Cobb, "Predictors of Change in Attachment Security during Adulthood," in W. Steven Rholes and Jeffry A. Simpson, eds., *Adult Attachment: Theory, Research, and Clinical Implications* (New York: Guilford Press, 2004), 134.

20 Patricia A. Frazier, Anne L. Byer, Ann R. Fischer, Deborah M. Wright, and Kurt A. Debord, "Adult Attachment Style and Partner Choice: Correlational and Experimental Findings," *Personal Relationships* 3, no. 2 (1996): 117–136.

21 Alicia F. Lieberman, Donna R. Weston, and Jeree H. Pawl, "Preventive Intervention and Outcome with Anxiously Attached Dyads," *Child Development* 62, no. 1 (1991): 199–209.

22 Reported in Jeremy Rifkin, *The Empathic Civilization: The Race to Global Consciousness in a World in Crisis* (New York: Tarcher/Penguin, 2009), 79–80.

23 Mikulincer and Shaver, *Attachment in Adulthood*.

24 Sue Johnson, "Extravagant Emotion: Understanding and Transforming Love Relationships in Emotionally Focused Therapy," in Diana Fosha, Dan Siegel, and Marion Solomon, eds., *The Healing Power of Emotion: Neurobiological Understandings and Therapeutic Perspectives* (New York: Norton, 2009), 257–279.

25 Sue Johnson, *Love Sense: The Revolutionary New Science of Romantic Relationships* (New York: Little, Brown, 2013), 54.

26 For more details about the Triple Warmer energy system, and additional techniques, see chapter 8 of Donna's *Energy Medicine,* rev. ed. (New York: Tarcher/Penguin, 2008).

27 W. Gerrod Parrott, *Emotions in Social Psychology* (New York: Psychology Press, 2001).

28 Robert Plutchik, *Emotions and Life: Perspectives from Psychology, Biology, and Evolution* (Washington, DC: American Psychological Association, 2002).

29 Siegel, *The Developing Mind,* 150.

30 Ibid., 103.

31 Siegel and Hartzell, *Parenting from the Inside Out,* chap. 7.

32 Ibid., 155.

33 Ibid.

Chapter 6

1 Roger Shattuck, *Proust* (London: Fontana, 1974), 131.

2 This concept is developed further in chapter 7 of Donna's *Energy Medicine,* rev. ed. (New York: Tarcher/Penguin, 2008).

3 David Feinstein, "What Does *Energy* Have to Do with Energy Psychology?" *Energy Psychology: Theory, Research, and Treatment* 4, no. 2 (2012): 59–80.

4 Helene M. Langevin and Jason A. Yandow, "Relationship of Acupuncture Points and Meridians to Connective Tissue Planes," *Anatomical Record* 269, no. 6 (2002): 257–265.

5 Marion Solomon and Stan Tatkin, *Love and War in Intimate Relationships* (New York: Norton, 2011).

6 Feinstein, "What Does *Energy* Have to Do with Energy Psychology?"

7 David Feinstein, "Acupoint Stimulation in Treating Psychological Disorders: Evidence of Efficacy," *Review of General Psychology* 2012, 16(4), 364–380.

8 Dawson Church and David Feinstein, "Energy Psychology in the Treatment of PTSD: Psychobiology and Clinical Principles," in Thijs Van Leeuwen and Marieke Brouwer, eds., *Psychology of Trauma* (Hauppauge, NY: Nova Science Publishers, 2013), 211–224.

9 Several organizations that provide training in energy psychology and list practitioners they have certified or consider to be competent can be found under the resources tab at http://www .energypsyched.com. As in choosing any professional for an important assignment, select carefully based on background, training, and reputation as well as rapport with you in your initial inquiries.

10 Informed guidelines for determining whether you need psychotherapy, and for finding a psychologist if you do, are provided by the American Psychological Association at http://www.apa.org/ helpcenter/choose-therapist.aspx. The principles are similar when seeking the services of other mental health professionals, such as psychiatrists, social workers, or marriage and family counselors.

11 Daniel G. Amen, *The Brain in Love* (New York: Three Rivers Press, 2007).

12 See http://www.eftuniverse.com/.

13 For an expanded presentation of the techniques excerpted in this section, see David Feinstein, Donna Eden, and Gary Craig, *The Promise of Energy Psychology: Revolutionary Tools for Dramatic Personal Change* (New York: Tarcher/Penguin, 2005). The approach used in that book and in this one is a variation on the popular EFT (Emotional Freedom Techniques) method. EFT is Gary Craig's

derivative of Roger Callahan's Thought Field Therapy (TFT). A four-hour seminar called *Introduction to Energy Psychology* is available on DVD through www.energypsyched.com.

14 Feinstein, Eden, and Craig, *The Promise of Energy Psychology*, 32.

15 Gary Craig, *The EFT Manual* (Fulton, CA: Energy Psychology Press, 2011), 70.

16 Roger Callahan, *Tapping the Healer Within: Using Thought-Field Therapy to Instantly Conquer Your Fears, Anxieties, and Emotional Distress* (New York: McGraw-Hill, 2002).

17 The Choices Method was developed by psychologist Patricia Carrington. You can learn more about this approach at http://masteringeft.com/masteringblog/introducing-the-choices-method/.

18 The teacher was Dawson Church.

Chapter 7

1 Erica Jong, *How to Save Your Own Life* (New York: Tarcher/Penguin, 2006), 263.

2 Robert Kegan, *The Emerging Self: Problem and Process in Human Development* (Cambridge, MA: Harvard University Press, 1982).

3 Dawson Church, *EFT for Love Relationships* (Fulton, CA: Energy Psychology Press, in press).

4 Ibid.

5 Fred Gallo, *Energy Diagnostic and Treatment Methods* (New York: Norton, 2000), 175–177.

6 David Feinstein, Donna Eden, and Gary Craig, *The Promise of Energy Psychology* (New York: Tarcher/Penguin, 2005). Nick Ortner has also written a superb introduction to acupoint tapping for the public, *The Tapping Solution: A Revolutionary System for Stress-Free Living* (Carlsbad, CA, 2013). Either will enhance your ability to use the method.

Chapter 8

1 John Gray, *Mars and Venus in the Bedroom: A Guide to Lasting Romance and Passion* (New York: HarperTorch, 2001), 7.

2 Alison Armstrong, "The Secret to Great Sex . . . Even When No One's in the Mood." In *The Art of Love* (teleseminar), moderated by Arielle Ford, 2012.

3 Sonja Lyubomirsky, "New Love: A Short Shelf Life," *New York Times*, December 1, 2012, http://www.nytimes.com/2012/12/02/opinion/sunday/new-love-a-short-shelf-life.html?pagewanted=1&emc=eta1&_r=0.

4 David Schnarch, *Intimacy and Desire: Awaken the Passion in Your Relationship* (New York: Beaufort, 2011), xvii.

5 Armstrong, "The Secret to Great Sex . . . Even When No One's in the Mood."

6 Ibid.

7 David Schnarch, *Passionate Marriage: Keeping Love and Intimacy Alive in Committed Relationships* (New York: Holt, 1997), chap. 1.

8 Schnarch, *Intimacy and Desire*, 19.

9 Ibid, 18.

10 Schnarch, *Passionate Marriage*, 55.

11 Ibid., 51.

12 Schnarch, *Intimacy and Desire*, 6–8.

13 Iris Krasnow, *Sex After . . . Women Share How Intimacy Changes as Life Changes* (New York: Gotham, 2014).

14   Nicole Daedone, *Slow Sex: The Art and Craft of the Female Orgasm* (New York: Grand Central Life and Style, 2011), 158.

15   Ibid., 159.

16   Schnarch, *Passionate Marriage*, 160.

17   Marianne Williamson, *Enchanted Love: The Mystical Power of Intimate Relationships* (New York: Simon and Schuster, 2001), 253–254.

18   Anaiya Sophia, *Sacred Sexual Union: The Alchemy of Love, Power, and Wisdom* (Rochester, VT: Destiny Books, 2013), 83.

19   Matthew J. Hertenstein et al., "The Communication of Emotion via Touch," *Emotion* 9 (2009): 566–573.

20   Schnarch, *Passionate Marriage*, 191.

21   Ibid., 191–192.

22   Ibid., 191.

23   Ellen Eatough, "Four Keys to Sexual Ecstasy: Experience Soulful Connection with Spine-Tingling Sex." CD seminar available from http://extatica.com.

24   Helen E. O'Connell, John M. Hutson, Colin R. Anderson, and Robert J. Plenter, "Anatomical Relationship between Urethra and Clitoris," *Journal of Urology* 159, no. 6 (1998): 1892–1897.

25   Ruth K. Westheimer, *Sex For Dummies: Dr. Ruth's Rx for a Pleasurable Sex Life* (Hoboken, NJ: Wiley, 2007).

26   Mantak Chia, Maneewan Chia, Douglas Abrams, and Rachel Carlton Abrams, *The Multi-Orgasmic Couple: Sexual Secrets Every Couple Should Know* (New York: HarperOne, 2000).

27   Judy Kuriansky, *The Complete Idiot's Guide to Tantric Sex*, 2nd ed. (Indianapolis, IN: Alpha Books, 2004). Also see *Tantra: The Art of Conscious Loving* (San Francisco: Mercury House, 1989), a less detailed but highly authoritative book by Kuriansky's teachers, Charles and Caroline Muir.

28   Chia et al., *The Multi-Orgasmic Couple*, 68. While the Central Meridian generally flows up the center of the body, it can change direction when the Microcosmic Orbit is activated. Taoist tradition maps the Microcosmic Orbit as moving up the spine and down the front of the body, but I (Donna) have seen it flow in the other direction as well. Circumstances seem to dictate the direction of its movement.

29   Ibid., 66.

30   Ibid., 71.

31   Ibid., xiii.

32   Kuriansky, *The Complete Idiot's Guide to Tantric Sex*, 5–6.

33   Ibid., 4.

34   The Spiritual Emergence Network was founded in 1980 by Christina and Stanislav Grof "in response to the lack of understanding and respect for psychospiritual growth in the mental health profession." While recognizing that a sudden spiritual awakening can be tumultuous and even traumatic, such episodes are viewed as normal, life-enhancing aspects of human development that can lead to "a greater capacity for wisdom, compassion . . . and a deeper sense of personal security and inner peace." Information and referrals to counselors who hold this perspective are available at http://www.spiritualemergence.info/.

35   Kuriansky, *The Complete Idiot's Guide to Tantric Sex*, 23.

36   Ibid., 24.

37 Ibid., xxi.

38 Marianne Brandon, *Monogamy: The Untold Story* (Santa Barbara, CA: Praeger, 2010), 131.

39 The role of the radiant circuits in immune function is discussed in chapter 8 of Donna's *Energy Medicine*, rev. ed. (New York: Tarcher/Penguin, 2008), and exercises for strengthening the radiant circuits are presented in chapter 7 of David Feinstein, Donna Eden, and Gary Craig, *The Promise of Energy Psychology: Revolutionary Tools for Dramatic Personal Change* (New York: Tarcher/Penguin, 2005).

40 Armstrong, "The Secret to Great Sex."

41 Mary Jo Rapini, "5 Ways to Keep the Sparks Flying in Your Marriage," 2013, http://www.yourtango.com/experts/mary-jo-rapini/married-sex-nothing-boring-or-snoring-about-it/page/3.

42 John Gray, *Mars and Venus in the Bedroom: A Guide to Lasting Romance and Passion* (New York: Harper-Torch, 2001), 245.

43 Eatough, "Four Keys to Sexual Ecstasy."

44 Esther Perel, "The Secret to Desire in a Long-Term Relationship," TED Talk, February 14, 2013, http://www.youtube.com/watch?v=saoRUmGTCYY&noredirect=1.

45 Esther Perel, *Mating in Captivity: Unlocking Erotic Intelligence* (New York: HarperPerennial, 2007), 212.

46 Eatough, "Four Keys to Sexual Ecstasy."

47 Ibid.

48 Ibid.

49 Daedone, *Slow Sex*, 47.

50 Donna Eden, *Energy Medicine for Women: Aligning Your Body's Energies to Boost Your Health and Vitality* (New York: Tarcher/Penguin, 2008), chap. 5.

51 Alan Batchelder was the therapist.

52 Williamson, *Enchanted Love*, 243.

53 Based on data for 2011 comparing the marriage rate with the rate of divorces and annulments, U.S. Centers for Disease Control and Prevention, http://www.cdc.gov/nchs/nvss/marriage_divorce_tables.htm.

54 Paul R. Amato and Denise Previti, "People's Reasons for Divorcing: Gender, Social Class, the Life Course, and Adjustment," *Journal of Family Issues* 24, no. 5 (2003): 602–626.

55 "Infidelity Statistics," 2012, http://www.statisticbrain.com/infidelity-statistics.

56 Eric Anderson, *The Monogamy Gap: Men, Love, and the Reality of Cheating* (New York: Oxford University Press, 2012), 4.

57 Ibid.

58 Louann Brizendine, *The Male Brain* (New York: Random House, 2010), 5.

59 John Lloyd, John Mitchinson, James Harkin, *1,227 Quite Interesting Facts to Blow Your Socks Off* (New York: Norton, 2013), 255.

60 Brizendine, *The Male Brain*, 4.

61 Ibid.

62 Ibid., chap. 3.

63 Ibid., 57.

64 Jan Havlicek, S. Craig Roberts, and Jaroslav Flegr, "Women's Preference for Dominant Male Odour: Effects of Menstrual Cycle and Relationship Status," *Biological Letters* 1, no. 3 (2005): 256–259.

65 Ibid.

66 Brizendine, *The Male Brain*, 59.

67 David Barash and Judith Eve Lipton, *The Myth of Monogamy: Fidelity and Infidelity in Animals and People* (New York: Holt, 2001), 57.

68 Ibid., 58.

69 Ibid., 1.

70 Stefan Beyst, *The Ecstasies of Eros* (1990–1992, translated 2007), http://d-sites.net/english/eros00 .htm#boven2.

71 Barash and Lipton, *The Myth of Monogamy*, 134.

72 Laura Betzig, "Sex, Succession, and Stratification in the First Six Civilizations: How Powerful Men Reproduced, Passed Power on to Their Sons, and Used Power to Defend Their Wealth, Women and Children," in Lee Ellis, ed., *Social Stratification and Socioeconomic Inequality*, vol. 1 (New York: Praeger, 1993), 37–74.

73 Christopher Opie, Quentin D. Atkinson, Robin I. M. Dunbar, and Susanne Shultz, "Male Infanticide Leads to Social Monogamy in Primates," *Proceedings of the National Academy of Sciences* 110, no. 33 (2013): 13328–13332.

74 Phil Gasper, "Is Biology Destiny?" *International Socialist Review* 38 (2004), online edition, http:// isreview.org/issues/38/genes.shtml.

75 Williamson, *Enchanted Love*, 230–231.

76 Sue Johnson, *Love Sense: The Revolutionary New Science of Romantic Relationships* (New York: Little, Brown, 2013), 21.

77 Laura Berman, *The Passion Prescription: Ten Weeks to Your Best Sex—Ever!* (New York: Hyperion, 2005).

78 Mary Jo Rapini, "5 Ways to Keep the Sparks Flying in Your Marriage," 2013, http://www.yourtango .com/experts/mary-jo-rapini/married-sex-nothing-boring-or-snoring-about-it.

79 "Paul Newman," *Wikipedia*, http://en.wikipedia.org/wiki/Paul_Newman.

80 Sophia, *Sacred Sexual Union*, 81–82.

Chapter 9

1 Marianne Williamson, *Enchanted Love: The Mystical Power of Intimate Relationships* (New York: Simon and Schuster, 2001), 28.

2 Bruce H. Lipton, *The Honeymoon Effect: The Science of Creating Heaven on Earth* (Carlsbad, CA: Hay House, 2013).

3 Ibid., 74–75.

4 Jett Psaris and Marlena S. Lyons, *Undefended Love* (Oakland, CA: New Harbinger, 2000), 9–10.

5 Ibid., 98.

6 Ronald D. Siegel, "West Meets East: Creating a New Wisdom Tradition," *Psychotherapy Networker* 35, no. 5 (2011): 20–27.

7 Ibid., 24.

8 Ibid., 24.

9 Ibid., 25.

10 Ronald D. Siegel, *The Mindfulness Solution: Everyday Practices for Everyday Problems* (New York: Guilford Press, 2010), 38.

11 Jeffrey M. Schwartz and Sharon Begley, *The Mind and the Brain: Neuroplasticity and the Power of Mental Force* (New York: HarperCollins, 2002).

12 Perla Kaliman et al., "Rapid Changes in Histone Deacetylases and Inflammatory Gene Expression in Expert Meditators," *Psychoneuroendocrinology*, 40 (2014): 96–107.

13 Christopher K. Germer and Ronald D. Siegel, *Mindfulness and Psychotherapy*, 2nd ed. (New York: Guilford Press, 2013).

14 Siegel, "West Meets East," 25.

15 Siegel, *The Mindfulness Solution*, vii.

16 We suggest you begin with the basic "Breath Awareness Meditation" and then experiment with others. "Stepping into Fear" will teach you how to meet your anxieties directly rather than to turn away from them. A powerful mediation (and perhaps scary in the amount of intimacy it can induce) for couples uses the simple title "Breathing Together."

17 David Feinstein, "The Psychological and Spiritual Challenges Inherent in Dying Well," in I. A. Serlin, *Whole Person Healthcare*, vol. 2: *Psychology, Spirituality, Health* (Westport, CN: Praeger, 2007), 235–262.

18 Gay Hendricks and Kathlyn Hendricks, *Conscious Loving: The Journey to Co-Commitment* (New York: Bantam, 1990), 111–118.

19 Ibid., 112.

20 Ibid., 112.

21 Ibid., 115.

22 Ibid., 118.

23 Mary Jo Rapini, "Guys, Some Things Are Better Left Unsaid," Expert's Blog, http://www.your tango.com.

24 Tricia J. Burke et al., "'You're Going to Eat That?': Relationship Processes and Conflict among Mixed-Weight Couples," *Journal of Social and Personal Relationships* 29, no. 8 (2012): 1109–1130.

25 Kahlil Gibran, *The Prophet* (Boston: Oneworld, 2008), 23.

26 Esther Perel, "The Secret to Desire in a Long-Term Relationship," TED Talk, February 14, 2013, http://www.youtube.com/watch?v=saoRUmGTCYY&noredirect=1.

27 David Schnarch, *Intimacy and Desire: Awaken the Passion in Your Relationship* (New York: Beaufort, 2009), 47.

Chapter 10

1 J. Denosky, *Mystical and Visionary Out of Body Experience: Travel in the Spiritual Worlds*, 2012, http://www.spiritualtravel.org/.

2 Ibid.

3 Anthony Dardis, *Mental Causation: The Mind-Body Problem* (New York: Columbia University Press, 2008).

4 David J. Chalmers, *The Character of Consciousness* (New York: Oxford University Press, 2010).

5 Thomas Moore, *Soul Mates: Honoring the Mysteries of Love and Relationship* (New York: HarperPerennial, 1994).

6 Carmen Harra, "The 10 Elements of a Soulmate," Huffington Post, July 17, 2013, http://www.huffingtonpost.com/dr-carmen-harra/elements-of-a-soulmate_b_3595992.html.

7 For a scientifically balanced explanation of the relationships among planetary alignments, the human psyche, and world events, see Richard Tarnas, *Cosmos and Psyche: Intimations of a New World View* (New York: Viking, 2006).

8   Generally attributed to the great Jesuit mystic Pierre Teilhard de Chardin.

9   Moore, *Soul Mates*, 45.

10 Ibid., 46.

11 Ibid., viii.

12 Ibid., xi.

13 Ibid., 3.

14 Thomas Moore, *The Re-Enchantment of Everyday Life* (New York: HarperPerennial, 1996), ix.

15 Ibid., 11.

16 Ibid., x.

17 Ibid.

18 Ibid.

19 Cited in Moore, *The Re-Enchantment of Everyday Life*, xviii.

20 Virginia A. Larson, "An Exploration of Psychotherapeutic Resonance," *Psychotherapy* 24 (1987): 321–324.

21 Molly Merrill Sterling and James F. T. Bugental, "The Meld Experience in Psychotherapy Supervision," *Journal of Humanistic Psychology* 33, no. 2 (1993): 38–48.

22 John O'Donohue, *To Bless the Space between Us* (New York: Doubleday, 2008), 32.

23 Marianne Williamson, *Illuminata: A Return to Prayer* (New York: Riverhead, 1994), 65–70.

24 A beautiful book that gives instruction for this is Gregg Braden's *Secrets of the Lost Mode of Prayer* (Carlsbad, CA: Hay House, 2006).

25 Jon Kabat-Zinn, *Wherever You Go, There You Are* (New York: Hyperion, 1994), 265–266.

26 Ronald Siegel, "West Meets East: Creating a New Wisdom Tradition," *Psychotherapy Networker* 35, no. 5 (2011): 20–27.

27 Carl G. Jung, "The Practice of Psychotherapy," in R. F. C. Hull, trans., *The Collected Works of Carl G. Jung, Volume 16*, 2nd ed. (Princeton, NJ: Princeton University Press, 1996), 42.

28 Robert Hoss and Lynn Hoss, *Dream To Freedom: A Handbook for Integrating Dreamwork and Energy Psychology* (Santa Rosa, CA: Energy Psychology Press, 2013).

29 Abraham Joshua Heschel, *The Sabbath* (New York: Farrar, Straus and Giroux, 1951), 8.

30 Ibid.

31 Ibid., 14.

32 Ibid., 15–16.

33 Wayne Muller, *Sabbath: Restoring the Sacred Rhythm of Rest* (New York: Bantam, 1999), 1.

34 Heschel, *The Sabbath*, 18.

35 Ibid., 21.

36 Ibid., 23.

37 Ibid., 3.

38 Ibid., 15.

39 Ibid., 14.

40 Ibid., 17.

Index

Page numbers in *italics* refer to illustrations.

Energetic attunement, 94
Energetic Stress Styles, 180. *See also*
   specific sensory styles
  aligning, 44–78
  assessing, 26–29, 45
  attachment style interaction
    with, 158
  attuning to partner's, 51
  best of each, 43
  biofield (aura) determination
    of, 21
  communication techniques for
    all, 51–74
  couple demonstrations of, 37–39
  distortions resulting from, 22–26
  gender and, 39
  interpersonal perils of each,
    35–36
  as not learned behavior, 37
  relationship style influenced by,
    157–59
  secondary modes in, 38
  sensory modes and, 21
  Stop technique when caught in,
    80–82
  of therapists, 38
  using strengths of, 45–47, 50–51
Energies. *See also* Sex, as energy
  medicine
  attachment, 147–78
  of attraction, 107–8
  awakening awareness of, 282
  dance between two, 29–30
  Eden's ability to see, 6, 18,
    107–8, 158
  gender and, 130–32
  of lust vs. romance, 110
  men and women's differing
    brains and, 107–44
  merging energy fields, 30
  mingling of, 341
  of new, stale and renewed
    relationships, 262
  of passion, 115
  physical connection for
    stimulating, 76–77
  scrambled, 214
  secure relating, 154
  STAR for colliding, 79–106,
    225–28
  tending hormones and, 127–30
  within and between us, 4–5

  use of, 2
Energies of love
  defined, 3
  overview, 10–13
  visual experience of, 337
Energy Dimension sections,
  about, 12
Energy exercises. *See* Energy
  techniques; Exercises
Energy medicine, 6. *See also* Sex, as
  energy medicine
Energy Medicine for Women
  (Eden), 286
Energy psychology, 6, 172, 191
  benefits of working as couple,
    192–93
  in conscious partnerships, 310,
    316–17
  counselors, 189
  emotional resolution approach
    in, 186
  learning from books, 190
  main interventions in, 183
  relationship areas improved by,
    187, 224–25
Energy structure, 4
  processing modes in, 18
Energy techniques. *See also*
    Acupoint tapping; Centering
    techniques; Communication
    techniques; "Do you mean"
    technique; Energetic Stress
    Styles; Harmony techniques;
    Sex, as energy medicine;
    STAR Pact
  for harmony, 65–78
  Heaven Rushing In, 77–78
  mental image, 255
  mindfulness, 180–82, 276,
    313, 315, 316–17,
    347–48
  for oxytocin and testosterone
    production, 125–27
  secure attachment, 170–78
  sexual energy principles and,
    280–85
  tearless trauma, 193
Entanglement, in physics, 112
Epicurus, 338
Eros, 3
Esalen Institute, 190
Estrogen, 109, 121, 123

Exercises. *See also* Centering
  techniques; Energy techniques
  Attach by Detaching, 161–62
  meridians in energy, 83
  Penetrating Flow, 279
  Tantric sexual practices, 275–78
  Taoist sexual, 273–74, *274*

Family of man, 335
Fate, 335
Fear
  anger and, 75–76
  of being on airplane, 209
  of future, 314
  of spiders, 206–7
Feeling band, biofield, 21
Feinstein, David
  appreciation volley example
    of, 71
  arguments between Eden and,
    1–2, 5, 179–80
  astrology sessions and, 334–35
  book-writing experiences of
    Eden and, 1–2, 179–80
  combined disciplines of Eden
    and, 18
  daily ritual of Eden and,
    342–44
  as digital, 103, 157–58,
    180, 319
  Eden as opposite of, xiii, 1
  Eden's attending Hypnosis class
    of, 17–18
  energy response to attractiveness,
    107–8
  relationship story of Eden and,
    331–35
  work of Eden and, 6
Females. *See* Women
Feminine qualities, balanced
  masculine and, 7–8
Fetal brain, 119
Field, Tiffany, 95
Fight or flight, 83, 95
  Triple Warmer Smoothie for
    turning off, 167–68, *168*
Figure-eight crossover patterns, 93
Fire element, 138–40
First aid, 216, 217
Fisher, Helen, 107, 108–9,
    111, 113, 114
5-to-1 ratio, 42

Five elements, 132–44
    earth, 140–41
    exploring, 133–34
    fire, 138–40
    metal, 141–43
    understanding own and
        partner's, 143–44
    water, 134–36
    wood, 136–38
    yin and yang, 132–33
Flooding, 80, 96, 105
Foreplay
    in bedroom, 284–85
    energies in sync as, 284
    holding hands as, 283
    kissing and, 267–68
    trust and safety as, 283–84
Foster boy, 223–24
"Four Keys to Sexual Ecstasy:
    Experience Soulful
    Connection with
    Spine-Tingling Sex," 268
Four Taps, 84–85, 85
Fredrickson, Barbara, 3
Free-floating anxiety, 208
Free love movement, 285–86
Freud, Sigmund, 5, 182, 186
Full-body orgasm, 272, 274

Gasper, Phil, 295
Gaze, gentle, 161, 162
Gender
    battle of the sexes, xiii–xiv
    biochemistry of, 125
    brain differences, 118–23
    in Energetic Stress Styles, 39
    energies and, 130–32
Generalization effect, 208
Genetics, infidelity and, 292
Gentle gaze, 161, 162
Gentle start-up, 66–69
Gibran, Kahlil, 323, 346
Global economy, women's
    empowerment and, 7–8
Good-enough parenting, 159
Goswami, Amit, 112
Gottman, John, 40–41, 66–67,
    70, 102
    divorce research of, 97
    on flooding, 80
    soft start-up technique of, 67
Governing Meridian, 272, 276

Grateful Dead, 349–50
Gratitude
    cultivating, 70–73
    expressing, 72
    gentle start-up using, 68
Gray, John, 123–24, 127, 129,
    259, 281
Great Virtues, 304
Guides, 348–49
Gunshot wound, 250–51

Habits. See Thought habits
Harlow, Harry, 149
Harmony techniques, 65–78
    High-Band It, 73
Harsh start-up, 69
Hartzell, Mary, 174, 176
Harvard Divinity School, 353
Healing
    catastrophe aftermath, 218–20
    of emotional wounds, 236–47
    previous marriage emotional
        issues, 247–48
    of sexual wounds, 285–88
"Healing Journey," 300
Heart
    brain in, 66
    emotional information of, 4–5
    notice breath, soften belly, open
        heart, 65–66
    Oxytocin Hearts, 126
Heart Chakra, 98
    with Acceptance Statement,
        198, 198
    in sexual energy medicine, 270
Heart Chakra Triple Warmer Tap,
    169, 169–70
HeartMath Institute, 4
Heaven Rushing In, 77–78
Hendricks, Gay, 75, 318–20
Hendricks, Kathlyn, 75, 318–20
Heschel, Abraham, 353, 354
Higamous, hogamous saying, 290
High-Band It, 73
High road, 174
Hook-up, 88, 88
    Three Chakra, 75, 76
Hoped-for-outcome rating, 242
Hormones. See also specific hormones
    bonding, 125, 127
    brain maturation, 121–22
    his/her, 123–25

of love, 109–13
    lust, 109
    menopause, 121–22
    monogamy, 112–13
    obsession-producing, 111
    orgasm, 113
    romance, 109–11
    stress-coping, 124
    tending energies and, 127–30
    women's dilemma regarding
        work and, 124–25
    yin and yang, 131–32
Horn, Paul, 299–308
Houston, Jean, 325
Hugs, 77
Hunger, in infants, 148
Hypnosis, 17–18
Hypothalamus, 120, 163

"I" instead of "you," 68
Illuminata: A Return to Prayer
    (Williamson), 345–46
Imagery
    calendar image, 252–53, 254–55
    envisioning relationship change,
        248–55
    Tantric practice using, 277–78
    technique, 255
Individuality, drive for, 261
Infants
    brain wiring in, 147–49
    energy in secure and insecure,
        150
    irritable, 159–60
    neglected or nurtured, 148
    parental attunement of, 160
    rhesus monkey, 149
Infidelity
    in men, 288–89
    overcoming biological
        programming for, 295
    in women, 290–92
Inherited aspects, of love
    aligning energetic styles, 44–78
    brain and energy differences
        between men and women,
        107–44
    defined, 10–11
    sensory styles, 17–43, 46
    STAR for energy collisions,
        79–106, 225–28
Inner guidance, 217